Deep Learning for Biomedical Applications

Artificial Intelligence (AI): Elementary to Advanced Practices

Series Editor:
Vijender Kumar Solanki,
Zhongyu (Joan) Lu,
and Valentina E. Balas

In the emerging smart city technology and industries, the role of artificial intelligence is getting more prominent. This AI book series will aim to cover the latest AI work, which will help the naïve user to get support to solve existing problems, and for the experienced AI practitioners, it will assist to shedding light for new avenues in the AI domains. The series will cover the recent work carried out in AI and its associated domains; it will cover Logics, Pattern Recognition, NLP, Expert Systems, Machine Learning, Block-Chain, and Big Data. The work domain of AI is quite deep, so it will be covering the latest trends which are evolving with the concepts of AI and it will be helping those who are new to the field, practitioners, students, as well as researchers to gain some new insights.

Cyber Defense Mechanisms
Security, Privacy, and Challenges
Gautam Kumar, Dinesh Kumar Saini, and Nguyen Ha Huy Cuong

Artificial Intelligence Trends for Data Analytics Using Machine Learning and Deep Learning Approaches
K. Gayathri Devi, Mamata Rath, and Nguyen Thi Dieu Linh

Transforming Management Using Artificial Intelligence Techniques
Vikas Garg and Rashmi Agrawal

AI and Deep Learning in Biometric Security
Trends, Potential, and Challenges
Gaurav Jaswal, Vivek Kanhangad, and Raghavendra Ramachandra

Enabling Technologies for Next Generation Wireless Communications
Edited by Mohammed Usman, Mohd Wajid, and Mohd Dilshad Ansari

Artificial Intelligence (AI)
Recent Trends and Applications
Edited by S. Kanimozhi Suguna, M. Dhivya, and Sara Paiva

Deep Learning for Biomedical Applications
Edited by Utku Kose, Omer Deperlioglu, and D. Jude Hemanth

For more information on this series, please visit: https://www.routledge.com/ Artificial-Intelligence-AI-Elementary-to-Advanced-Practices/book-series/ CRCAIEAP

Deep Learning for Biomedical Applications

Edited by
Utku Kose, Omer Deperlioglu,
and D. Jude Hemanth

CRC Press
Taylor & Francis Group
Boca Raton London New York

CRC Press is an imprint of the
Taylor & Francis Group, an **informa** business

MATLAB® is a trademark of The MathWorks, Inc. and is used with permission. The MathWorks does not warrant the accuracy of the text or exercises in this book. This book's use or discussion of MATLAB® software or related products does not constitute endorsement or sponsorship by The MathWorks of a particular pedagogical approach or particular use of the MATLAB® software

First edition published 2021
by CRC Press
6000 Broken Sound Parkway NW, Suite 300, Boca Raton, FL 33487-2742

and by CRC Press
2 Park Square, Milton Park, Abingdon, Oxon, OX14 4RN

© 2021 Taylor & Francis Group, LLC

CRC Press is an imprint of Taylor & Francis Group, LLC

Library of Congress Cataloging-in-Publication Data
Names: Kose, Utku, 1985- editor. | Deperlioglu, Omer, 1967- editor. |
Hemanth, D. Jude, editor.
Title: Deep learning for biomedical applications / edited by Utku Kose,
Omer Deperlioglu, and D. Jude Hemanth.
Description: Boca Raton : CRC Press, 2021. | Series: Artificial
intelligence (AI): elementary to advanced practices | Includes
bibliographical references and index.
Identifiers: LCCN 2021001265 (print) | LCCN 2021001266 (ebook) |
ISBN 9780367422509 (hardback) | ISBN 9780367855611 (ebook)
Subjects: LCSH: Diagnostic imaging—Data processing. | Image analysis. |
Artificial intelligence—Medical applications.
Classification: LCC RC78.7.D53 D424 2021 (print) | LCC RC78.7.D53 (ebook)
| DDC 616.07/54—dc23
LC record available at https://lccn.loc.gov/2021001265
LC ebook record available at https://lccn.loc.gov/2021001266

ISBN: 978-0-367-42250-9 (hbk)
ISBN: 978-1-032-03323-5 (pbk)
ISBN: 978-0-367-85561-1 (ebk)

Typeset in Times
by codeMantra

Contents

Foreword

As the most recent, advanced formation of Machine Learning, Deep Learning plays an essential role in solving present real-world problems. As today's problems generally require a detailed analysis of intense data, Deep Learning has been a vital tool for unstoppable improvements in the field of Artificial Intelligence. It seems that the future world will be comprised of smart devices that create smart environments. Due to the emergence of intelligent systems used to solve specific problems, the future world will include common smart objects that can improve the standard of human life. One important criterion to achieve this at this point is building necessary background computational solutions that are generally provided by mathematically and logically strong systems. It is very important to establish these smart systems in the fields that play vital roles in the well-being of humankind. Biomedical is among these fields, where advances in terms of Artificial Intelligence directly affect the way of present and future biomedical developments. From medical diagnosis to treatment, from IoT-based healthcare tools and robotic systems to decision-support-oriented managerial systems, Artificial Intelligence has become a dominant factor in finding critical solutions to improve health-oriented life standards. As the most cutting-edge solutions are provided by the Deep Learning side, it is important to feed the literature with the most recent research reports.

This book, titled *Deep Learning for Biomedical Applications*, is one of the most recent reference works containing the most recent knowledge about what is currently ongoing in the literature of Deep Learning and Biomedical. Some trendy topics like medical diagnosis and intelligent medical image analysis are attracting much interest in the literature, but there are many more different topics that are widely discussed. In this context, this book covers a variety of topics including precision medicine, genomics, gait recognition, and public health. Moreover, critical topics such as image segmentation-oriented diagnosis of diseases (especially cancer) are also covered extensively in the chapters ahead. International coverage of the whole book is also another advantage so that you are able to understand international trends in the research on Deep Learning and Biomedical issues. Eventually, I would like to thank dear editors Dr. Kose, Deperlioglu, and Hemanth for providing us such a timely and well-structured book.

As my final words, I also wish that every reader enjoys their reading while learning about the current state of the literature of biomedical, which is highly supported by advanced, careful solutions of Deep Learning.

Dr. José-Antonio Marmolejo-Saucedo
Universidad Panamericana, Mexico

Preface

The beginning of the 21st century has brought many rapid developments in the context of data processing. Not only software solutions, but also hardware-based components of computer systems have gained great momentum in terms of lower costs with higher computational capacities. As a result, computational approach to deal with real-world problems has gone through revolutionary-level improvements to transform even daily life. Nowadays, intense use of data processing methods and Artificial Intelligence takes place even in our mobile phones and home environments. From a general perspective, it is possible to indicate that the dominance of Artificial Intelligence has already started to make its impacts on different communities. It is clear that this rise has been supported by many alternative technologies such as electronics, mechanics, and communication. However, the future technology trends tend to be covering essentials of Artificial Intelligence-based solutions.

The year 2020 has been a very different time period for humankind so far. Emerging around September 2019, the fatal disease, COVID-19 has become a pandemic in 2020. The sudden global state of emergency was still active while we were writing these chapters in November 2020. Except for the precautions taken by governments, the medical staff is at the center of combat against COVID-19. Thanks to predictive and descriptive methods provided by Artificial Intelligence, there has been remarkable research interest in diagnosing, tracking, and treating COVID-19. At this point, Deep Learning, which is the most recent method of Artificial Intelligence, has been widely used in the context of medical imaging and massive data-based applications. By referring to the beginning of the first paragraph, we can indicate that Deep Learning has been among the outcomes of rapid developments for data processing solutions. As a sub-method of Machine Learning, Deep Learning employs newer types of neural networks that are capable of dealing with details of data to reach high accuracy levels in findings. Therefore, it is already a remarkable method that has been applied in the context of medical/ biomedical applications.

This book *Deep Learning for Biomedical Applications* is a carefully prepared edited work that hits at different sides of biomedical applications including the use of Deep Learning. We have tried to cover different topics to satisfy every reader's desires in the context of Deep Learning solutions for the biomedical field. As Deep Learning is very effective in medical image-based operations, readers will be able to see many examples of image processing-oriented solutions achieved by Deep Learning techniques. In this context, all readers are welcome to read the chapters targeting precision medicine (Chapter 1), embryo grade prediction (Chapter 2), biometric gait features analysis (Chapter 3), medical image analysis/segmentation-based works – especially aiming tumor detection – (Chapters 4–7, Chapters 10, 11, 13, 15, and 16), Deep Learning for healthcare/public health (Chapters 8 and 12), genomics (Chapter 9), and even Cesarean data classification (Chapter 14). It is remarkable that all chapters employ different usages of Deep Learning techniques and the associated data processing methods for effective outcomes of biomedical problems.

As editors, we would like to thank the respectful authors for providing their valuable research findings to the scientific audience and wish all readers to enjoy their fly over the clouds of Deep Learning. All ideas and suggestions are welcome, and they can be sent to our contact points. Stay safe and healthy!

Dr. Utku Kose
Suleyman Demirel University, Turkey
http://www.utkukose.com
Dr. Omer Deperlioglu
Afyon Kocatepe University, Turkey
deperlioglu@aku.edu.tr
Dr. D. Jude Hemanth
Karunya Institute of Technology and Sciences, India
judehemanth@karunya.edu

MATLAB® is a registered trademark of The MathWorks, Inc. For product information, please contact:

The MathWorks, Inc.
3 Apple Hill Drive
Natick, MA 01760-2098 USA
Tel: 508-647-7000
Fax: 508-647-7001
E-mail: info@mathworks.com
Web: www.mathworks.com

Editors

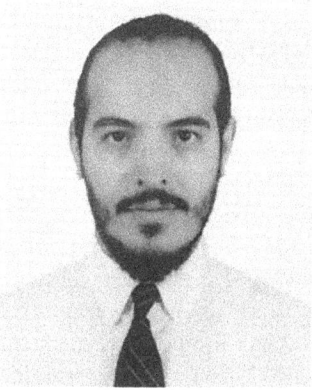

Utku Kose received a B.S. degree in 2008 from computer education of Gazi University, Turkey, as a faculty valedictorian. He received a M.S. degree in 2010 from Afyon Kocatepe University, Turkey, in the field of computer and a D.S./Ph.D. degree in 2017 from Selcuk University, Turkey, in the field of computer engineering. Between 2009 and 2011, he worked as a research assistant in Afyon Kocatepe University. He also worked as a lecturer and vocational School – vice director in Afyon Kocatepe University between 2011 and 2012, as a lecturer and research center director in Usak University between 2012 and 2017, and as an assistant professor in Suleyman Demirel University between 2017 and 2019. Currently, he is an associate professor in Suleyman Demirel University, Turkey. He has more than 100 publications including articles, authored and edited books, proceedings, and reports. He is also on editorial boards of many scientific journals and serves as one of the editors of the Biomedical and Robotics Healthcare book series by CRC Press. His research interest includes artificial intelligence, machine ethics, artificial intelligence safety, optimization, the chaos theory, distance education, e-learning, computer education, and computer science.

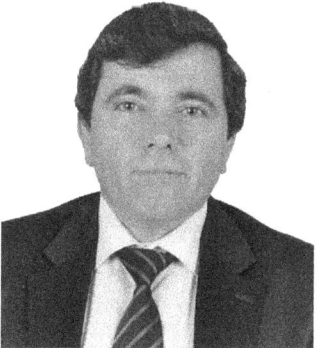

Omer Deperlioglu received his Ph.D. degree from Gazi University, Department of Computer Science, Ankara, Turkey, in 2001. In 2012, he joined the Department of Computer Science, Afyon Kocatepe University, as an associate professor, where he served as the head of the department. His current research interests include Artificial Intelligence applications, signal processing, and image processing in Biomedical engineering. He has published 10 books, 40 articles, and more than 50 papers and attended more than 40 conferences. He was a member of the International Technical Committee in six conferences and workshops. He is serving as an editorial board member of several international journals including associate editor of IET, *The Journal of Engineering*. He is also a book series editor – Biomedical and Robotics Healthcare (CRC Press).

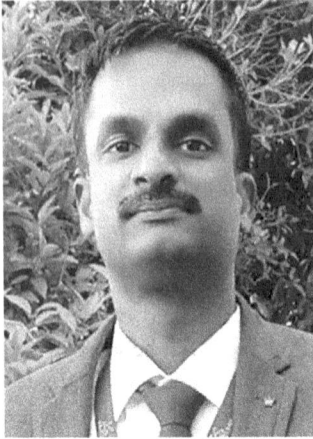

D. Jude Hemanth received his B.E. degree in ECE from Bharathiar University in 2002, M.E. degree in communication systems from Anna University in 2006, and Ph.D. from Karunya University in 2013. His research areas include Computational Intelligence and Image Processing. He has authored more than 130 research papers in reputed SCIE indexed International Journals and Scopus indexed International Conferences. His Cumulative Impact Factor is more than 180. He has published 33 edited books with reputed publishers such as Elsevier, Springer, and IET.

He has been serving as associate editor/scientific editor of SCIE Indexed International Journals such as *Journal of Intelligent and Fuzzy Systems*, and *Mathematical Problems in Engineering*, IET *Quantum Communications and Dyna* (Spain). He serves as an editorial board member/ guest editor of many journals with leading publishers such as Elsevier (*Soft Computing Letters*), Springer (*Multidimensional Systems and Signal Processing, SN Computer Science, Sensing and Imaging*), and Inderscience (*IJAIP, IJICT, IJCVR, IJBET*). He is the series editor of "Biomedical Engineering" book series in Elsevier and "Robotics & Healthcare" book series with CRC Press.

He has received a project grant with 35,000 UK Pound from Government of UK (GCRF scheme) with collaborators from University of Westminster, UK. He has also completed one funded research project from CSIR, Govt. of India, and one ongoing funded project from DST, Govt. of India. He also serves as the "Research Scientist" of Computational Intelligence and Information Systems (CI2S) Lab, Argentina; LAPISCO Research Lab, Brazil; RIADI Lab; Tunisia and Research Centre for Applied Intelligence, University of Craiova, Romania.

He has also been the organizing committee member of several international conferences across the globe including Portugal, Romania, UK, Egypt, China, etc. He has delivered more than 100 Keynote Talks/Invited Lectures in International Conferences/Workshops. He also holds a professional membership with IEEE Technical Committee on Neural Networks (IEEE Computational Intelligence Society) and IEEE Technical Committee on Soft Computing (IEEE Systems, Man, and Cybernetics Society).

Currently, he is working as an associate professor in the Department of ECE, Karunya University, Coimbatore, India.

Contributors

Aditya Pratap Acharya
Machine Intelligence & Bio-Motion
    Research Lab
Department of CSE
National Institute of Technology
Rourkela, India

Q. U. Ain
Department of Chemistry
Government College Women University
    Faisalabad
Faisalabad, Pakistan

Abdelmageed Algamdi
Department of Computer and
    Information Systems
University of Bisha
Saudi Arabia

Gokhan Altan
Department of Computer Engineering
Iskenderun Technical University
Merkez Kampüs, Turkey

Sezin Barin
Department of Biomedical Engineering
Afyon Kocatepe University
Afyonkarahisar, Turkey

Mohammed El Amine Bechar
Biomedical Engineering Laboratory
University of Tlemcen
Tlemcen, Algeria

Subrato Bharati
Institute of ICT
Bangladesh University of Engineering
    and Technology
Dhaka, Bangladesh

Said Khalfa Mokhtar Brika
Department of Administrative Sciences
University of Bisha
Bisha, Saudi Arabia

X. Chen
Department of Statistics and
    Department of Molecular and
    Cellular Biochemistry
University of Kentucky
Lexington, Kentucky

Khalil Chergui
Department of Management Sciences
University of Oum El Bouaghi
Oum El Bouaghi, Algeria

Emre Dandıl
Department of Computer Engineering
Bilecik Seyh Edebali University
Bilecik, Turkey

Inês Domingues
Medical Physics, Radiobiology and
    Radiation Protection Group
IPO Porto Research Centre
    (CI-IPOP)
Porto, Portugal

Kurubaran Ganasegeran
Clinical Research Center
Seberang Jaya Hospital, Ministry of
    Health Malaysia
Penang, Malaysia

Arepalli Peda Gopi
Department of IT
Vignan's Nirula Institute of Technology
    & Science for Women
Guntur, India

Gür Emre Güraksin
Department of Biomedical
    Engineering
Afyon Kocatepe University
Afyonkarahisar, Turkey

Ita Fauzia Hanoum
DR Sardjito Hospital
Indonesia

Sumit Hazra
Machine Intelligence & Bio-Motion
    Research Lab
Department of CSE
National Institute of Technology
Rourkela, India

Filbert H. Juwono
Department of Electrical and
    Computer Engineering
Curtin University Malaysia
Miri, Malaysia

A. Karacı
Department of Computer Engineering
University of Kastamonu
Kastamonu, Turkey

H. Ajay Kumar
Department of Electronics and
    Communication Engineering
Mar Ephraem College of Engineering
    and Technology
Tamil Nadu, India

S. N Kumar
Department of Electrical and
    Electronics Engineering
Amal Jyothi College of Engineering
Kanjirapally, Kerala

Utku Kose
Department of Computer Engineering
Suleyman Demirel University
Isparta, Turkey

Kusum Lata
Department of Electronics and
    Communication Engineering
The LNM Institute of Information
    Technology
Jaipur, India

Adam Musa
Department of Administrative Sciences
University of Bisha
Saudi Arabia

Anup Nandy
Machine Intelligence & Bio-Motion
    Research Lab
Department of CSE
National Institute of Technology
Rourkela, India

V. Lakshman Narayana
Department of IT
Vignan's Nirula Institute of Technology
    & Science for Women
Guntur, India

Panca Dewi Pamungkasari
Graduate School of Environment and
    Information Sciences
Yokohama National University
Yokohama, Japan

R. S. M. Lakshmi Patibandla
Department of IT
Vignan's Foundation for Science,
    Technology, and Research
Guntur, India

Prajoy Podder
Institute of ICT
Bangladesh University of Engineering
    and Technology
Dhaka, Bangladesh

Mohammad Atikur Rahman
Department of Electrical and Electronic
    Engineering
Ranada Prasad Shaha University
Narayanganj, Bangladesh

B. Tarakeswara Rao
Department of CSE
Kallam Haranadha Reddy Institute of
Technology
Guntur, India

M. A. Rather
Division of Fish Genetics and
Biotechnology
Sher-e-Kashmir University of
Agricultural Sciences and
Technology
Rangil-Gandarbal, India

R. A. Rayan
Department of Epidemiology
Alexandria University
Alexandria, Egypt

Shota Saito
Yokohama National University /
SkillUp AI Co. Ltd.
Yokohama, Japan

T. K. Saj Sachin
Center for Computational Engineering
& Networking (CEN)
Amrita School of Engineering
Amrita Vishwa Vidyapeetham
Coimbatore, India

Sandeep Saini
Department of Electronics and
Communication Engineering
The LNM Institute of Information
Technology
Jaipur, India

Jins Sebastin
Amal Jyothi College of Engineering
Kanjirapally, Kerala

Nesma Settouti
Biomedical Engineering Laboratory
University of Tlemcen
Tlemcen, Algeria

Shinichi Shirakawa
Graduate School of Environment and
Information Sciences
Yokohama National University
Yokohama, Japan

K. P. Soman
Center for Computational Engineering
& Networking (CEN)
Amrita School of Engineering
Amrita Vishwa Vidyapeetham
Coimbatore, India

V. Sowmya
Center for Computational Engineering
& Networking (CEN)
Amrita School of Engineering
Amrita Vishwa Vidyapeetham
Coimbatore, India

Safiye Pelin Taş
Department of Biomedical
Engineering
Afyon Kocatepe University
Afyonkarahisar, Turkey

Kento Uchida
Yokohama National University
Yokohama, Japan

Süleyman Uzun
Department of Computer
Engineering
Sakarya University of Applied Science
Sakarya, Turkey

Fethia Yahiaoui
Department of Management Sciences
University of Oum El Bouaghi
Oum El Bouaghi, Algeria

I. Zafar
Department of Bioinformatics
and Computational Biology
Virtual University of Pakistan
Lahor, Pakistan

1 Precision Medicine and Omics in the Context of Deep Learning

I. Zafar
Virtual University of Pakistan

M. A. Rather
Sher-e-Kashmir University of Agricultural
Sciences and Technology

Q. U. Ain
Government College Women University Faisalabad

R. A. Rayan
Alexandria University

CONTENTS

1.1 INTRODUCTION

With immense development of high-throughput techniques in the field of bioinformatics and other computational sciences like next-generation sequencing, microarrays analysis, drug discovery, gene expression, and profiling, etc., it led to a dramatic growth and analysis of big data in the field of biomedical information and integration of natural science to know the structural and functional characteristics of an object (Cook et al., 2016). Utilization of advanced tools and techniques derived the innovation of omics data sets and provided the opportunity to operate the cost-effective analysis on various features in the domain of genomics, proteomics, transcriptomics, and metabolomics within a short time frame. These techniques have transformed system in the field of bioinformatics and allowed further extensive insights for examining molecular pathways and gene ontological systems. A complete access through developed tools or algorithms of deep learning (DL) in the field of information technology is highly promising among numerous challenges in data-driven methods to deal with biomedical data, upcoming disorders, inference of diagnosis, precision medicine (PM), and purpose of individualized therapies (Grapov et al., 2018).

DL is a subcategory of machine learning (ML) algorithms marked with applying artificial neural networks (ANN). ANNs are data-driven techniques from biologic neural networks as they are developed from integrated artificial neurons that get input, translate data, and deliver output (could act as an input for another neuron). DL is an interesting technique for encoding and learning from complicated and disparate data. DL technologies have reached substantial advances in the standard obstacles of artificial intelligence (AI), such as recognizing image or speech and processing language (Lecun et al., 2015).

The proper representation of data is an extensive way for performance and reliability based on deliberated algorithms for ML and is known as features (Goodfellow et al., 2016). The term features is developed by expert individuals based on market need or nature of task via identifying the domains which are suitable for assigned tasks. However, for understanding or finalizing this type of big data task, DL provides novel insight via emerging with developed sophisticated algorithms for parallel, distributed, and cloud computing. Therefore, the interest for ML increases very rapidly in the field of data science integrated with biological science to solve problem of big data; a flow chart of information is mentioned in Figure 1.1.

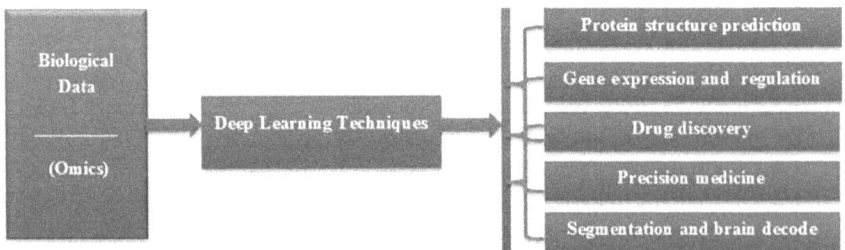

FIGURE 1.1 Illustration of omics data using DL techniques to handle PM.

In some context, DL involved with wide-ranging field to provide the opportunity for resolving high-throughput tasks with great promises, where many other techniques like platform of AI are already struggling (LeCun et al., 2015). DL provides wide-ranging applications or advantages in the field of computational science like image processing, speech reorganization (Chorowski et al., 2015), natural language processing (Kiros et al., 2015), language translations (Luong et al., 2015). In ML, DL provides various opportunities in medical science such as detection of lapses from electroencephalography signals, utilization of image processing for reorganizations of finger joints, etc. Utilization of DL is based on developed algorithms, methods, and techniques; here we will discuss some beneficial techniques of DL for exploring multiple tasks via providing cost, time, space, and complexity benefits, and dealing with different types of problems. This chapter examines the principal applications of DL techniques in analyzing omics data with stressing on the kinds of analysis, constraints, and potential for PM.

Our main objective is to highlight the growing attention for promising DL techniques to establish analytic frameworks and recognize complicated trends in clinical and medical imaging based on omics techniques integrated with wide-ranging molecular databases. This chapter summarizes the major applications of DL techniques in biomedical studies, highlighting PM applications. It reviews some principle applications and issues addressed by DL in analyzing medical images and omics data. It also discusses applications to enhance detecting, sorting, and managing complex disorders in the contact of time, space, and complexity.

1.2 DEEP LEARNING TECHNIQUES AND METHODS

In the field of bioinformatics and computational biology, DL technologies are being applied increasingly for analyzing omics data and manipulate the data based on different information retrieval techniques algorithms' to solve complex biological problem via performing different functions on databases like retrieving, updating, managing, deleting data with logical consequences of efficiency, sensitivity, or specificity. DL algorithms provide opportunity over bioinformatics to deal very comprehensively among omics challenges with advantages of time, space, cost, and complexity such as adopting PM techniques, enabling early diagnosis, sorting of disorders, and individualized treatments for every patient according to their biochemical history (Min et al., 2017) as shown in Figure 1.2.

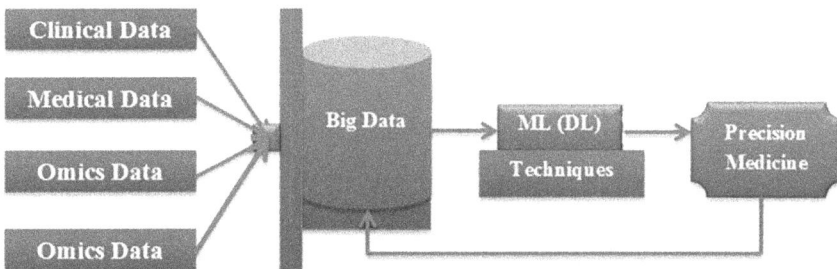

FIGURE 1.2   Omics, big data, and DL techniques for PM.

In context of DL, deep learning networks (DLN) are a subset of ML algorithms to identify a mathematic function f which maps several inputs, (*x*), to their related outputs, (*y*), like [$y=f(x)$]. Some examples for DL techniques in the context of omics for PM are deep feed-forward (DFF) neural network, convolutional neural network (CNN), recurrent neural network (RNN), long-/short-term memory (LSTM), deep belief network (DBN), and autoencoder (AE). The implementation of DL in the field of data-driven is based on developed tools, techniques, methods, and algorithms. Here we will discuss some beneficial techniques of DL for exploring multiple tasks (understating the relation between PM and Omics) via providing cost, time, space, and complexity benefits on different types of problems.

1.2.1 Deep Neural Networks

The classification of ML algorithms provides the opportunity to design the deep neural networks (DNNs) that used to map the number of inputs via determining the mathematical function for corresponding outputs then with weight then equation will be. This simple network based on the simplest DL architecture can be defined through composition of nonlinear transformation techniques to identify the hidden layers for activation of filtration system among the provided data during updating of machine training; a detailed overview is shown in Figure 1.3. Furthermore, training data based on supervised learning called batch because it usually operates iterative function to complete the task with the help of statistical calculations, if in any iteration batch loses their function then it uses the process of weight (*w*) updating to minimize the issue in next iteration based on roles of back-propagation algorithm (LeCun et al., 1989); therefore weight (*w*) progression parameters provide best approximation results to deal corresponding outputs.

1.2.2 Convolutional Neural Network

A CNN involves input, output, and several hidden layers, finally extended as a building block like fully connected, pooling, and convolutional layers with processes of transfer learning to enhance their performance from target domains. With the

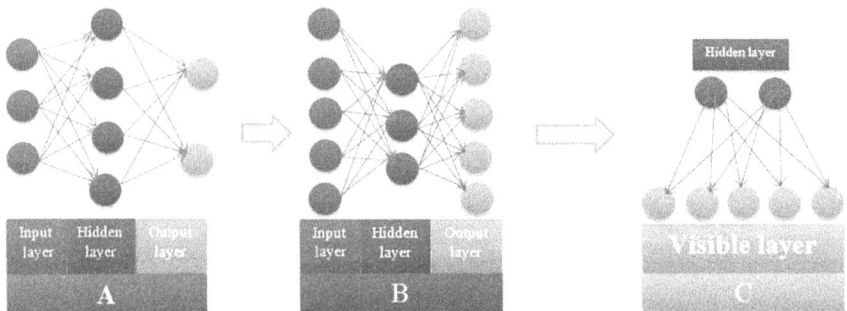

FIGURE 1.3 Representation of DNN structures: (a) MLP contains only one hidden layer. (b) Layout of auto-encoder structure. (c) A typical RBM structure.

explanations of CNNs in medical science, it works as an extensive dimensionality reduction method to take image as input (disease) or classify this as output (healthy patient) according to classification score. In DL, CNN employs a convolution approach to classification from DNNs and most adequate to deal with high multi-dimensional data sets via pretrained approaches (Deng et al., 2009) such as visual imagery concepts in medical science (Valueva et al., 2020). The extensive character-istics of CNN are very broad due to its shared weightage framework, and this shared phenomenon is known as space invariant ANNs (Zhang, 1988). In the current trend of technology CNN is used for broad range of fields to provide potential applica-tions like image classification and recognition (Ciregan et al., 2012), medical imaging and analysis, natural language processing (Kiros et al., 2015), recommender systems (Ongsulee, 2017), drug discovery (Wallach et al., 2015), valuation of health risk, and aging biomarkers (Pyrkov et al., 2018), etc.

1.2.3 RECURRENT NEURAL NETWORK

An RNN originates from ANN and is specifically designed to work with sequence pre-diction and sequential data problems where the association is shaped among nodes to a direct graph. RNNs can practice their inner state (memory) to proceed variable length input sequences (Dupond, 2019) and also use reverse propagation over every interval that has extended the primary choice at step t1, distressing the outcome to be reached a second later at time step t as mentioned in Figure 1.4. This type of network systems has dual input sources, the current and the past, which commonly combined to explore how they return information to new data. RNN has a numerous of applications used for biological computational fields such a protein homology modeling and detection with-out alignment (Hochreiter et al., 2007), human behavioral understanding, bidirectional process to predicting subcellular localization of proteins (Thireou et al., 2007), and prediction in clinical events or medical care pathways (Choi et al., 2016).

1.2.4 LONG-/SHORT-TERM MEMORY

The RNN, hidden Markov models, and numerous other sequence learning tech-niques were used to address some issues like vanishing gradient and relative insen-sitivity to gap length, etc., for that reason in the field of DL, the variant of RNN was intended to observe the best operative solutions based on artificial RNN architecture (Hochreiter, 1997). The architecture of LSTM is simplified in a single unit having three types of gates such as input and output, and forgets in computer memory to

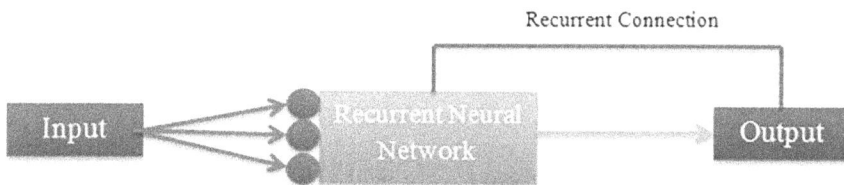

FIGURE 1.4 Detailed architecture of RNN algorithm with loop.

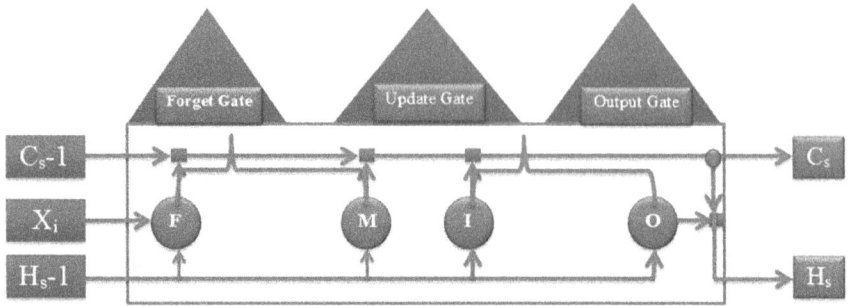

FIGURE 1.5 LSTM blocks, where Xi for input system, Cs-1 for cell states, Hs-1 for hidden states, F for forget gate, M for memory cell, I for input gate, and O for output gate.

process single and complete sequence data as mentioned in Figure 1.5 and example of this algorithm are imaging analysis, speech recognition, and videos transforming. The flow of data is passed among cell via remembering the value over long duration of time intervals for regulating the input and output series of information. The main objective of this technique is to understand or learn further constant errors which are growing drastically by backpropagation though layers and time.

1.2.5 DEEP BELIEF NETWORK

With the advanced development in the field of ML, the initiation of DL has great advantages such as many tools and graphically connects methods for combining the big data from chunks. A DBN is composed of manifold layers of latent variables and controlled Boltzmann machine (Hinton, 2009) as a core component and known as a class of DNN or generative graphical model used for supervised and unsupervised learning (Fischer and Igel, 2012). DBN can be trained greedily to generate probabilistic (probability and statistics) values, rearrange from query in early stage or after learning; it improves skills with supervision to perform classification of data (Hinton et al., 2006). Finally, DBN has two types of layers, amalgamation of visible and hidden, utilized to play a vital role in numerous real life applications via forming bipartite graph such as discovery of potential drugs (Ghasemi et al., 2018), PM, and electrophysiological detection of human brain functions (Movahedi et al., 2017).

1.2.6 AUTOENCODER

In general, an AE is a class of ANN based on unsupervised manner trying to learn series of data coding distribution from wide-ranging data sets (Rumelhart et al., 1985). The main objective of AE algorithm is to learn about representation of data in a specific way by training the network to reduce the noise and perform the active contribution as dimensionality reduction networks without new engineering (Salakhutdinov & Hinton, 2006) to meet with original inputs. According to the empower of AE, several variants (contractive autoencoders, sparse, and denoising) and methods (vanilla, multilayer, convolutional, and regularized AE) are available

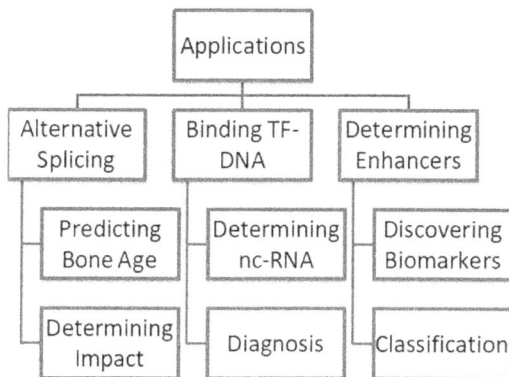

FIGURE 1.6   Some DL applications in omics for PM.

for effective classification of task (Vincent et al., 2010). AE involved with generative variants and methods to show applications in many fields to solve numerous applied problems such as information retrieval technique and semantic hashing (Salakhutdinov & Hinton, 2009), face recognitions (Hinton et al., 2011), and drug discovery in computational fields (Zhavoronkov et al., 2019).

1.3   USING DEEP LEARNING TO ANALYZE OMICS DATA

DL tools, techniques, methods, and algorithms, which are functionally driven from computational technologies, provide a key role to solve, retrieve, explore complicated, diverse, and high-dimensional data sets in the order of omics (Zhang et al., 2019). Figure 1.6 shows an overview of the major applications of DL in PM.

1.3.1   DL IN GENOMICS

Genomics is a field of science derived from molecular biology for the study of entire genome from individual organisms and provides opportunity for the analysis of whole genome, editing, mapping, and functioning. According to empower of genome analysis or interaction of big data, genomics can be divided into three major parts: structural, functional, and regulatory genomics.

Application of DL in genomics is a rapidly growing area that directly primed for genomic analysis and revolution via understanding of genome biology. The potential of DL algorithms is holding a large amount of genomic data that is spreading to all aspects of genomics research. Therefore, genomics applies some advance methods for manipulation of data and exploration of sequences of DNA to investigate the composition and mechanism of genomes properties like genetic regulation, and gene modifications on structural and functional levels that can be related with many disorders. From several time periods, DL techniques have been adopted to apply on genomics data for solving many challenges or issues; for example, using CNNs in DL methods to determine the flow of indels (insertion or deletion of nucleotides among sequences) and single-nucleotide polymorphisms (SNP) (Poplin et al., 2018). In the same way other methods (DFF, ResNets, and CNN) are also applied to solve the genetic variations-related problems or calculate the pathogenic penalties (Qi et al., 2018; Quang et al., 2015; Zhou & Troyanskaya, 2015). DFFs and sparse autoencoders algorithms are also used to purse the effect of genetic variations on gene modification and expression levels (Xie et al., 2017).

Today, in the era of genomics, gene editing is a very hot topic used to alter the DNA at cell to individual levels using CRISPR technology with very cost-effective approaches for targeted sequences. In the domain of functional genomics, DL methods are used to calculate the regulatory motifs of protein and regulatory domains of DNA and enhancer's sequences (transcription factors) from genomic resources (Oubounyt et al., 2019) like chromatin accessibility, histone alterations, etc. (Li et al., 2018). The combinations of CNN and LSTM algorithmic networks are used to purse the results of gene promoters (Wang et al., 2018). In addition CNN method in DL has advantages or used to identify the splice junctions (Zuallaert et al., 2018). Finally, we conclude that DL technologies and methods interacting with omics data can potentially handle many computational challenges or issues that we are facing today with cost-effective improved outputs.

1.3.2 DL in Genome-Wide Association Studies

In the recent era, genome-wide association studies (GWAS) provide the novel insight to detect the mainstream functionality of new genetic variants which are directly involved to influence the risk mechanism of several complex diseases such as cancer, cardiovascular, and miscommunication of immune system also known as autoimmune diseases. It also provides the opportunity for screening of genomic locations (loci) which correlated to alleles, phenotypes, genotypes test, and their disorders. GWAS studies determine SNPs in genetic regions that are integrated with frameworks for predicting risk factors characteristically investigated through polygenic risk method (Wei et al., 2009), as well as many SNPs and involved effects should be examined at once. However, there are some challenges or issues still identified for approaching GWAS study to handle combined effects of multiple genetic disorders associated with other environmental factors such as identification of SNPs on a genome-wide scale in the contexts of genotype and determination of billions of SNPs in thousands of topics. Therefore such processes are facing many challenges like failure to decrease the loosed heritability, handling phenomenon of epistasis in genetics, and detailed assumption for a global linear association models (Purcell et al., 2009). Among these challengers many standard statistical approaches like logistic regression and multiple linear analyses are not suited to take benefits of time, space, and complexity in genome-wide data sets.

Here, ML in the context of DL provides promising networks or methods to analyze large number of data sets which are correlated with many possible genetic variables as model complex relationships like usage of obesity classification model as a binary phenotypic system (Montañez et al., 2018). Thus far, the predictive capabilities of such type genetic markers are very weak because these makers are founded on individual locus. Recently, using advanced methods like stacked sparse autoencoders in epistatic phenomenon of mutation and its effects of SNPs could identify the preterm birth processes in American and African females (Fergus et al., 2020). This method has shown highly achieved results for classifying or capturing valid interactions of DNA loci using blackbox techniques. The chosen SNPs lose the dimension of GWAS; hence examining their impacts on phenotype is further challenging and for this type of challenges a new approach of DL is used to arrest the problem using PGMRA (online web based server for phenotypic and genotypic relation analysis for one-to-many or many-to-many in GWAS). The PGMRA is a DL approach based on supervised or unsupervised learning or apply multiple domains on phenotype-genotype data sets to analyze their relations through using semisupervised interactions or nonnegative matrix factorization as an artificial environment (AE) for optimizing multiobjective tasks (Arnedo et al., 2013; Hinton & Salakhutdinov, 2006). In PGMRA, for optimizing the solutions, every layer has a unique procedure for learning and represents the input for the subsequent layer, after which its outcomes are defined and could reduce the lacking heritability and recognize the epistatic sets of markers, which constitute the phenotypic and genotypic structure of disease and traits (Arnedo et al., 2014).

1.3.3 DL in Transcriptomics

Transcriptomics optimizes the level of expression for the entire RNA transcripts created in a cell. Transcriptomics raw data are often analyzed to produce expression matrices carrying an expression level estimate for every transcript or gene along with multiple conditions and samples that are usually the input for DL techniques. DL has been used with success in a wide ranging of applications or models in transcriptomics or provides potential benefits via predicting the ratio of phenotypes (e.g., disease stage, progression, type, and subtypes) and detecting complex signal from multiple genes by means of entire transcriptomes. For instance, the major aim of data in gene expression is exploring alternative splicing that is compiling various isoforms of the transcripts using the same gene. However, CNNs have determined real splice junctions from false positives created while aligning RNA sequence (RNA-seq) reads (Zhang et al., 2018).

In DL, there are three main supervised learning methods that are used for transcriptome-based data sets like feedforward neural network for predicting gene expression level values based on approximation theorem, 2-dimensional CNN (2D CNN) for conversion in image like data from transcriptome data sets, and in the last, the third algorithm, the graph convolutional network for illustrating chemical structures and predicting the feasibility of transcriptomic data.

Other advantages of DL in transcriptomic are estimating the new RNA types like noncoding RNAs (ncRNAs) and characterizing their expression. An RNN is an algorithm which involves distinguishing the coding and noncoding region of RNAs or provides applications to determine ncRNAs with no prior knowledge (Hill et al., 2018). Furthermore, DFF technique was proposed to predict long ncRNAs (lncRNAs) where they achieved a significant 99% precision rate implementing as source repository (Tripathi et al., 2016). Long intergenic ncRNAs (lincRNAs), a class of lncRNAs that are transcribed in intergenic regions, have also been satisfactorily anticipated by inputting an AE with prior lincRNAs knowledge (Yu et al., 2017).

1.3.4   DL in Epigenomics

In this era, there is a great importance to deal with genomic data; before this, dealing with genomic data using suitable methods was very limited to deal with genotype, nucleotide sequencing from individual organism. Later, advanced technology such as ML or DL played vital role to detect specific structure, characteristics, and association of specific molecular marker and gave a new insight for identification of genomic regions mutually called epigenomics. The epigenomics big data interpretation and underlined problems are very difficult task to handle, due to its large size, complexity, or other lack of biological knowledge factors. To support unravel this big data, we focus on advanced ML models which are actively involved to resolve these challenges. Epigenomics examines alterations in DNA which comprises markers that could modify expressing a gene with no changes in the sequence of DNA. There are several epigenetic markers such as methylating DNA, altering histone, and uniquely aligning of nucleosomes. Methylating DNA might be the highly examined alteration in epigenetics where it examines methylation patterns which, as in gene expression templates, could determine biomarkers or classify the flow of disease.

In epigenetics research, broad-range of applications (bioinformatics complex data, epigenome mapping, disease detection, environmental exposure detection and biological investigations) had done using DL techniques. DL techniques could precisely estimate the sequences identified via proteins linked to RNA and DNA by CNNs (Alipanahi et al., 2015). A major benefit of such a technique is combining data from various methods in epigenomics research. Meanwhile, the methylating DNA state was precisely estimated by sequence data (Wang et al., 2016). Altering histone, likewise, methylating DNA does not impact DNA sequence yet could alter its accessibility to the transcriptional tools. CNNs could build an algorithm to estimate such histone alterations (Yin et al., 2019). CNN could derive expressing a gene from histone alterations data; however, LSTM could estimate differential gene expression, as well from these data (Grau et al., 2013; Singh et al., 2016).

1.3.5   DL in Proteomics and Metabolomics

Proteomics covers a group of methods to measure levels of expression, posttranslational alterations, or mapping of proteins in biological samples or cells. Metabolomics examines an entire metabolome, which are small molecule that take part in metabolic reactions. The methods utilized by such omics-streams are like nuclear magnetic resonance (NMR) or mass spectrometry (MS), challenging to researchers to assign raw instrumental signals to metabolites or proteins (Min et al., 2017).

In proteomics, the highly frequent empirical approach is cutting proteins into small peptides (chains of amino acids) and examining them in an MS. The MS output signals are determined via comparison to peptide templates preserved in databases. Yet, such databases are imprecise. Hence, an application uses an LSTM network to estimate peptide MS/MS spectra (Zhou et al., 2017). Recognizing peptide spectra in advance enables assigning MS/MS spectra to peptides and matching them to the hypothetical spectra. De novo peptide sequencing, another proteomics application, could characterize proteins where a model integrated LSTMs and CNN to achieve this hard job successfully (Tran et al., 2017). After sequencing the peptides' group in a proteomics sample, the following obstacle is determining the original proteins of these peptides; therefore, a CNN was used to get improved outcomes than before (Kim et al., 2017). DL could use amino acid sequences to estimate the secondary structures of a protein (Spencer et al., 2015).

NMR technique is needed to produce data in both metabolomics and proteomics. Yet, it has a technical constraint of retrieving several noise signals that should be cleared to enhance precision. Such an essential step was automated by using CNNs to eliminate noise peaks from NMR spectra, hence enhancing the function (Kobayashi et al., 2018). Using DL techniques with metabolomics data is difficult since they cannot determine certain elements that affect particular samples needed in such studies. However, several DL techniques have been designed and achieved interesting outcomes. For example, integrating mean decrease accuracy metric with DNNs could identify NMR-derived metabolomics data, surpassing other ML techniques (Asakura et al., 2018; Date & Kikuchi, 2018).

1.4　DEEP LEARNING APPLICATIONS IN PRECISION MEDICINE

Ultimately, PM targets shifting from common interventions for the wide public to tailored personalized therapeutic plans and interventions according to every patient's molecular background, or build preventive medicine protocols depending on predicting vulnerability to disorders (Ashley, 2016; Chen & Snyder, 2013). Omics data facilitate examining disorders from many parallel dimensions such as sequencing DNA, expressing genes, and medical imaging and recognizing the modified components of these complicated biological operations. Multiple ML-derived techniques have been used in medicine (Rajkomar et al., 2019). Despite ML has shown to be valuable in several applications of PM, it has some drawbacks which could be addressed via DL models. For example, ML function relies heavily on preprocessing data for retrieving characteristics; however, DL architectures involve such retrieving characteristics (Eraslan et al., 2019).

1.4.1　FINDING BIOMARKER AND CLASSIFYING PATIENTS

Recognizing novel biomarkers for early disorders' detection, classification, and treatment response are among the popular applications of omics techniques in biomedical research. A huge quantity of public omics data particularly in cancer, like the Cancer Genome Atlas (TCGA), has enabled recognizing novel biomarkers with both DL and non-DL methods (Weinstein et al., 2013). Promising research was able to classify breast cancer samples, via data on gene expression, from the TCGA database into diseased or healthy (Danaee et al., 2017). This technique determined a group of responding genes that could be valuable biomarkers for cancer. TCGA data on gene expression have been as well applied to precisely distinguish samples into various kinds of cancers (Lyu & Haque, 2018). Meanwhile, an AE was applied to classify healthy and diseased subjects with breast cancer through methylating data, and CNN also was applied to classify various kinds of cancers by their methylating characteristics, reaching highly promising outcomes (Chatterjee et al., 2018; Si et al., 2016). Many omics such as methylating data, RNA-seq, or miRNA-seq have been integrated to classify hepatic cancer patients into various surviving clusters (Chaudhary et al., 2018).

Data from TCGA applied to train AE framework; however, this technique is expected to improve by further clinical data. Likewise, omics data from TCGA were integrated to categorize bladder cancer patients by their probabilities to survive where an AE technique applied to segregate patients into two surviving groups which determined biomarkers related to rates of survival (Poirion et al., 2018). DFFs have also been applied to predict Alzheimer's disease biomarkers (Zafeiris et al., 2018). Another technique to classify kinds of cancers according to somatic mutations where statistical methods were integrated with a DFF and such a technique was trained and evaluated using data from TCGA on 12 kinds of cancer (Yuan et al., 2016).

1.4.2 MEDICAL IMAGING

Medical imaging is a major shifting technology from classical medicine toward PM. For example, the initial step in detecting dermatological tumors is dermatologists' visual inspections. Therefore, detecting dermatological tumors is a conventional image recognition issue where scientists have used ML and image recognition techniques. Recently, CNN was trained with thousands of medical images to digitally classify cancerous dermatological lesions where the outcomes were comparable to a board of professional dermatologists (Esteva et al., 2017). In the upcoming years, for the promising findings, these studies are to be turned into mobile applications for precisely detecting cancerous dermatological lesions (Brinker et al., 2018).

Computed tomography (CT) can diagnose many disorders via 3D anatomical images. Several DL techniques might facilitate applying CT imaging to PM. For example, CNNs are planned to classify instantly CT images into the various anatomical structures of a human that would be the initial step in several CT-derived diagnosis schemes (Roth, Lee, et al., 2015). Other examples are scoring calcium in a coronary artery or segmenting the pancreas (Roth, Farag, et al., 2015; Wolterink et al., 2016).

Ultrasound (US), another imaging technology, has several applications in medicine, for example, in detecting cardiac dysfunctions applying DBNs to monitor left ventricle endocardium, for diagnosing various cardiomyopathies (Carneiro & Nascimento, 2013). Meanwhile, CNN was used for identifying the contents of a carotid plaque (Lekadir et al., 2017). A DL technique was designed for identifying hepatic US images to diagnose and stratify hepatic disorders (Biswas et al., 2018).

Several DL techniques have been used with X-ray images. For example, CNN was applied to identify vessel regions, an essential step to diagnosing coronary artery disorders (Nasr-Esfahani et al., 2016). Evaluating the age of the bone is a popular method in determining defects in growth, and now, it is accomplished manually by comparing databases' X-ray images, though DL algorithms were used to automate such a procedure (Lee & Kim, 2018).

Ultimately, face images are being used, having highly positive outcomes, to detect disorders automatically. Lately, a model was proposed for analyzing face to characterize genetic syndrome where CNNs and images of patients' faces were used to measure analogies of facial characteristics to several syndromes surpassing professionals in diagnosing jobs (Gurovich et al., 2019).

1.4.3 DIAGNOSING CANCER

In cerebral tumors, segmenting tumor is required to determine the size and the morphology of the tumor and then make diagnosis and treatment. Physicians often make such segmenting manually through images got from magnetic resonance imaging (MRI). Yet, this important job is subjective and highly time-consuming. Hence, great attention to automating segmenting tumor using MRI data has been given; such a job is challenging since MRI data comprise heterogeneous 3D images that vary, for each tumor, among patients, based on the applied process or the used device (Işın et al., 2016). Many researchers applied CNNs to solve this issue (Naceur et al., 2018).

Examining histopathological images is a highly prevalent test to detect tumors. Similarly, to segmenting cerebral tumors, examining images is done manually by pathologists, which is consuming time; hence, automating such a procedure became necessary. A CNN-derived scheme was applied to detect tumors in breast and prostate; however, it gave initial outcomes, and more studies are required (Litjens et al., 2016). Various DL algorithms were integrated to use histopathological images for classifying subtypes of breast cancer, and a ResNet was used to classify colorectal lesions (Korbar et al., 2017; Xie et al., 2019).

1.5 CONCLUSIONS

Omics techniques are transforming biomedical research and presenting innovative challenging analyses to bioinformatics. In PM, DL is an attractive technology to explore such diverse and complicated big data. This chapter examined some promising DL techniques in analyzing omics data and PM. So far, supervised learning has the most booming DL applications in biomedical research. Since the quality of learning relies upon the quality of the data feed, care should be given to the training sets. Although, using DL techniques in omics and PM is an innovative domain, there are several challenges. Generally, there is no solely applicable technique; hence, selecting and using DL techniques would be challenging. For the insufficient data, conventional analytical techniques would be credible and superior. A drawback for DL is the rising difficulty in designing models and the needed computational context. However, there are growing research attempts to address the main limitations. For the future, the growing accessibility to a greater amount of omics data, medical imaging, and health records is sparking the potential applications of DL techniques in PM.

REFERENCES

Alipanahi, B., Delong, A., Weirauch, M. T., & Frey, B. J. (2015). Predicting the sequence specificities of DNA- and RNA-binding proteins by deep learning. *Nature Biotechnology*, 33(8), 831–838. Doi: 10.1038/nbt.3300.

Arnedo, J., del Val, C., de Erausquin, G. A., Romero-Zaliz, R., Svrakic, D., Cloninger, C. R., & Zwir, I. (2013). PGMRA: A web server for (phenotype×genotype) many-to-many relation analysis in GWAS. *Nucleic Acids Research*, 41(W1), W142–W149. Doi: 10.1093/nar/gkt496.

Arnedo, J., Svrakic, D. M., del Val, C., Romero-Zaliz, R., Hernández-Cuervo, H., Fanous, A. H., Pato, M. T., Pato, C. N., de Erausquin, G. A., Cloninger, C. R., & Zwir, I. (2014). Uncovering the hidden risk architecture of the schizophrenias: Confirmation in three independent genome-wide association studies. *American Journal of Psychiatry*, 172(2), 139–153. Doi: 10.1176/appi.ajp.2014.14040435.

Asakura, T., Date, Y., & Kikuchi, J. (2018). Application of ensemble deep neural network to metabolomics studies. *Analytica Chimica Acta*, 1037, 230–236. Doi: 10.1016/j.aca.2018.02.045.

Ashley, E. A. (2016). Towards precision medicine. *Nature Reviews Genetics*, 17(9), 507–522. Doi: 10.1038/nrg.2016.86.

Biswas, M., Kuppili, V., Edla, D. R., Suri, H. S., Saba, L., Marinhoe, R. T., Sanches, J. M., & Suri, J. S. (2018). Symtosis: A liver ultrasound tissue characterization and risk stratification in optimized deep learning paradigm. *Computer Methods and Programs in Biomedicine*, 155, 165–177. Doi: 10.1016/j.cmpb.2017.12.016.

Brinker, T. J., Hekler, A., Utikal, J. S., Grabe, N., Schadendorf, D., Klode, J., Berking, C., Steeb, T., Enk, A. H., & Kalle, C. von. (2018). Skin cancer classification using convolutional neural networks: Systematic review. *Journal of Medical Internet Research*, 20(10), e11936. Doi: 10.2196/11936.

Carneiro, G., & Nascimento, J. C. (2013). Combining multiple dynamic models and deep learning architectures for tracking the left ventricle endocardium in ultrasound data. *IEEE Transactions on Pattern Analysis and Machine Intelligence*, 35(11), 2592–2607. Doi: 10.1109/TPAMI.2013.96.

Chatterjee, S., Iyer, A., Avva, S., Kollara, A., & Sankarasubbu, M. (2018). Convolutional neural networks in classifying cancer through DNA methylation. *ArXiv:1807.09617* [Cs, q-Bio, Stat]. http://arxiv.org/abs/1807.09617.

Chaudhary, K., Poirion, O. B., Lu, L., & Garmire, L. X. (2018). Deep learning–based multi-omics integration robustly predicts survival in liver cancer. *Clinical Cancer Research*, 24(6), 1248–1259. Doi: 10.1158/1078-0432.CCR-17-0853.

Chen, R., & Snyder, M. (2013). Promise of personalized omics to precision medicine. *WIREs Systems Biology and Medicine*, 5(1), 73–82. Doi: 10.1002/wsbm.1198.

Choi, E., Bahadori, M. T., Schuetz, A., Stewart, W. F., & Sun, J. (2016, December). Doctor ai: Predicting clinical events via recurrent neural networks. In *Machine Learning for Healthcare Conference* (pp. 301–318), Proceedings of Machine Learning Research, ML Research Press, Los Angeles, CA.

Chorowski, J. K., Bahdanau, D., Serdyuk, D., Cho, K., & Bengio, Y. (2015). Attention-based models for speech recognition. In *Advances in Neural Information Processing Systems* (pp. 577–585), Neural Information Processing System Foundation, Inc., Quebec.

Ciregan, D., Meier, U., & Schmidhuber, J. (2012, June). Multi-column deep neural networks for image classification. In *2012 IEEE Conference on Computer Vision and Pattern Recognition* (pp. 3642–3649). IEEE, Providence, Rhode Island.

Cook, C. E., Bergman, M. T., Finn, R. D., Cochrane, G., Birney, E., & Apweiler, R. (2016). The European bioinformatics institute in 2016: Data growth and integration. *Nucleic Acids Research*, 44(Database issue), D20–D26. Doi: 10.1093/nar/gkv1352.

Danaee, P., Ghaeini, R., & Hendrix, D. A. (2017). A deep learning approach for cancer detection and relevant gene identification. *Pacific Symposium on Biocomputing. Pacific Symposium on Biocomputing*, 22, 219–229. Doi: 10.1142/9789813207813_0022.

Date, Y., & Kikuchi, J. (2018). Application of a deep neural network to metabolomics studies and its performance in determining important variables. *Analytical Chemistry*, 90(3), 1805–1810. Doi: 10.1021/acs.analchem.7b03795.

Deng, J., Dong, W., Socher, R., Li, L. J., Li, K., & Fei-Fei, L. (2009, June). Imagenet: A large-scale hierarchical image database. In *2009 IEEE Conference on Computer Vision and Pattern Recognition* (pp. 248–255). IEEE, Miami, FL.

Dupond, S. (2019). A thorough review on the current advance of neural network structures. *Annual Reviews in Control*, *14*, 200–230.

Eraslan, G., Avsec, Ž., Gagneur, J., & Theis, F. J. (2019). Deep learning: New computational modelling techniques for genomics. *Nature Reviews Genetics*, 20(7), 389–403. Doi: 10.1038/s41576-019-0122-6.

Esteva, A., Kuprel, B., Novoa, R. A., Ko, J., Swetter, S. M., Blau, H. M., & Thrun, S. (2017). Dermatologist-level classification of skin cancer with deep neural networks. *Nature*, 542(7639), 115–118. Doi: 10.1038/nature21056.

Fergus, P., Montañez, C. C., Abdulaimma, B., Lisboa, P., Chalmers, C., & Pineles, B. (2020). Utilizing deep learning and genome wide association studies for epistatic-driven preterm birth classification in African-American women. *IEEE/ACM Transactions on Computational Biology and Bioinformatics*, 17(2), 668–678. Doi: 10.1109/TCBB.2018.2868667.

Fischer, A., & Igel, C. (2012, September). An introduction to restricted Boltzmann machines. In *Iberoamerican Congress on Pattern Recognition* (pp. 14–36). Springer, Berlin.

Ghasemi, F., Mehridehnavi, A., Perez-Garrido, A., & Perez-Sanchez, H. (2018). Neural network and deep-learning algorithms used in QSAR studies: Merits and drawbacks. *Drug Discovery Today*, 23(10), 1784–1790.

Goodfellow, I., Bengio, Y., & Courville, A. (2016). Machine learning basics. *Deep Learning*, *1*, 98–164.

Grapov, D., Fahrmann, J., Wanichthanarak, K., & Khoomrung, S. (2018). Rise of deep learning for genomic, proteomic, and metabolomic data integration in precision medicine. *Omics: A Journal of Integrative Biology*, 22(10), 630–636. Doi: 10.1089/omi.2018.0097.

Grau, J., Boch, J., & Posch, S. (2013). TALENoffer: Genome-wide TALEN off-target prediction. *Bioinformatics*, 29(22), 2931–2932. Doi: 10.1093/bioinformatics/btt501.

Gurovich, Y., Hanani, Y., Bar, O., Nadav, G., Fleischer, N., Gelbman, D., Basel-Salmon, L., Krawitz, P. M., Kamphausen, S. B., Zenker, M., Bird, L. M., & Gripp, K. W. (2019). Identifying facial phenotypes of genetic disorders using deep learning. *Nature Medicine*, 25(1), 60–64. Doi: 10.1038/s41591-018-0279-0.

Hill, S. T., Kuintzle, R., Teegarden, A., Merrill, E., Danaee, P., & Hendrix, D. A. (2018). A deep recurrent neural network discovers complex biological rules to decipher RNA protein-coding potential. *Nucleic Acids Research*, 46(16), 8105–8113. Doi: 10.1093/nar/gky567.

Hinton, G. E. (2009). Deep belief networks. *Scholarpedia*, 4(5), 5947.

Hinton, G. E., & Salakhutdinov, R. R. (2006). Reducing the dimensionality of data with neural networks. *Science*, 313(5786), 504–507. Doi: 10.1126/science.1127647.

Hinton, G. E., Krizhevsky, A., & Wang, S. D. (2011, June). Transforming auto-encoders. In *International Conference on Artificial Neural Networks* (pp. 44–51). Springer, Berlin.

Hinton, G. E., Osindero, S., & Teh, Y. W. (2006). A fast learning algorithm for deep belief nets. *Neural Computation*, 18(7), 1527–1554.

Hochreiter, S. & Schmidhuber J. (1997). Long short-term memory. *Neural Computation*, 9(8), 1735–1780.

Hochreiter, S., Heusel, M., & Obermayer, K. (2007). Fast model-based protein homology detection without alignment. *Bioinformatics*, 23(14), 1728–1736.

Işın, A., Direkoğlu, C., & Şah, M. (2016). Review of MRI-based brain tumor image segmentation using deep learning methods. *Procedia Computer Science*, *102*, 317–324. Doi: 10.1016/j.procs.2016.09.407.

Kim, M., Eetemadi, A., & Tagkopoulos, I. (2017). DeepPep: Deep proteome inference from peptide profiles. *PLOS Computational Biology*, 13(9), e1005661. Doi: 10.1371/journal.pcbi.1005661.

Kiros, R., Zhu, Y., Salakhutdinov, R. R., Zemel, R., Urtasun, R., Torralba, A., & Fidler, S. (2015). Skip-thought vectors. In *Advances in Neural Information Processing Systems* (pp. 3294–3302), Neural Information Processing System Foundation, Inc., Quebec.

Kobayashi, N., Hattori, Y., Nagata, T., Shinya, S., Güntert, P., Kojima, C., & Fujiwara, T. (2018). Noise peak filtering in multi-dimensional NMR spectra using convolutional neural networks. *Bioinformatics*, 34(24), 4300–4301. Doi: 10.1093/bioinformatics/bty581.

Korbar, B., Olofson, A. M., Miraflor, A. P., Nicka, C. M., Suriawinata, M. A., Torresani, L., Suriawinata, A. A., & Hassanpour, S. (2017). Deep learning for classification of colorectal polyps on whole-slide images. *Journal of Pathology Informatics*, 8, 30. Doi: 10.4103/jpi.jpi_34_17.

Lecun, Y., Bengio, Y., & Hinton, G. (2015). Deep learning. *Nature*, 521(7553), 436–444. Doi: 10.1038/nature14539.

Lee, J. H., & Kim, K. G. (2018). Applying deep learning in medical images: The case of bone age estimation. *Healthcare Informatics Research*, 24(1), 86–92. Doi: 10.4258/hir.2018.24.1.86.

Lekadir, K., Galimzianova, A., Betriu, À., del Mar Vila, M., Igual, L., Rubin, D. L., Fernández, E., Radeva, P., & Napel, S. (2017). A convolutional neural network for automatic characterization of plaque composition in carotid ultrasound. *IEEE Journal of Biomedical and Health Informatics*, 21(1), 48–55. Doi: 10.1109/JBHI.2016.2631401.

Li, Y., Shi, W., & Wasserman, W. W. (2018). Genome-wide prediction of cis-regulatory regions using supervised deep learning methods. *BMC Bioinformatics*, 19(1), 202. Doi: 10.1186/s12859-018-2187-1.

Litjens, G., Sánchez, C. I., Timofeeva, N., Hermsen, M., Nagtegaal, I., Kovacs, I., Hulsbergen-van de Kaa, C., Bult, P., van Ginneken, B., & van der Laak, J. (2016). Deep learning as a tool for increased accuracy and efficiency of histopathological diagnosis. *Scientific Reports*, 6, 26286. Doi: 10.1038/srep26286.

Luong, M. T., Pham, H., & Manning, C. D. (2015). Effective approaches to attention-based neural machine translation. *arXiv preprint arXiv:1508.04025*.

Lyu, B., & Haque, A. (2018). Deep learning based tumor type classification using gene expression data. *BioRxiv*, 364323. Doi: 10.1101/364323.

Min, S., Lee, B., & Yoon, S. (2017). Deep learning in bioinformatics. *Briefings in Bioinformatics*, 18(5), 851–869. Doi: 10.1093/bib/bbw068.

Montañez, C. A. C., Fergus, P., Montañez, A. C., & Chalmers, C. (2018). Deep learning classification of polygenic obesity using genome wide association study SNPs. *ArXiv*:1804.03198 [Cs, q-Bio]. http://arxiv.org/abs/1804.03198.

Movahedi, F., Coyle, J. L., & Sejdić, E. (2017). Deep belief networks for electroencephalography: A review of recent contributions and future outlooks. *IEEE Journal of Biomedical and Health Informatics*, 22(3), 642–652.

naceur, M. B., Saouli, R., Akil, M., & Kachouri, R. (2018). Fully automatic brain tumor segmentation using end-to-end incremental deep neural networks in MRI images. *Computer Methods and Programs in Biomedicine*, 166, 39–49. Doi: 10.1016/j.cmpb.2018.09.007.

Nasr-Esfahani, E., Samavi, S., Karimi, N., Soroushmehr, S. M. R., Ward, K., Jafari, M. H., Felfeliyan, B., Nallamothu, B., & Najarian, K. (2016). Vessel extraction in X-ray angiograms using deep learning. In *2016 38th Annual International Conference of the IEEE Engineering in Medicine and Biology Society (EMBC)* (pp. 643–646). IEEE, Orlando, FL.

Ongsulee, P. (2017, November). Artificial intelligence, machine learning and deep learning. In *2017 15th International Conference on ICT and Knowledge Engineering (ICT&KE)* (pp. 1–6). IEEE.

Oubounyt, M., Louadi, Z., Tayara, H., & Chong, K. T. (2019). DeePromoter: Robust promoter predictor using deep learning. *Frontiers in Genetics*, 10. Doi: 10.3389/fgene.2019.00286.

Poirion, O. B., Chaudhary, K., & Garmire, L. X. (2018). Deep learning data integration for better risk stratification models of bladder cancer. AMIA Joint Summits on translational science proceedings. *AMIA Joint Summits on Translational Science*, 2017, 197–206.

Poplin, R., Chang, P.-C., Alexander, D., Schwartz, S., Colthurst, T., Ku, A., Newburger, D., Dijamco, J., Nguyen, N., Afshar, P. T., Gross, S. S., Dorfman, L., McLean, C. Y., & DePristo, M. A. (2018). A universal SNP and small-indel variant caller using deep neural networks. *Nature Biotechnology*, 36(10), 983–987. Doi: 10.1038/nbt.4235.

Purcell, S. M., Wray, N. R., Stone, J. L., Visscher, P. M., O'Donovan, M. C., Sullivan, P. F., … Stanley Center for Psychiatric Research and Broad Institute of MIT and Harvard. (2009). Common polygenic variation contributes to risk of schizophrenia and bipolar disorder. *Nature*, 460(7256), 748–752. Doi: 10.1038/nature08185.

Pyrkov, T. V., Slipensky, K., Barg, M., Kondrashin, A., Zhurov, B., Zenin, A., … Fedichev, P. O. (2018). Extracting biological age from biomedical data via deep learning: Too much of a good thing? *Scientific Reports*, 8(1), 1–11.

Qi, H., Chen, C., Zhang, H., Long, J. J., Chung, W. K., Guan, Y., & Shen, Y. (2018). MVP: Predicting pathogenicity of missense variants by deep neural networks. *BioRxiv*, 259390. Doi: 10.1101/259390.

Quang, D., Chen, Y., & Xie, X. (2015). DANN: A deep learning approach for annotating the pathogenicity of genetic variants. *Bioinformatics (Oxford, England)*, 31(5), 761–763. Doi: 10.1093/bioinformatics/btu703.

Rajkomar, A., Dean, J., & Kohane, I. (2019). Machine learning in medicine. *New England Journal of Medicine*. https://www.nejm.org/doi/10.1056/NEJMra1814259.

Roth, H. R., Farag, A., Lu, L., Turkbey, E. B., & Summers, R. M. (2015). Deep convolutional networks for pancreas segmentation in CT imaging. *Medical Imaging 2015: Image Processing*, 9413, 94131G. Doi: 10.1117/12.2081420.

Roth, H. R., Lee, C. T., Shin, H.-C., Seff, A., Kim, L., Yao, J., Lu, L., & Summers, R. M. (2015). Anatomy-specific classification of medical images using deep convolutional nets. *2015 IEEE 12th International Symposium on Biomedical Imaging (ISBI)*, 101–104. Doi: 10.1109/ISBI.2015.7163826.

Rumelhart, D. E., Hinton, G. E., & Williams, R. J. (1985). *Learning Internal Representations by Error Propagation (No. ICS-8506)*. California University, San Diego La Jolla Institute for Cognitive Science, La Jolla, CA, USA.

Salakhutdinov, R., & Hinton, G. (2009). Semantic hashing. *International Journal of Approximate Reasoning*, 50(7), 969–978.

Salakhutdinov, R., & Hinton, G. E. (2006). Reducing the dimensionality of data with neural networks. *Science*, 313(5786), 504–507.

Si, Z., Yu, H., & Ma, Z. (2016). Learning deep features for DNA methylation data analysis. *IEEE Access*. Doi: 10.1109/ACCESS.2016.2576598.

Singh, R., Lanchantin, J., Robins, G., & Qi, Y. (2016). DeepChrome: Deep-learning for predicting gene expression from histone modifications. *Bioinformatics*. http://agris.fao.org/agris-search/search.do?recordID=US201900253083.

Spencer, M., Eickholt, J., & Cheng, J. (2015). A Deep learning network approach to ab initio protein secondary structure prediction. *IEEE/ACM Transactions on Computational Biology and Bioinformatics*, 12(1), 103–112. Doi: 10.1109/TCBB.2014.2343960

Thireou, T., & Reczko, M. (2007). Bidirectional long short-term memory networks for predicting the subcellular localization of eukaryotic proteins. *IEEE/ACM Transactions on Computational Biology and Bioinformatics*, 4(3), 441–446.

Tran, N. H., Zhang, X., Xin, L., Shan, B., & Li, M. (2017). De novo peptide sequencing by deep learning. *Proceedings of the National Academy of Sciences*, 114(31), 8247–8252. Doi: 10.1073/pnas.1705691114.

Tripathi, R., Patel, S., Kumari, V., Chakraborty, P., & Varadwaj, P. K. (2016). DeepLNC, a long non-coding RNA prediction tool using deep neural network. *Network Modeling Analysis in Health Informatics and Bioinformatics*, 5(1), 21. Doi: 10.1007/s13721-016-0129-2.

Vincent, P., Larochelle, H., Lajoie, I., Bengio, Y., Manzagol, P. A., & Bottou, L. (2010). Stacked denoising autoencoders: Learning useful representations in a deep network with a local denoising criterion. *Journal of Machine Learning Research*, *11*(12), 3371–3408.

Wallach, I., Dzamba, M., & Heifets, A. (2015). AtomNet: A deep convolutional neural network for bioactivity prediction in structure-based drug discovery. *arXiv preprint arXiv:1510.02855*.

Wang, M., Tai, C., E, W., & Wei, L. (2018). DeFine: Deep convolutional neural networks accurately quantify intensities of transcription factor-DNA binding and facilitate evaluation of functional non-coding variants. *Nucleic Acids Research*, 46(11), e69. Doi: 10.1093/nar/gky215.

Wang, Y., Liu, T., Xu, D., Shi, H., Zhang, C., Mo, Y.-Y., & Wang, Z. (2016). Predicting DNA methylation state of CpG dinucleotide using genome topological features and deep networks. *Scientific Reports*, 6(1), 1–15. Doi: 10.1038/srep19598.

Wei, Z., Wang, K., Qu, H.-Q., Zhang, H., Bradfield, J., Kim, C., Frackleton, E., Hou, C., Glessner, J. T., Chiavacci, R., Stanley, C., Monos, D., Grant, S. F. A., Polychronakos, C., & Hakonarson, H. (2009). From disease association to risk assessment: An optimistic view from genome-wide association studies on type 1 diabetes. *PLOS Genetics*, 5(10), e1000678. Doi: 10.1371/journal.pgen.1000678.

Weinstein, J. N., Collisson, E. A., Mills, G. B., Shaw, K. R. M., Ozenberger, B. A., Ellrott, K., Shmulevich, I., Sander, C., & Stuart, J. M. (2013). The cancer genome atlas Pan-Cancer analysis project. *Nature Genetics*, 45(10), 1113–1120. Doi: 10.1038/ng.2764.

Wolterink, J. M., Leiner, T., de Vos, B. D., van Hamersvelt, R. W., Viergever, M. A., & Išgum, I. (2016). Automatic coronary artery calcium scoring in cardiac CT angiography using paired convolutional neural networks. *Medical Image Analysis*, 34, 123–136. Doi: 10.1016/j.media.2016.04.004.

Xie, J., Liu, R., Luttrell, J. I., & Zhang, C. (2019). Deep learning based analysis of histopathological images of breast cancer. *Frontiers in Genetics*, 10. Doi: 10.3389/fgene.2019.00080.

Xie, R., Wen, J., Quitadamo, A., Cheng, J., & Shi, X. (2017). A deep auto-encoder model for gene expression prediction. *BMC Genomics*, 18(9), 845. Doi: 10.1186/s12864-017-4226-0.

Yin, Q., Wu, M., Liu, Q., Lv, H., & Jiang, R. (2019). DeepHistone: A deep learning approach to predicting histone modifications. *BMC Genomics*, 20(Suppl 2), 193. Doi: 10.1186/s12864-019-5489-4.

Yu, N., Yu, Z., & Pan, Y. (2017). A deep learning method for lincRNA detection using auto-encoder algorithm. *BMC Bioinformatics*, 18(15), 511. Doi: 10.1186/s12859-017-1922-3

Yuan, Y., Shi, Y., Li, C., Kim, J., Cai, W., Han, Z., & Feng, D. D. (2016). DeepGene: An advanced cancer type classifier based on deep learning and somatic point mutations. *BMC Bioinformatics*, 17(17), 476. Doi: 10.1186/s12859-016-1334-9.

Zafeiris, D., Rutella, S., & Ball, G. R. (2018). An artificial neural network integrated pipeline for biomarker discovery using Alzheimer's Disease as a case study. *Computational and Structural Biotechnology Journal*, 16, 77–87. Doi: 10.1016/j.csbj.2018.02.001.

Zhang, W. (1988, September). Shift-invariant pattern recognition neural network and its optical architecture. In *Proceedings of Annual Conference of the Japan Society of Applied Physics*, IOP Press, Tokyo.

Zhang, Y., Liu, X., MacLeod, J., & Liu, J. (2018). Discerning novel splice junctions derived from RNA-seq alignment: A deep learning approach. *BMC Genomics*, 19(1), 971. Doi: 10.1186/s12864-018-5350-1.

Zhang, Z., Zhao, Y., Liao, X., Shi, W., Li, K., Zou, Q., & Peng, S. (2019). Deep learning in omics: A survey and guideline. *Briefings in Functional Genomics*, 18(1), 41–57. Doi: 10.1093/bfgp/ely030.

Zhavoronkov, A., Ivanenkov, Y. A., Aliper, A., Veselov, M. S., Aladinskiy, V. A., Aladinskaya, A. V., … Volkov, Y. (2019). Deep learning enables rapid identification of potent DDR1 kinase inhibitors. *Nature Biotechnology*, *37*(9), 1038–1040.

Zhou, J., & Troyanskaya, O. G. (2015). Predicting effects of noncoding variants with deep learning-based sequence model. *Nature Methods*, 12(10), 931–934. Doi: 10.1038/nmeth.3547.

Zhou, X.-X., Zeng, W.-F., Chi, H., Luo, C., Liu, C., Zhan, J., He, S.-M., & Zhang, Z. (2017). pDeep: Predicting MS/MS spectra of peptides with deep learning. *Analytical Chemistry*, 89(23), 12690–12697. Doi: 10.1021/acs.analchem.7b02566.

Zuallaert, J., Godin, F., Kim, M., Soete, A., Saeys, Y., & De Neve, W. (2018). SpliceRover: Interpretable convolutional neural networks for improved splice site prediction. *Bioinformatics (Oxford, England)*, 34(24), 4180–4188. Doi: 10.1093/bioinformatics/bty497.

2 Embryo Grade Prediction for *In-Vitro* Fertilization

Panca Dewi Pamungkasari
Yokohama National University

Kento Uchida
Yokohama National University

Shota Saito
Yokohama National University / SkillUp AI Co. Ltd.

Filbert H. Juwono
Curtin University Malaysia

Ita Fauzia Hanoum
DR Sardjito Hospital

Shinichi Shirakawa
Yokohama National University

CONTENTS

2.1   INTRODUCTION

The applications of convolutional neural network (CNN) to biomedical imaging have emerged in several medical processes such as radiology (Yamashita, Nishio, Do, & Togashi, 2018) and lung cancer detection (Xiong, et al., 2019). The CNNs in those applications need medical images as input and output the predictions automatically. However, the biomedical images are often not suitable for direct use in the system due to some disturbances, such as noise contamination. Therefore, a preprocessing stage is important to reduce the effects of the disturbances. The typical preprocessing stage, such as denoising and edge extraction, can be in the form of image processing filters. In particular, it has been shown in Calderon, et al. (2018) that the performance of CNN for X-ray images can be improved by the preprocessing process, such as denoising, contrast enhancement, and edge enhancement.

In this article, we aim to use CNN to perform an automated grading of embryo image for the *in-vitro* fertilization (IVF) process.[1] We exploit the use of several image processing filters as the preprocessing stage where the adequate filters are selected through a binary vector. Furthermore, we consider a multivariate Bernoulli distribution to generate the binary vector, and the distribution parameter is optimized instead of the binary vector. This problem transformation is known as *stochastic relaxation* which has been used in one-shot neural architecture search (Shirakawa, Iwata, & Akimoto, 2018) and embedded feature selection (Saito, Shirakawa, & Akimoto, 2018). The conceptual diagram of the proposed method is depicted in Figure 2.1. Before going to our proposed method, a brief discussion of IVF will be presented.

2.2   IVF PROCEDURE

According to the World Health Organization (WHO), infertility is defined as "the failure to achieve a clinical pregnancy after 12 months or more of regular unprotected sexual intercourse." Many possible medical reasons underlie the problem of infertility. The source of infertility can come from the male or female, or both (Anwar & Anwar, 2016). The infertility in female can be caused by imperfect ovulation, problems in the ovum and sperm transport, and implantation issues. On the other hand, the sources of male infertility include imperfect spermatogenesis, transport issues, and ineffective sperm delivery. After the infertility factor is determined, a reproductive treatment can be used to facilitate the pregnancy process. IVF is the most common assisted reproductive treatment which has been done since decades ago. The first successful IVF baby was born in 1978, and since then, over eight million babies have been born from IVF.

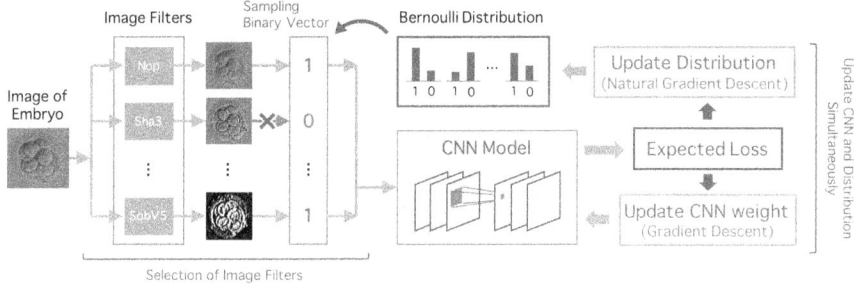

FIGURE 2.1 Proposed joint optimization of image processing filter selection and CNN weights scheme.

The basic concept of IVF is to inseminate sperm and eggs which are collected from the ovaries via "in-vitro" process, i.e., outside the human body, usually in a lab. Note that IVF is the most common fertility treatment utilized by patients today. However, IVF requires high fees as well as physical readiness and mental readiness. The success rate of IVF is still very low and influenced by age and reproductive health conditions of the couple, including the quality of the embryos (Pierce & Mocanu, 2018).

During IVF, ovarian stimulation is used to mature multiple eggs as follicles in a single cycle. Follicle stimulating hormone (FSH) and luteinizing hormone (LH) constitute gonadotropins that are used for the hyper-stimulation of ovaries in IVF and are required to stimulate follicular growth and ovulation (Ginsburg & Racowsky, 2012). FSH, as its name would suggest, helps stimulating the follicles in female while LH activates the follicles to make the eggs mature and then create the progesterone hormone. Ovum pick-up is egg retrieval using a needle which is guided by an ultrasound-transvaginal to go through the vaginal and inside to the ovary. The mature eggs are fertilized by using the conventional IVF technique or intracytoplasmic sperm injection (ICSI) technique. In the conventional IVF technique, the sperm should inseminate the egg by itself while ICSI is the process of injecting a single sperm into an egg. The fertilized eggs are referred to as zygotes. The zygote develops into an embryo by dividing one cell into eight cells until day 3. The embryo structure called morula occurs on day 4, and the blastocyst is shaped on day 5. The last procedure of IVF is called embryo transfer (ET) where the embryo is transferred to the uterus. This process is simple as it does not need anesthesia procedure. It is common to carry out ET on day 3 or day 5 of embryo growth and ET is often performed two or three days after fertilization. Moreover, ET is performed using a soft catheter which is placed in the uterine cavity via the cervix under ultrasound guidance.

2.3 EMBRYO ASSESSMENT

As mentioned above, ET can be performed using day 3 or day 5 embryos. In particular, the embryologist will make the decision whether the embryos should be transferred to the uterus or kept cultured until the blastocyst phase based on the quality of day 3 embryos (Sasikala, et al., 2015). Therefore, the embryo-grading assessment on

TABLE 2.1

Embryo-Grading Introduced by Veeck (1999) and the Modified Grading Used in this Research Work

Grade (Veeck, 1999)	Modified Grade	Number of Cells	Blastomere	Fragmentation
1	Excellent	7–8 cells	Similar	Less than 5%
2	Moderate	7–8 cells	Similar	5%–15%
3	Poor	6–8 cells	Fairly similar	15%–25%
4	Poor	4–6 cells	Fairly similar	25%–30%
5	Poor	4–5 cells	Not similar	More than 30%

We also show the third-day embryo morphological criterion.

day 3 embryos is a crucial stage for the IVF process. The embryo-grading assessed on day 3 embryos is based on the cell numbers, percentage of fragmentation, and blastomere size. For this grading task, we use day 3 embryo images instead of day 5 embryo images, which were obtained from an infertility clinic in Indonesia between 2016 and 2018. From now on, for the sake of simplicity, we will just use the term "embryo" to denote the "day 3 embryo."

According to the standard morphological criterion (Veeck, 1999), the grades of the embryos can be classified into five categories. However, as the size of the data set is limited, we modified the classification to only three categories (grades): excellent, moderate, and poor. The grade modification was done by an experienced embryologist and the result is presented in Table 2.1.

2.4   CNN AND ITS APPLICATION TO EMBRYO GRADING

The CNN is an effective and popular machine learning model for image recognition tasks such as image classification. The CNN consists of several layers where the feature in the output of preceding layer is extracted and transformed. A typical structure of the CNN is repetition of the convolution layers and the pooling layers before the fully connected layers. The convolution layer and the pooling layer extract the structural feature through the operation to the patches of the input feature map, while the fully connected layer extracts the real-valued feature from the whole of the input features. In the convolution layer, an input feature map is transformed by the convolutional operation, where the weighted sum of the patch of the input feature map with weight parameters is inputted to an activation function to obtain the transformed feature map. In the pooling layer, the patch of the input feature map is applied to an operation such as taking the maximum and the average of the patch. The fully connected layer computes the output of the activation function inputted the weighted sum of the whole input features. The performance of the CNN is greatly affected by its architecture (composition of basic layers). Because the proper architecture varies according to the given task, several architectures have been proposed (Simonyan & Zisserman, 2015; He, Zhang, Ren, & Sun, 2016; Szegedy, et al., 2015).

The optimization of the weights of the CNN, called as *training*, is basically performed by an optimization algorithm based on the gradient descent so as to decrease the loss calculated with the training data set. Those gradient-based algorithms are usually more efficient than the optimization algorithms which do not utilize the information of the gradient.

Several applications of machine learning methods to biomedical image processing tasks have been proposed. In Khan, Gould, and Salzmann (2015), a conditional random field (CRF) was applied to cell counting in embryonic images, which has become a basic element for cell embryo analysis algorithms. However, the features necessary to predict the shape and number of cells were integrated with other image features. Moreover, the simultaneous interactions of embryos over time and space are too complex to obtain sufficient performance by the CRF. In Khan, Gould, and Salzmann (2016), the number of cell is predicted via the CNN combined with CRF framework, which makes consistency between neighbor frames using temporal information. They exploited 265 raw microscopy images of day 3 human embryos and utilized the CNN following AlexNet architecture (Krizhevsky, Sutskever, & Hinton, 2012), which contains five convolutional and three fully connected layers. The experiments have indicated that this scheme improves the accuracy by around 16.12% compared with the cell counting result in Khan, Gould, and Salzmann (2015), which was previously the state-of-the-art method. In Chen, et al. (2019), two approaches of the transfer learning, fine-tuning, and extraction are applied to the embryo-grading prediction from the raw microscopic images on day 5 after fertilization. Although both models utilize the weights of the CNN previously trained with ImageNet data set for object classification, the fine-tuning approach further updates the weight using the embryo image data set while the extraction approach does not update the transferred weight and treats the transferred part as a feature extractor. The overall predictive accuracy of the model with fine-tuning is 75.36%, which is a little bit better than the model with extraction. For the assessment of the embryo quality on day 5, STORK, which is a framework with CNN based on Google's Inception-V1 architecture (Szegedy, et al., 2015), is proposed in Khosravi, et al. (2019). The embryo images for the training were provided from an embryology laboratory and were classified as good quality or poor quality based on their pregnancy rate. The data set consists of the embryo images captured with different focal depths. The performance of STORK is evaluated with a test set randomly selected from good-quality images and poor-quality images, where the accuracy reaches 96.94%.

2.5   JOINT OPTIMIZATION OF IMAGE PROCESSING FILTER SELECTION AND CNN WEIGHTS

2.5.1   IMAGE PROCESSING FILTERS

The target of image processing is the enhancement of the features in the image. The enhancement includes noise removal, image sharpening, image smoothing, and edge detection. We will briefly discuss several image processing used in this article.

Image processing filters are linear or nonlinear operations applied to spatial regions in the image selected by a window. The image processing filters used in our scheme are categorized as the statistical image filter or the linear image filter. The statistical image filter returns the statistical value of the pixel values in the window. The linear filter returns the weighted sum of the pixel values in the window using the kernel. More precisely, when the pixel values in the image and the kernel are denoted as x and K, respectively, the weighted sum $g(i,j)$ in the window centered around (i,j) is derived as

$$g(i,j) = \sum_{i=-w}^{w} \sum_{j=-h}^{h} x_{i+w,j+h} K_{w,h} \qquad (2.1)$$

where the width and height of the kernel are given by $2w+1$ and $2h+1$, respectively. The details of each filter can be seen in Jain, Kasturi, and Schunck (1995) and Gonzalez and Woods (2002).

2.5.1.1 Median Filter

The median filter is a kind of statistical image filter that is commonly used for eliminating salt-and-pepper noise. The principle is to replace a pixel value with the median value of the surrounding pixels. We explain the working principle of the median filter with an example shown in Figure 2.2. Let us consider the 3×3 window with the gray value of "2" in the center. We then sort the pixel values into ascending order and find the median value, that is, "5." We then replace the center value with "5." Note that if the number of pixels is even, we can use the average of the two middle values after sorting. The filtered image is obtained by applying the above operation to all spatially divided areas around each pixel.

2.5.1.2 Gaussian Filter

The Gaussian filter can be categorized as a linear filter. It is known to be effective in removing the Gaussian noise. The kernel is determined based on the two-dimensional Gaussian distribution centered around the origin whose probability density function is given by

$$p(i,j) = \frac{1}{2\pi\sigma^2} \exp\left(-\frac{i^2 + j^2}{2\sigma^2}\right) \qquad (2.2)$$

where σ denotes the standard deviation. Since the position on the image is discrete, the kernel value is obtained by discrete approximation. As a result, the 3×3 kernel (with $\sigma = 1$) is derived as

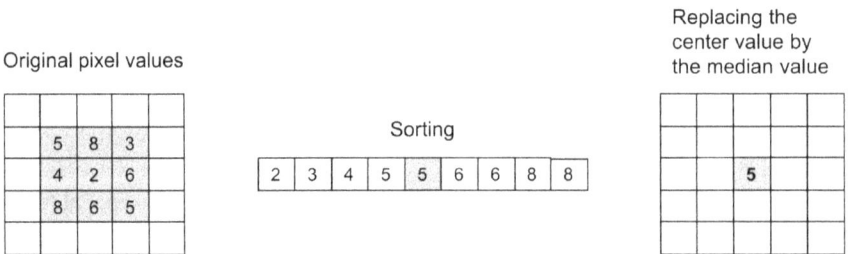

FIGURE 2.2   An example of image processing with median filter.

$$K = \frac{1}{16} \begin{bmatrix} 1 & 2 & 1 \\ 2 & 4 & 2 \\ 1 & 2 & 1 \end{bmatrix}$$

and the 5×5 kernel is derived as

$$K = \frac{1}{273} \begin{bmatrix} 1 & 4 & 7 & 4 & 1 \\ 4 & 16 & 26 & 16 & 4 \\ 7 & 26 & 41 & 26 & 7 \\ 4 & 16 & 26 & 16 & 4 \\ 1 & 4 & 7 & 4 & 1 \end{bmatrix}$$

We note that we used OpenCV (Bradski, 2008) for the implementation of filters and the standard deviation is computed as $\sigma = 0.3 \times ((s-1)/2 - 1) + 0.8$, where s is the width and height of the kernel. The detailed information is written in the OpenCV document.

2.5.1.3 Sobel Filter

The Sobel filter is a linear filter and is used to detect the edges of an image. The design principle of the Sobel filter is the calculation of the derivation along the vertical or horizontal axis. The derivation of a two-dimensional function $f(x,y)$ is approximated by central difference as

$$\frac{\partial f}{\partial x} \approx f(x+h,y) - f(x-h,y),$$

where h is set to be one. Different from basic implementation, which is known as the Prewitt filter, the centerline is enhanced by multiplying the kernel value by two. The vertical and horizontal 3×3 kernels are obtained as

$$K = \begin{bmatrix} -1 & -2 & -1 \\ 0 & 0 & 0 \\ 1 & 2 & 1 \end{bmatrix},$$

and

$$K = \begin{bmatrix} -1 & 0 & 1 \\ -2 & 0 & 2 \\ -1 & 0 & 1 \end{bmatrix}$$

Meanwhile, the 5×5 kernels are given by

$$K = \begin{bmatrix} -1 & -4 & -6 & -4 & -1 \\ -2 & -8 & -12 & -8 & -2 \\ 0 & 0 & 0 & 0 & 0 \\ 2 & 8 & 12 & 8 & 2 \\ 1 & 4 & 6 & 4 & 1 \end{bmatrix},$$

and

$$K = \begin{bmatrix} -1 & -2 & 0 & 2 & 1 \\ -4 & -8 & 0 & 8 & 4 \\ -6 & -12 & 0 & 12 & 6 \\ -4 & -8 & 0 & 8 & 4 \\ -1 & -2 & 0 & 2 & 1 \end{bmatrix}$$

2.5.1.4 Laplacian Filter

The Laplacian filter is a linear image filter which is used to detect the edge in the image. The mask is derived from the Laplacian operator, which is a second derivative operation for functions accepting two-dimensional variables. Consider a function $f(x,y)$, which provides the pixel value of the position (x,y). The discrete form of the Laplacian of $f(x,y)$ is given by the partial derivatives of x- and y-directions as

$$\frac{\partial^2 f}{\partial x^2} \approx f(x+1,y) + f(x-1,y) - 2f(x,y), \tag{2.3}$$

$$\frac{\partial^2 f}{\partial y^2} \approx f(x,y+1) + f(x,y-1) - 2f(x,y) \tag{2.4}$$

The implementation can be performed by summing up the two equations

$$\nabla^2 f \approx \left[f(x+1,y) + f(x-1,y) + f(x,y+1) + f(x,y-1) \right] - 4f(x,y) \tag{2.5}$$

Moreover, adding the implementation of the Laplacian operation along the diagonal axis, we obtained the 3×3 kernel as

$$K = \begin{bmatrix} -1 & -1 & -1 \\ -1 & 8 & -1 \\ -1 & -1 & -1 \end{bmatrix}$$

Similarly, we can obtain the 5×5 kernel as

$$K = \begin{bmatrix} -1 & -1 & -1 & -1 & -1 \\ -1 & -1 & -1 & -1 & -1 \\ -1 & -1 & 24 & -1 & -1 \\ -1 & -1 & -1 & -1 & -1 \\ -1 & -1 & -1 & -1 & -1 \end{bmatrix}$$

2.5.1.5 Sharpening Filter

The sharpening filter is a kind of linear filter for edge detection. The 3×3 kernel is given by

$$K = \begin{bmatrix} -1 & -1 & -1 \\ -1 & 9 & -1 \\ -1 & -1 & -1 \end{bmatrix}$$

The 5×5 kernel is given by

$$K = \begin{bmatrix} -1 & -1 & -1 & -1 & -1 \\ -1 & -1 & -1 & -1 & -1 \\ -1 & -1 & 25 & -1 & -1 \\ -1 & -1 & -1 & -1 & -1 \\ -1 & -1 & -1 & -1 & -1 \end{bmatrix}$$

Although the kernel is similar to that of the Laplacian filter, the filtered images are different. For example, when considering an one-color image, the filtered image with the sharpening filter is the same as the original image while the filtered image with Laplacian filter becomes an image whose pixel values are zero.

2.5.1.6 Blur Filter

Blur filter is a linear filter for noise reduction. The 3×3 kernel we used is given by

$$K = \frac{1}{9} \begin{pmatrix} 1 & 1 & 1 \\ 1 & 1 & 1 \\ 1 & 1 & 1 \end{pmatrix}$$

and the 5×5 kernel is given by

$$K = \frac{1}{25} \begin{pmatrix} 1 & 1 & 1 & 1 & 1 \\ 1 & 1 & 1 & 1 & 1 \\ 1 & 1 & 1 & 1 & 1 \\ 1 & 1 & 1 & 1 & 1 \\ 1 & 1 & 1 & 1 & 1 \end{pmatrix}$$

This filter performs the averaging of the pixel values in the window. Compared with the kernel of the Gaussian filter, the kernel value does not get smaller as the distance from the center becomes greater.

2.5.2 PROPOSED ALGORITHM

Same as the purpose of general supervised learning, we aim to obtain a model that maps an input image x to a target value y for any given pair of data (x, y). In the training procedure, we optimize the weight of the model to minimize the loss function $\mathcal{L}$ constructed with the training data set $D = \{X, Y\}$, where $X = \{x_1, \ldots, x_N\}$ is the set of the N images and $Y = \{y_1, \ldots, y_N\}$ is the set of the N corresponding target values.

We consider the preprocessing stage consisting of d image processing filters $(\psi_1, \cdots, \psi_d)$ that generate the filtered images of an image x as $\bar{x} = (\psi_1(x), \cdots, \psi_d(x))$. As introduced in the previous section, the filters have different functions and purposes. Therefore, some filters may not be suitable and lead to the performance deterioration of the CNN. Then we consider a selection process where a binary vector $M \in \mathcal{M} = \{0,1\}^d$ determines which filters are inputted to the CNN. More precisely, each filtered image is multiplied by the corresponding element of the binary vector, and the CNN receives the selected filtered image as $(m_1\psi_1(x),\cdots,m_d\psi_d(x))$. We aim to develop an algorithm so that the binary vector, which is responsible for filter selection, is able to select the best combination of filters while training the CNN.

We consider the loss function $\mathcal{L}(W,M)$ to be minimized with respect to (w.r.t.) M and W, where W is the weight of the CNN. We note that $\mathcal{L}(W,M)$ is not differentiable w.r.t. the binary vector M. Then the objective function is transformed using a technique called *stochastic relaxation* as discussed below so as to optimize the filter selection process by a gradient-based method. The multivariate Bernoulli distribution is considered as a law of the binary vector, i.e., $p_\theta(M) = \prod_{i=1}^{d} \theta_i^{m_i}(1-\theta_i)^{1-m_i}$, where

$\theta_i \in [0,1]$ is the selection probability of the i-th image processing filter, i.e., the probability that $m_i = 1$. Then we transform the target problem into the optimization of θ instead of M. The transformed objective function is obtained by taking the expectation of the $\mathcal{L}(W,M)$ over the distribution, i.e., $\mathcal{G}(W,\theta) = E_{p_\theta}[\mathcal{L}(W,M)]$. The transformed objective function is differentiable w.r.t. both W and θ. The minimization of $\mathcal{G}(W,\theta)$ is the same as the minimization of $\mathcal{L}(W,M)$ in the sense that the Bernoulli distribution parametrized by the optimal solution θ^* of $\mathcal{G}(W,\theta)$ generates the optimal solution of $\mathcal{L}(W,M)$ with probability of 1.

We apply the optimization algorithm proposed by (Shirakawa, Iwata, & Akimoto, 2018) and (Saito, Shirakawa, & Akimoto, 2018). For the update of W, we consider the Euclidian gradient of transformed objective function w.r.t. W, which is derived as $\nabla_W \mathcal{G}(W,\theta) = \sum_{M\in\mathcal{M}} \nabla_W \mathcal{L}(W,M)p_\theta(M)$. For the update of θ, we consider the natural gradient w.r.t. θ, which is the steepest direction of θ w.r.t. the Kullback-Leibler divergence (Amari, 1998). The natural gradient is given by

$$\tilde{\nabla}_\theta \mathcal{G}(W,\theta) = \sum_{M\in\mathcal{M}} \mathcal{L}(W,M)\tilde{\nabla}_\theta \ln p_\theta(M)p_\theta(M),$$

where $\tilde{\nabla}_\theta = F(\theta)^{-1}\nabla_\theta$, and $F(\theta)$ is the Fisher information matrix of p_θ. We train the model by iteratively updating W and θ until a certain threshold is reached.

In practice, we approximate the gradients using the Monte-Carlo method of λ samples $(M_1,\ldots,M_\lambda)$ drawn from the distribution p_θ. Further, N minibatch data sample $\mathcal{Z}$ is used to approximate the loss function as $\mathcal{L}(W,M) \approx \bar{\mathcal{L}}(W,M;\mathcal{Z}) = \frac{1}{N}\sum_{z\in\mathcal{Z}} \ell(W,M;z)$,

where $\ell(W,M;z)$ is the loss of a datum z. Then, we approximate the Euclidian gradient as

$$\nabla_W \mathcal{G}(W,\theta) \approx \frac{1}{\lambda}\sum_{i=1}^{\lambda} \nabla_W \bar{\mathcal{L}}(W,M_i;\mathcal{Z}) \tag{2.6}$$

Back-propagation can be used to compute $\nabla_W \mathcal{L}(W,M_i;\mathcal{Z})$ the same way as in general training scheme of CNN, and any stochastic gradient descent algorithm can be used to optimize W.

Similarly, we approximate the natural gradient w.r.t. θ using λ samples and minibatch data $\mathcal{Z}$. We note that the natural gradient of the log-likelihood of the Bernoulli distribution can be analytically derived as $\tilde{\nabla} \ln p_\theta(M) = M - \theta$. Therefore, we approximate the natural gradient w.r.t. θ as $\tilde{\nabla}_\theta \mathcal{G}(W,\theta) \approx \dfrac{1}{\lambda} \displaystyle\sum_{i=1}^{\lambda} \mathcal{L}(W,M_i;\mathcal{Z})(M_i - \theta)$. Moreover, we apply the ranking-based utility transformation to the loss value as done by Shirakawa, Iwata, and Akimoto (2018) and Saito, Shirakawa, and Akimoto (2018). We set the utility value as $u_i = 1$ for best $\lceil \lambda/4 \rceil$ samples, $u_i = -1$ for the worst $\lceil \lambda/4 \rceil$ samples, and $u_i = 0$ for others. Thanks to this utility transformation, the algorithm obtains the invariance to the non-decreasing transformation of $\mathcal{L}$. As a result, the update rule of θ is constructed as

$$\theta^{(t+1)} = \theta^{(t)} + \frac{\eta_\theta}{\lambda} \sum_{i=1}^{\lambda} u_i \left(M_i - \theta^{(t)} \right) \tag{2.7}$$

where η_θ is the learning rate for θ. It is worth mentioning that we change the minimization problem to the maximization problem due to the use of ranking-based utility. In practice, we restrict θ within $\left[1/d, 1-1/d \right]^d$ to prevent the distribution becoming a degenerate distribution. The overall training procedure is described in Algorithm 2.1.

Algorithm 2.1   The Training Procedure of the Proposed Method

---
Algorithm 2.1: The training procedure of the proposed method.

Input: Training data $\mathcal{D} = \{X,Y\}$ and hyperparameters $\{\lambda, \eta_\theta\}$
Output: Optimized parameter of W and θ

1 **begin**
2   Initialize the connection weights of CNN and Bernoulli distribution parameter as $W^{(0)}$ and $\theta^{(0)}$
3    $t \leftarrow 0$
4   **while** *not stopping criterion is satisfied* **do**
5   Get N mini-batch samples from $\mathcal{D}$
6   Sample $M_1, \ldots, M_\lambda$ from $p_{\theta^{(t)}}$
7   Compute the loss $\mathcal{L}(W, M_i)$ for each sample
8   Update the distribution parameter to $\theta^{(t+1)}$ using (2.7)
9   Force $\theta^{(t+1)} \in [1/d, 1 - 1/d]^d$
10   Update the connection weights to $W^{(t+1)}$ using (2.6) by any SGD
11      $t \leftarrow t + 1$

For test phase, the binary vector with highest likelihood $\hat{M} = \arg\max_{M \in \mathcal{M}} p_\theta(M)$ is chosen to predict new data. This binary vector $\hat{M}$ is obtained as $m_i = 1$ for $\theta_i \geq 0.5$ and $m_i = 0$ otherwise. Finally, the prediction of the target value of the new image can be obtained by the CNN and the image processing filters selected by $\hat{M}$.

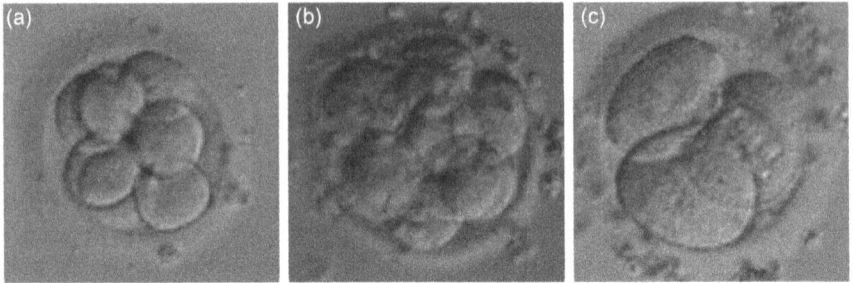

FIGURE 2.3 Images of embryo and their grades. From (a–c): excellent, moderate, and poor grades.

2.6 EXPERIMENT AND RESULTS

2.6.1 DATA SET

Our data set consists of 1,386 embryo images which can be broken down into 245 excellent grade embryo images, 599 moderate grade embryo images, and 533 images for poor grade embryo. The images were obtained from 238 anonymous patients where about four embryos were contributed by each patient. The embryo samples, each represents excellent grade, moderate grade, and poor grade, are shown in Figure 2.3. Prior to the experiment, we resized the images as 128×128 and converted them to gray scale. The training and test data sets consist of 80% and 20% of the images, respectively, which are allocated randomly.

2.6.2 EXPERIMENTAL SETTINGS

The architecture of the CNN used in this experiment was VGG-Net architecture (Simonyan & Zisserman, 2015) with 16 convolutional layers and 3×3 kernel with some modifications. More precisely, batch normalization was inserted both in the convolutional layers and the fully connected layers. In addition, the dropout (Srivastava, Hinton, Krizhevsky, Sutskever, & Salakhutdinov, 2014) in the fully connected layers was removed and the global average pooling (Lin, Chen, & Yan, 2014) was inserted before the first fully connected layer. We chose soft-max cross-entropy loss function as the task is to perform classification.

The simulation parameters are as follows: The size of minibatch was set to $N = 64$, the total number of epochs was 3,000 (i.e., 54,000 iterations approximately), the hyperparameters of the proposed method were set to $\lambda = 2$ and $\eta_\theta = 1 / 15$. The weight parameters, W, were initialized according to He's initialization (He, Zhang, Ren, & Sun, 2015) and Nesterov's accelerated stochastic gradient method (Sutskever, Martens, Dahl, & Hinton, 2013) with momentum of 0.9 was used as the optimizer for W. We also added the weight decay of 10^{-4} to the loss. The initial learning rate for W was set to be 0.1 and then divided by 10 at $1/2$ and $3/4$ of the total number of epochs. Further, all elements of initial distribution parameter $\theta_i^{(0)}$ were set to be 0.5. These settings are based on Shirakawa, Iwata, and Akimoto (2018).

TABLE 2.2

Image Processing Filters Prepared for Embryo Grading Prediction Task

Filter	-	3×3 Kernel	5×5 Kernel
		Abbreviation	
No filter (original image)	Nop	–	–
Blur filter	–	Blur3	Blur5
Gaussian filter	–	Gau3	Gau5
Sharpening filter	–	Sha3	Sha5
Laplacian filter	–	Lap3	Lap5
Vertical-Sobel filter	–	SobV3	SobV5
Horizontal-Sobel filter	–	SobH3	SobH5
Median filter	–	Med3	Med5

We prepared 15 types of image processing filters for this experiment, including no operation (Nop) filter. The types of filters are summarized in Table 2.2. The filtered images were standardized by subtracting the mean from each pixel values and then dividing them by the standard deviation. Data augmentation in terms of random flipping, random shifting, and random rotation was also applied.

We compared the following four models/scenarios as follows:

1. *No filters*: The original images were used, i.e., no image processing filters were applied (naive CNN).
2. *All filters*: All image processing filters discussed in Chapter 2.5.1 were used.
3. *Random*: Filter selection with a fixed selection probability of 0.5 (optimization of θ was not applied) was used.
4. *Joint optimization*: The proposed model employing joint optimization of image processing filter selection and CNN weights was used.

2.6.3 RESULTS AND DISCUSSION

We performed five trials in the experiment. Each scenario was performed with different random seeds. Figure 2.4 shows the transition of the median value and

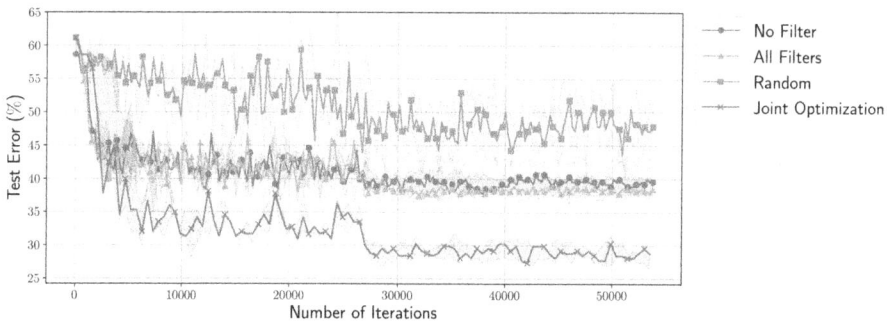

FIGURE 2.4   Test error transitions in each scenario.

inter-quartile ranges of the test error in each scenario. It can be seen that our proposed method achieved the lowest median value of the test error (28.78%) at the final iteration. When compared with No Filter and All Filters, our proposed method successfully reduced the test error by more than 8%. It means that redundant image processing filters can have adverse effects while the performance of the CNN with appropriate filter selection can be improved. Meanwhile, the worst performance was given by the Random scenario, where randomly selected image processing filters were used. It is worth mentioning that all scenarios had relatively the same training time. Therefore, we can claim that our proposed method improves the prediction performance without a sharp increase in the computational cost.

We show the confusion matrices of test data set for each scenario in Figure 2.5. These confusion matrices were obtained in the trial with the median test error for each scenario. It can be seen that our scenario achieved the highest recall for moderate and poor grades. Meanwhile, we had relatively the same accuracy values for all scenarios for the excellent grade, which infers that incorrect prediction tended to occur for the excellent embryos. More precisely, the excellent embryos tended to be predicted as moderate. On the other hand, the probability that excellent embryos were graded as poor, or vice versa, was very low for the model using our proposed method.

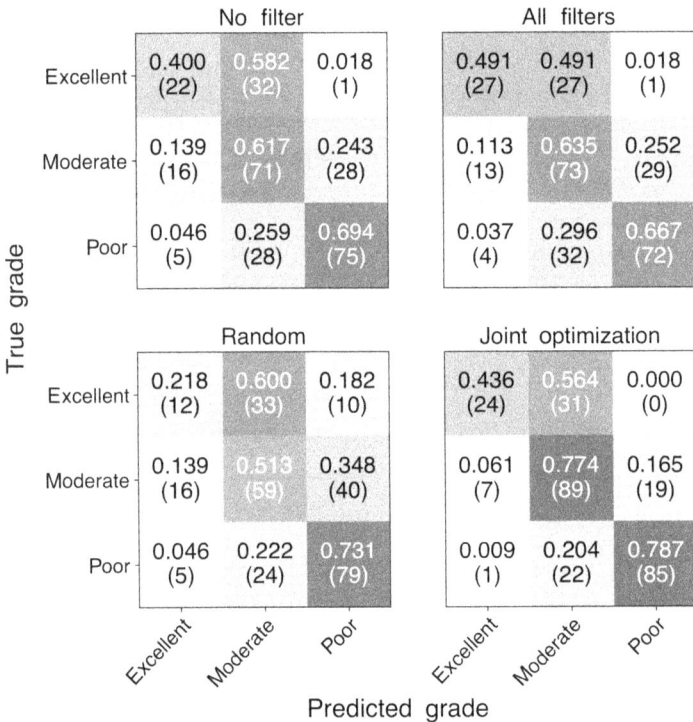

FIGURE 2.5 Confusion matrices of the test data. Note that the numbers written outside the parentheses show the ratio of the data classified into each category. The numbers written inside the parentheses depict the absolute numbers.

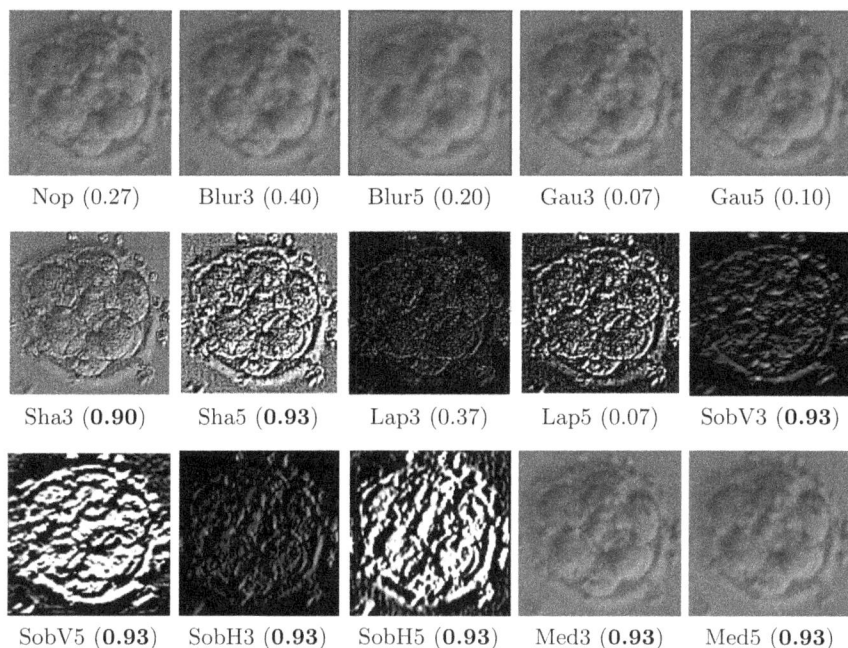

| Nop (0.27) | Blur3 (0.40) | Blur5 (0.20) | Gau3 (0.07) | Gau5 (0.10) |

| Sha3 (**0.90**) | Sha5 (**0.93**) | Lap3 (0.37) | Lap5 (0.07) | SobV3 (**0.93**) |

| SobV5 (**0.93**) | SobH3 (**0.93**) | SobH5 (**0.93**) | Med3 (**0.93**) | Med5 (**0.93**) |

FIGURE 2.6   Examples of filtered images of the embryo data set. The numbers in the parentheses show the selection probability and the one higher than 0.8 is written in bold. We report the values obtained in the trial recorded the median of the test error.

From the embryologist's point of view, it does not give adverse effect as embryos with excellent and moderate grades are allowed to be transferred to the uterus. As a result, the main important task for the system is to grade the poor embryos correctly.

The filtered images and their selection probabilities obtained in the trial with median test error are shown in Figure 2.6. We denote the selection probability in boldface when it is higher than 0.8. From the figure, it can be seen that the probability for Nop (original image) to be selected was relatively low. This implies that the use of image processing filters is useful to improve the prediction performance. The filters with selection probability higher than 0.8 were as follows: Sha3, Sha5, SobV3, SobV5, SobH3, SobH5, Med3, Med5. Referring to Table 2.2, Med3 and Med5 filters can eliminate small fragmentation well while Sha3 and Sha5 filters can be used to emphasize the fragmentation. The remaining filters are useful to count the number of embryos and the similarity of the blastomeres.

We also report the receiver operating characteristic (ROC) curves in Figure 2.7 and the area under curve (AUC) values in Table 2.3 for each scenario. In Table 2.3, we can see that the AUC for the poor grade is high while AUC for the moderate grade is relatively low in all scenarios. Considering that the accuracy for the moderate grade in the confusion matrix is not low, and the confidence of the prediction for the moderate grade may be relatively low. On the other hand, the AUC for excellent grade is not low, which indicates the confidence in the prediction with the excellent grade embryo is higher than that with the moderate grade embryo.

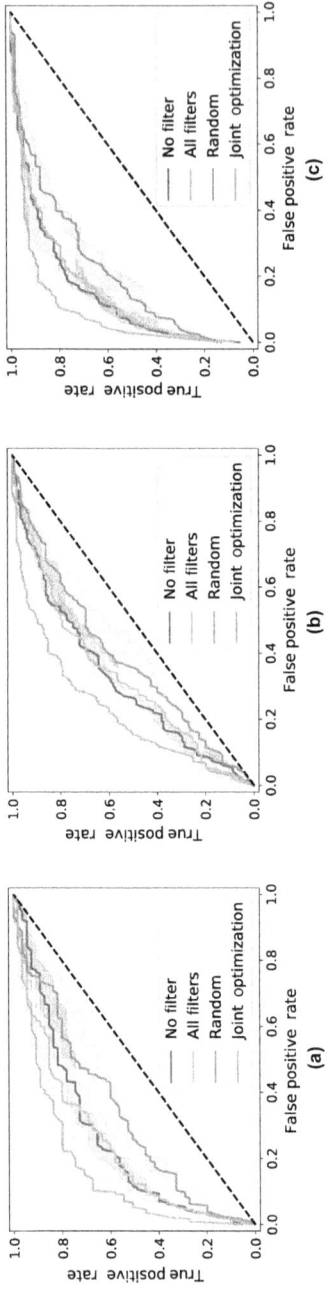

FIGURE 2.7 ROC of each scenario for each embryo grade. The (a–c) figures show the ROCs for the excellent, moderate, and poor embryos, respectively.

TABLE 2.3
AUC of Each Scenario for Each Embryo Grades

	Excellent	Moderate	Poor
No Filter	0.728	0.678	0.853
	(0.705, 0.774)	(0.661,0.697)	(0.841, 0.866)
All Filters	0.747	0.683	0.851
	(0.732, 0.786)	(0.644, 0.700)	(0.826, 0.853)
Random	0.673	0.616	0.776
	(0.617,0.696)	(0.573,0.635)	(0.774,0.830)
Joint Optimization	0.840	0.770	0.909
	(0.829, 0.854)	(0.762,0.796)	(0.903, 0.910)

We report the median and interquartile values of five trials.

TABLE 2.4
AUC of the Proposed Method with Different Procedure of Making Prediction

	Excellent	Moderate	Poor
Deterministic	0.840	0.770	0.909
(threshold 0.5)	(0.829, 0.854)	(0.762, 0.796)	(0.903, 0.910)
Deterministic	0.834	0.764	0.908
(threshold 0.2)	(0.820, 0.984)	(0.760, 0.796)	(0.902, 0.910)
Deterministic	0.840	0.772	0.909
(threshold 0.8)	(0.831, 0.850)	(0.762, 0.796)	(0.904, 0.910)
Stochastic	0.841	0.775	0.910
(#sample 100)	(0.830, 0.853)	(0.765, 0.795)	(0.905. 0.911)

We perform training five times with different random seeds. The reported values are the median and interquartile values of AUC calculated with the same five trained models.

Finally, we investigate the stability of the performance of proposed method. When the selection probabilities of several image processing filter are around 0.5, the performance may greatly change based on when the training is terminated. To evaluate the stability, we change the procedure for making prediction in two ways as (a) changing the threshold for determining the image processing filters in test phase, and (b) making ensemble of predictions using several binary vectors generated according to the selection probability. Therefore, we additionally evaluate the AUC values of the proposed method using the threshold of 0.2 and 0.8 and the ensemble using 100 predictions. Table 2.4 shows the AUC values of each model. Focusing the models with different thresholds, the AUC values are almost same and the performance degradation has not occurred. This means that the selection probabilities of the image processing filters with positive and negative influence are significantly high and low, respectively. On the other hand, the ensemble does not lead to significant improvement of the performance on the embryo prediction task. We consider that the ensemble may be useful when applying the proposed method to more difficult problems where the selection probabilities are not well optimized.

2.7   CONCLUSION

We have proposed the joint optimization of the CNN and selection of image process-ing filters used in preprocessing process. We consider a binary vector to select the image processing filters and introduced the multivariate Bernoulli distribution to gen-erate the binary vector. Under the stochastic relaxation, we transformed the objective function into the expected loss over the distribution. Then we consider optimizing the weight of CNN and the parameter of the distribution. The gradient directions w.r.t. the CNN weights and the distribution parameter are estimated using Monte Carlo estimation with the minibatch loss, and the joint optimization of the CNN weight and distribution parameter by the gradient-based method was developed.

The proposed method is then implemented for predicting embryo grades, which is one of the important stages in IVF treatment. The data set contained 254 embryo images with excellent grade, 599 images with moderate grade, and 533 poor grade embryo images. Based on their morphological criteria, these embryo images were classified by an embryologist into their appropriate grades. The proposed method has successfully reduced the test error by at least 8% compared to the naïve CNN and the CNN without using image processing filter selection.

Although most of the prepared filters in the experiment have linear operation and can be well performed by a convolution operation, our proposed method has improved the performance of the CNN. We consider this happens because the embryo data set is not large enough for the CNN to optimize its weight sufficiently. Therefore, apply-ing the proposed method on a large data set is one of the future works. In addition, the evaluation of our proposed method with nonlinear and nondifferentiable image processing is another important future work.

NOTE

1   This article is an extension of (Uchida, et al., 2019).

REFERENCES

Amari, S. (1998). Natural gradient works efficiently in learning. *Neural Computation, 10*(2), 251–276.

Anwar, S., & Anwar, A. (2016). Infertility: A review on causes, treatment and management. *Women's Health & Gynecology, 2*(6), 1–5.

Bradski, G. (2008). The OpenCV library. *Dr. Dobb's Journal of Software Tools.*

Calderon, S., Fallas, F., Zumbado, M., Tyrrell, P. N., Stark, H., Emersic, Z., … Solis, M. (2018). Assessing the impact of the deceived no local means filter as a preprocessing stage in a convolutional neural network based approach for age estimation using digital hand X-ray images. In *2018 25th IEEE International Conference on Image Processing (ICIP)*, (pp. 1752–1756). IEEE, Athens.

Chen, T. J., Zheng, W. L., Liu, C. H., Huang, I., Lai, H. H., & Liu, M. (2019). Using deep learn-ing with large dataset of microscope images to develop an automated embryo grading system. *Fertility & Reproduction, 01*(01), 51–56.

Ginsburg, E. S., & Racowsky, C. (2012). *In Vitro Fretilization: A Comprehensive Guide.* New York: Springer.

Gonzalez, R. C., & Woods, R. E. (2002). *Digital Image Processing* (2 ed.). Upper Saddle River, NJ: Prentice Hall.

He, K., Zhang, X., Ren, S., & Sun, J. (2015). Delving deep into rectifiers: Surpassing human-level performance on imagenet classification. *Proceedings of IEEE International Conference on Computer Vision (ICCV)*, (pp. 1026–1034), IEEE, Santiago.

He, K., Zhang, X., Ren, S., & Sun, J. (2016). Deep residual learning for image recognition. *Proceedings of IEEE Conference on Computer Vision and Pattern Recognition (CVPR)*, 770–778.

Jain, R., Kasturi, R., & Schunck, B. G. (1995). *Machine Vision*. New York: McGraw-Hill.

Khan, A., Gould, S., & Salzmann, M. (2015). Automated monitoring of human embryonic cells up to the 5-cell stage in time-lapse microscopy images. *Proceedings of the 12th IEEE International Symposium in Biomedical Imaging*, (pp. 389–393), Brooklyn, New York.

Khan, A., Gould, S., & Salzmann, M. (2016). Deep convolutional neural networks for human embryonic cell counting. *Proceedings of The European Conference on Computer Vision*, 339–348.

Khosravi, P., Kazemi, E., Zhan, Q., Malmsten, J. E., Toschi, M., Zisimopoulos, P., ... Zaninovic, N. (2019). Deep learning enables robust assessment and selection of human blastocysts after *in vitro* fertilization. *NPJ Digital Medicine, 2*, 1–9.

Krizhevsky, A., Sutskever, I., & Hinton, G. E. (2012). ImageNet classification with deep convolutional neural networks. *Proceedings of the 25th International Conference on Neural Information Processing Systems, 1*, 1097–1105.

Lin, M., Chen, Q., & Yan, S. (2014). Network in network. *International Conference on Learning Representation (ICLR)*. arXiv preprint arXiv:1312.4400.

Pierce, N., & Mocanu, E. (2018). Female age and assisted reproduction technology. *Global Reproduction Health, 3*(2), e9.

Saito, S., Shirakawa, S., & Akimoto, Y. (2018). Embedded feature selection using probabilistic model-based optimization. *Proceedings of the Genetic and Evolutionary Computation Conference Companion*, (pp. 1922–1925), Kyoto.

Sasikala, N., Rajapriya, A., Mahalakshmi, S., Janani, D., Archana, B., & Parameaswari, P. (2015). Blastocyst culture depends on quality of embryos on day 3, not quantity. *Middle East Fertility Society Journal, 20*(4), 224–230.

Shirakawa, S., Iwata, Y., & Akimoto, Y. (2018). Dynamic optimization of neural network structures using probabilistic modeling. *Proceedings of 32nd AAAI Conference on Artificial Intelligence (AAAI)*, (pp. 4074–4082), New Orleans, LA.

Simonyan, K., & Zisserman, A. (2015). Very deep convolutional networks for large-scale image recognition. *Proceedings of International Conference on Learning Representations (ICLR)*, San Diego, CA.

Srivastava, N., Hinton, G., Krizhevsky, A., Sutskever, I., & Salakhutdinov, R. (2014). Dropout: A simple way to prevent neural networks from overfitting. *Journal of Machine Learning Research, 15*, 1929–1958.

Sutskever, I., Martens, J., Dahl, G., & Hinton, G. (2013). On the importance of initialization and momentum in deep learning. *Proceedings of the 30th International Conference on Machine Learning (ICML)*, (pp. 1139–1147), JMLR.org, Atlanta, GA.

Szegedy, C., Liu, W., Jia, Y., Sermanet, P., Reed, S., Anguelov, D., ... Rabinovich, A. (2015). Going deeper with convolutions. *Proceedings of IEEE Conference on Computer Vision and Pattern Recognition (CVPR)*, (pp. 1–9), Boston, MA.

Uchida, K., Saito, S., Pamungkasari, P. D., Kawai, Y., Hanoum, I. F., H. Juwono, F., & Shirakawa, S. (2019). Joint optimization of convolutional neural network and image preprocessing selection for embryo grade prediction in *in vitro* fertilization. *Advances in Visual Computing, 2*, 14–24.

Veeck, L. (1999). *An Atlas of Human Gametes and Conceptuses: An Illustrated Reference for Assisted Reproductive Technology.* New York: The Parthenon Publishing Group.

Xiong, J., Li, X., Lu, L., Schwartz, L. H., Fu, X., Zhao, J., & Zhao, B. (2019). Implementation strategy of a CNN model affects the performance of CT assessment of EGFR mutation status in lung cancer patients. *IEEE Access, 7,* 64583–64591.

Yamashita, R., Nishio, M., Do, R. K., & Togashi, K. (2018). Convolutional neural networks: An overview and application in radiology. *Insights into Imaging, 9*(4), 611–629.

3 Biometric Gait Features Analysis Using Deep Learning Approaches

*Sumit Hazra, Acharya Aditya Pratap,
and Anup Nandy*
National Institute of Technology

CONTENTS

3.1 INTRODUCTION: BACKGROUND

Physiotherapists routinely observe gaits in clinical practice. Human strolling is a perplexing procedure which requires a lot of equalization and coordination. The analysis of human motion also known as human gait is a subject of broad research. The efficient and systematic movement of limbs bringing about bipedal motion called as gait is viewed as noteworthy biometric attribute with applications in sensitive domains such as surveillance security, medical implications, etc. Acquisition of data for carrying out analysis on human gait is done utilizing Kinect v2.0 sensors, which is a vision-based technique. The second version of the Kinect, i.e., Kinect v2.0, offers a superior resolution with respect to the first version, i.e., Kinect v1.0 sensors. Also, Kinect v2.0 provides an expanded view in contrary to the original Kinect technology. Further, since Kinect v2.0 operates by taking into consideration the time-of-flight principle, it offers notable improvement in the accuracy of depth sensing as compared to the former version which utilized structured light for third-dimension reconstruction. Despite the camera and the human subject are being inaccessible enough from one another, this biometric gives near accurate results. The video-based stride investigation is computationally intensive as it involves a lot of other procedures such as image segmentation, tracking, and silhouette extraction algorithms. This again is attributed to the essential requirement of pre-processing the raw data obtained. As the analysis generally needs the human subject as the region of interest, extraction of only the object involves image segmentation. Furthermore, the motion analysis for feature extractions involves tracking and silhouette or frames extraction algorithms. The wearable sensor-based methodologies for gait analysis may pull in wrong outcomes because of elements like dislodging of sensors during strolling and hence causing discomfort, blunders in estimation of sensor readings, etc. (Han and Bhanu 2005), in their work first proposed a spatial-temporal representation of the gait sequence known as Gait Energy Images (GEIs). This GEI concept further came into widespread use for gait analysis domain work which we also use in our research for two-dimensional Convolution Neural Network (2D CNN). As GEI is an average of the frames extracted, the analysis of the walking patterns of human subjects becomes much more easy and precise. For extraction of features, Dadashi, Araabi, and Soltanian-Zadeh (2009) proposed the matching pursuit algorithm along with the Independent Component Analysis Technique for the selection of the best features. The Independent Component Analysis Technique generates essentially contributing components of features for any kind of analysis and also helps in the removal of artifacts. These artifacts, if not examined and obliterated intricately, generate erroneous outcomes. Bashir, Xiang, and Gong (2008) examined and proposed a factual learning hypothesis-based feature selection procedure for GEIs after the utilization of cross-validation strategies.

Talking about the contribution/objectives of our research, the aim is to make an usable solution for people recognition and tracking which involves extraction of spatio-temporal features of human gait from Color Depth videos procured by means of Kinect V2.0 sensors. Two methodologies are followed for the extraction of features. In one approach, a stick model is created utilizing the body aspect ratios of the people. The model is generated with the help of the distance metric measured between the boundary coordinates and the centroids of the regions of the human body, using the body segment ratios. Generally, for this work, focus is laid on the lower portion of the human body. Then for using as gait features, the hip joint angles are obtained from the generated model. In the other approach, the number of frames constituting a single gait cycle is determined using autocorrelation technique. Following which the frames corresponding to a single gait cycle are extracted and the GEIs of the subjects are obtained from these frames. Convolution Neural Network technique is applied on the obtained GEIs leading to automatic feature extraction. Features are extracted from each of the layers of the 2D CNN model used. The features thus acquired from both the strategies are examined and reliability tested utilizing T-test, K-S test, Pearson's r test and energy distance test. The outcomes are seen to be encouraging and the exhibitions are shown with legitimate graphical portrayals and tabular charts for better understanding. The outcomes put forth a clear picture about the relevance of features for clinical gait analysis in the biomedical domain. Also, the expertise knowledge gained from this work ensures data reliability and makes gait analysis from vision-based technique much more convenient.

3.2 LITERATURE REVIEW

There has been a significant rise in the activities taking place in the gait analysis research domain since a few years now. Advancements in technology and availability of devices which are of higher configurations, better processing speeds and cheaper costs act as an impetus to this very cause. Based on some of the earlier works carried out for the purpose of people identification and tracking from color or depth images (Haritaoglu, Harwood, and Davis 2000; Foresti, Marcenaro, and Regazzoni 2002), utilization of algorithms for the purpose of obtaining the region of interests has become a cynosure. The discovery of RGB-D cameras such as Microsoft Kinect has been extremely helpful in the research domains of computer vision, artificial intelligence on a large scale. This is because both color and depth images are available on the same instrument. Also these cameras are user-friendly and available at cheaper rates when compared to other 3D cameras such as Long-Wave Infrared cameras. The applicability of these new cameras for human pose estimations is well explained in works such as Krishnamurthy (2011) and Guan et al. (2007), respectively. Human detection mainly involves two methodologies. The first technique is based on machine learning methods, such as multi-class Support Vector Machines, which use features like Histogram of Oriented Gradients (Spinello and Arras 2011) or AdaBoost (Davis and Keck 2005; Ikemura and Fujiyoshi 2010; Correa et al. 2012) for the classification of objects as to whether they belong to the human race or not. The other usable approach is template matching that is employed in systems such as Xia, Chen and Aggarwal (2011). The spatial pose model for estimating joints of the body can be classified into two groups. One is based on models which are tree-structured and graphical (Pishchulin et al. 2013; Felzenszwalb and Huttenlocher 2005; Andriluka, Roth, and Schiele 2009, 2010; Ramanan, Forsyth, and Zisserman 2005; Yang and Ramanan 2012; Johnson and Everingham 2010) which extract the relationship between the adjacent joints in a Kinect chain. The other models are nontree (Karlinsky and Ullman 2012; Dantone et al. 2013; Lan and Huttenlocher 2005), which add additional edges to the tree structure to obtain specific features such as occlusion, symmetry, and relationships which are not of short-range. In order to comprehend the worldwide spatial dependencies by implementing systems and networks with enormous receptive fields, the use of CNN was discussed in Pfister, Charles, and Zisserman (2015). It was recommended in Newell, Yang, and Deng (2016) that quick supervisions are in every case better for a stacked hourglass architecture. Given the location and scale of person of interest, the number of persons assumed for all of these is one. Again, in order to acquire dependable perceptions of body parts locally, Convolutional Neural Networks (CNNs) are used, which further aided in estimating the joints of the body with more precision and accuracy (Chu et al. 2017; Wei et al. 2016; Belagiannis and Zisserman 2017; Tompson et al. 2014; Ke et al. 2018; Yang et al. 2017; Tang, Yu, and Wu 2018). In this chapter, color depth videos are dealt with and spatio-temporal features of gait are extracted from them. Various machine and deep learning techniques like 2D CNN, etc., are also applied. The reliability and applicability of features in the near future for clinical gait analysis are analyzed with the application of different statistical techniques.

3.3 METHODOLOGY PROPOSED AND ADOPTED

The workflow diagram for this work is presented in Figure 3.1. Two approaches are proposed and discussed in this chapter. Spatio-temporal features of gait are obtained from color depth videos using Kinect v2.0 sensors. The features include the pattern of the hip angles with gait speeds of 3 and 5 km/h and the ones extracted through the application of 2D CNN. Ten subjects are advised to walk on a treadmill at 3 and 5 km/h, with the Kinect V2.0 camera placed at an approximate distance of 2.5 m from the treadmill. The video is captured at 29–30 fps wherein the features are extracted from each frame, examined separately. All the frames obtained undergo further processing. Also, we ensure that the experimental set-up is occlusion-free. Finally, the features undergo various statistical techniques for reliability testing, as discussed in Section 3.4. The features extracted are the hip angles obtained from a generated stick model and the ones automatically obtained after applying 2D CNN, from Color Depth videos.

3.3.1 Acquiring Information for Depth Video

The Kinect v2.0 sensor is kept at a distance 2.5 m from the treadmill and the subject. A system possessing 8 GB RAM and Intel i5 core processor is used to acquire the Color Depth videos of the subjects moving on the treadmill at 3 and 5 km/h,

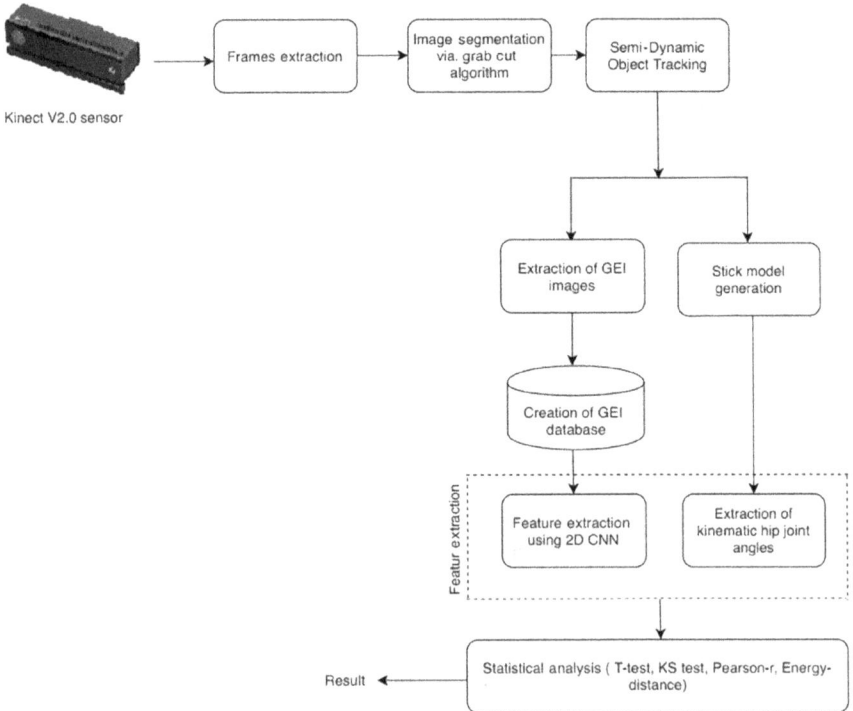

FIGURE 3.1   Proposed workflow.

respectively, one by one. The recorded video is stored in .xef file formats through Kinect Studio v2.0. Hence to store the videos in .avi or .mp4 formats which are much more user-friendly, a screen recorder is used. Gait features are extracted from the depth video utilizing two methodologies: First, utilizing the body viewpoint proportion of subjects, a stick model is created and then the extracted joint angles are used as the features for our analysis. In the second method, features are extracted automatically after the application of 2D CNN on GEIs, which are then analyzed.

3.3.2 CALCULATION AND EXTRACTION OF REGIONS OF INTEREST

The first step in our workflow is the detection of regions of interest (ROI) in the acquired images, known as ROIs. Hence the parts of an image that a human subject populates and provides significant information are obtained.

   a. *Segmentation of acquired images*: A foreground object indicates an object or region of interest in an image. The term "background" refers to all pixels in the image that are not part of the foreground object. The procedure of separating the foreground and background parts in an image is termed as image segmentation. Hence, the color depth image undergoes pre-processing, followed by the extraction of the ROI using Kinect v2.0 sensors. For the extraction of ROIs from depth images, various techniques such as histogram analysis, thresholding and other background subtraction algorithms are usually used. GrabCut algorithm is used for background subtraction in our work. "GrabCut" is an advanced segmentation technique that utilizes both region and boundary information of an image. It stores the information that it requires with the help of a graph. Based on a Min-Cut/Max-Flow algorithm, the graph is segmented and hence the image. With the help of the algorithm, a matting procedure is additionally incorporated, which is utilized to compute the alpha matte for limits of regions which are segmented. Thus, the challenge of isolating an object from the background in an image is met, given certain conditions. A color depth image assigns various colors depending on how much distant an object is from the camera irrespective of the variation in the lighting condition. Hence utilizing this feature, the algorithm uses a single rectangle around the object to distinguish between the background and the inner portion of rectangle which involves both the object (foreground) and some portion of the background as well. These constraints are initial solution to the algorithmic problem, leading to an iterative method which concludes by assigning a label to each image pixel which is either "Background" or "Foreground."
   b. *Creation of bounding box for dynamic object tracking*: As a result of the strategy discussed in the previous section, the area of the floor is also obtained additionally between the human subject on the treadmill and the Kinect sensor besides the required object, in the image frame. As the human subject is our only focus, whose spatio-temporal features of gait are to be obtained, the human is explicitly extricated. It is done with the assumption that if the subject is standing with his back upright, the distance from the

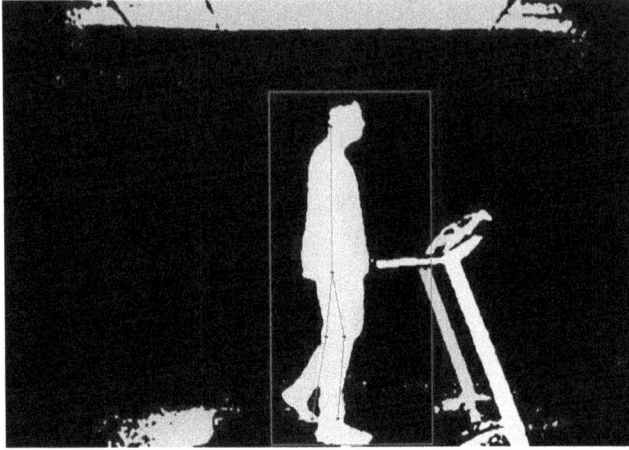

FIGURE 3.2 Bounding box and skeletal frame generation on the extracted frame.

head to the feet will be the maximum patch of pixels with almost the same depth. Then, a semi-dynamic [can be enlarged or reduced in size along its width] bounding box is fit around the human subject to ease the task of extraction. All the objects inside the bounding box are considered as the ROI, though the main ROI is the human subject on the treadmill. Taking into consideration the 3D nature of human beings, the ROI has the same color with the least deviation. The maximum separation is measured, and then its midpoint is assumed to be the body's center when observed in the vertical direction. The semi-dynamic nature is introduced by calculating the maximum width on pixels. If it is more than the width of the bounding box calculated initially, the width is enlarged and vice-versa. This is the basic underlying principle of our proposed semi-dynamic object-tracking algorithm. Figure 3.2. shows an extracted image with a rectangular bounding box around the subject on the treadmill along with the stick model generation, which is explained explicitly in Section 3.3.3a.

3.3.3 Extracting Features from Acquired Depth Images from Kinect V2.0 Sensors

The extracted bounding box will contain ROI, from where we extract the features via two techniques explained in the following sections:

a. *Generation of Proposed Stick Model and Extraction of Features*: As an outcome of the step discussed in the previous section, the region of interest is obtained. It undergoes further processing. Following the ratio of the human body determined anatomically (Winter 2009), the image is decayed into three regions, namely, head node, body torso and the leg region, which are not dependent on each other. Thus, using the body segment ratios, the heights of the three regions are calculated. From each independent region, human gait patterns are obtained. The boundary coordinates for the head node, body torso and the lower limb are found out as we are focusing mainly on the lower portion of the human body starting from the hip. Euclidean distance between the coordinates of the boundaries and the centroid of each part of the human body is calculated. The features obtained are the kinematic hip joint angles. The generated stick model is shown in Figure 3.2. Calculations for the hip angle feature from the corresponding stick model are explicitly explained both diagrammatically (Figure 3.3a and b) as well as mathematically in Equations (3.1–3.4). Figure 3.4 gives a plot of the hip angles for a subject running at 3 km/h.

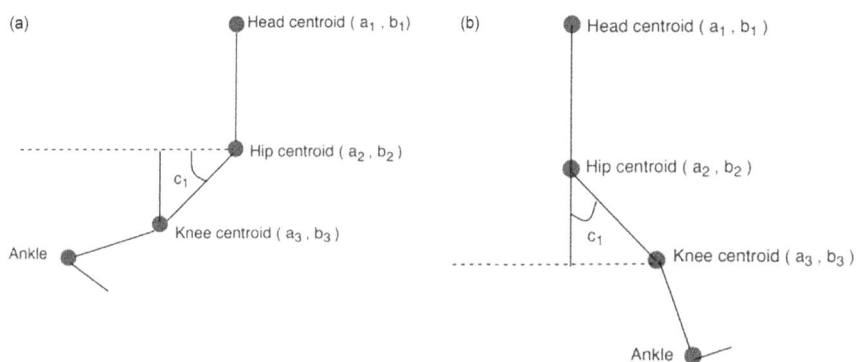

FIGURE 3.3 Hip angle calculations from the proposed stick model.

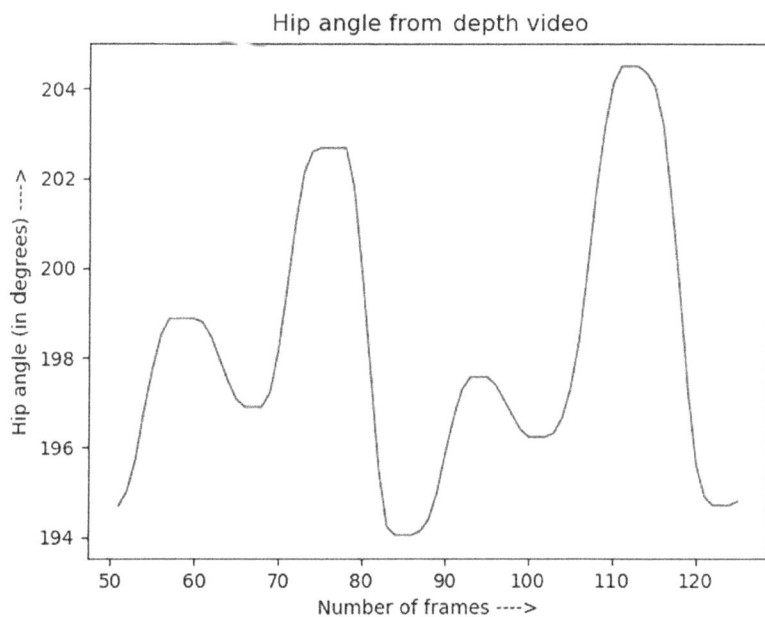

FIGURE 3.4 Hip angles for two gait cycles obtained for a subject moving at 3 km/h.

- *Case 1: When knee centroid is behind the hip centroid:*

$$Hip_\theta = 90° + c_1 \tag{3.1}$$

$$c_1 = \tan^{-1}\left(b_3 - b_2\right)\Big/\left(a_3 - a_2\right) \tag{3.2}$$

where
$c_1 =$ an angle as shown in Figure 3.3a.
Hip_θ = is the hip joint angle.

- *Case 2: When knee centroid is ahead of the hip centroid:*

$$c_1 = \tan^{-1}\left(a_3 - a_2\right)\Big/\left(b_3 - b_2\right) \tag{3.3}$$

$$Hip_\theta = 180° + c_1 \tag{3.4}$$

where c_1 and Hip_θ have the same significances and meanings as in *Case 1*.

b. *Implementation of two-dimensional convolution neural network models for extraction of features*: An indispensable piece of the traditional pattern classification problems is feature extraction. In this section, GEIs, which are used as features for further analysis, are discussed herewith. As we are well aware of the fact that a gait pattern provisions spatio-temporal information of human walking, various elements namely view angles, the speed at which a subject is walking, etc., are taken into consideration, as they increase the variance within a class. In order to reduce any kind of confusion regarding subject identification, a gait feature which is unique and distinct such as GEI is used. Averaging all the frames that constitute one complete gait cycle results in a frame known as the GEI frame. Hence the computational expense is also reduced as the procedure involves averaging. The gait cycle is measured by finding out the correlation coefficient between the extracted frames.

- *Gait period calculation*: The entire motion from the occurrence of a gait event to the re-occurrence of the same gait event by the same leg is known as a gait cycle. The number of frames constituting a full gait cycle defines a gait period. It is known that a video is a sequence of frames, and hence from the captured depth videos, silhouette frames of the human subject's movements are extracted. Then, the correlation coefficient of the first frame with all the remaining frames is calculated. Also, pixel matrix in an image is converted into a single column vector. In our work gait period is calculated by a correlation-based approach with the formula as stated below:

$$Co_{coeff} = \frac{\sum_{l=1}^{T}\left(GP_l - \overline{GP}\right)\left(NG_L - \overline{NG}\right)}{\sqrt{\sum_{l=1}^{T}\left(GP_l - \overline{GP}\right)^2}\sqrt{\sum_{l=1}^{T}\left(NG_L - \overline{NG}\right)^2}} \tag{3.5}$$

where

Co_{coeff} = correlation coefficient

GP = first frame of gait sequence or pattern

NG = next frame of the gait sequence or pattern

T = total number of frames in the gait sequence

Correlation coefficient is calculated for all the frames extracted from the acquired depth videos. Figure 3.5 depicts the correlation coefficient values versus the number of frames. The curve has peaks at subsequent locations which are where the coefficients have maximum values. These maxima are indicated by red dots and the number of frames between two successive maxima constitutes a gait period. The peaks are determined based on the knowledge of simple convex property and speed at which a human subject walks. This entire procedure known as autocorrelation is repeated for all the ten subjects running at 3 and 5 km/h on the treadmill. The length of a gait cycle is the average of all the gait periods when only a particular speed is considered; after the ROI is obtained in the previous step, autocorrelation.

- *GEI*: For the entire feature extraction process, it is of utmost necessity that sufficient amount of gait information of a subject is retained. As GEI is the temporal normalized mean of the frames in a gait period, the purpose is rightfully served. GEIs for a subject walking at a speed of 3 and 5 km/h on the treadmill are shown in Figures 3.6a and b. The mathematical formulation for GEI is

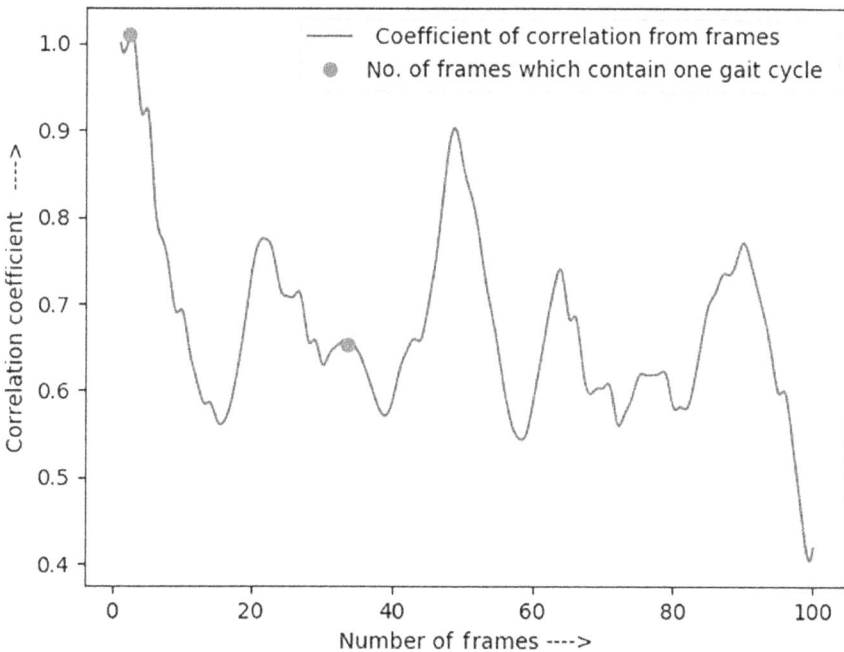

FIGURE 3.5   Correlation coefficient plot for a subject running at 3 km/h is carried out.

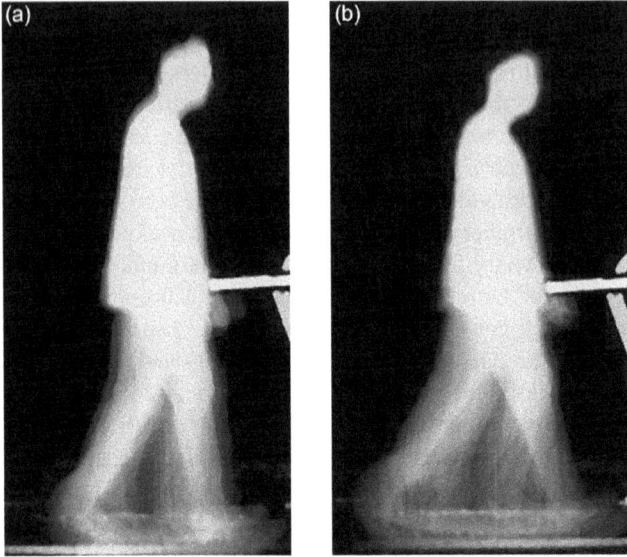

FIGURE 3.6 Sample GEI images of a subject walking at the desired speeds.

$$\text{GEI}(u, v) = \frac{\sum_{r=1}^{GC} F_t(u, v)}{GC} \tag{3.6}$$

where

$F_t(u, v) = t^{th}$ frame in a gait period or cycle GC (Gait Cycle).

u & v = the corresponding pixel coordinates of the image frames.

Figures 3.6a and b clearly give a visual understanding that the main trunk of the body does not show any variation. Hence, that part does not provide any important information. This further allows the subtraction of each and every frame without any kind of significant loss. Thus, the GEIs are extracted and given as inputs to the 2D CNN model for automatic feature extraction.

- *Architectural overview*: The 2D CNN architecture that is implemented is the AlexNet architecture. Classification of images is carefully handled in this work. As there are ten subjects, corresponding to them there are ten different classes. The input GEI image belongs to one of the ten different classes. The output is a vector which has ten numbers. The "k^{th}" element of the output vector denotes the probabilistic value by which an image is classified into the "k^{th}" class. Thus, the output vector possesses elements which sum up to 1. The dimension of each of the images in our dataset is 224×224. Our 2D CNN model consists of five convolutional layers and three dense connected layers. Interesting and the essential features of an image are obtained with the help of the convolution filters present and implemented in the model. A single convolutional layer generally possesses various equally sized kernels. The first convolution layer of AlexNet contains 96, 11 ×11 ×3 sized kernels. In this work the kernels used have equal measurements in terms of width and height whereas the depth is equivalent to the count of channels. Overlapping max-pooling layers succeed the first two convolutional layers. There exists a direct connection between the next set of convolution layers wherein the last convolutional layer is followed by an overlapping max-pooling layer. The next two fully connected layers take as input the results of the max-pooling layer that follows the fifth convolution layer. A softmax classifier is fed with 6 class labels by the second fully connected layer. The GEIs are fed into the 2D CNN model. Our own created data set consisting of 30 GEIs (Figure 3.7) is used for prediction and cross-validation.

Figure 3.8 depicts the 2D CNN architecture used in our research. The first max-pooling layer of the 2D CNN fetches 96 features. Various features thus extracted from different layers of the CNN model undergo statistical tests for further analysis.

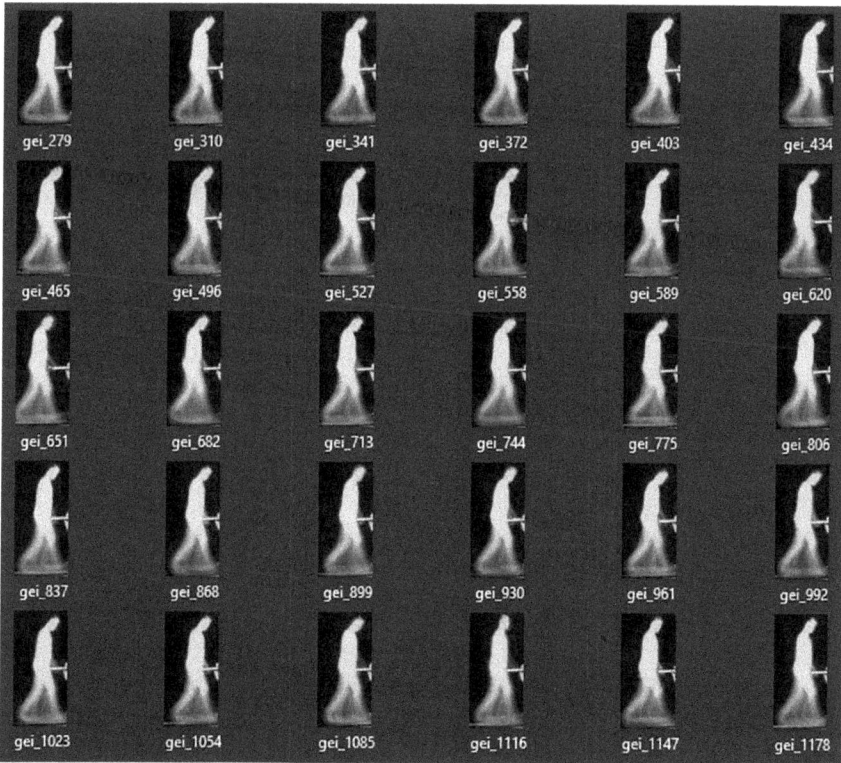

FIGURE 3.7 Generated GEI data set for cross-validation.

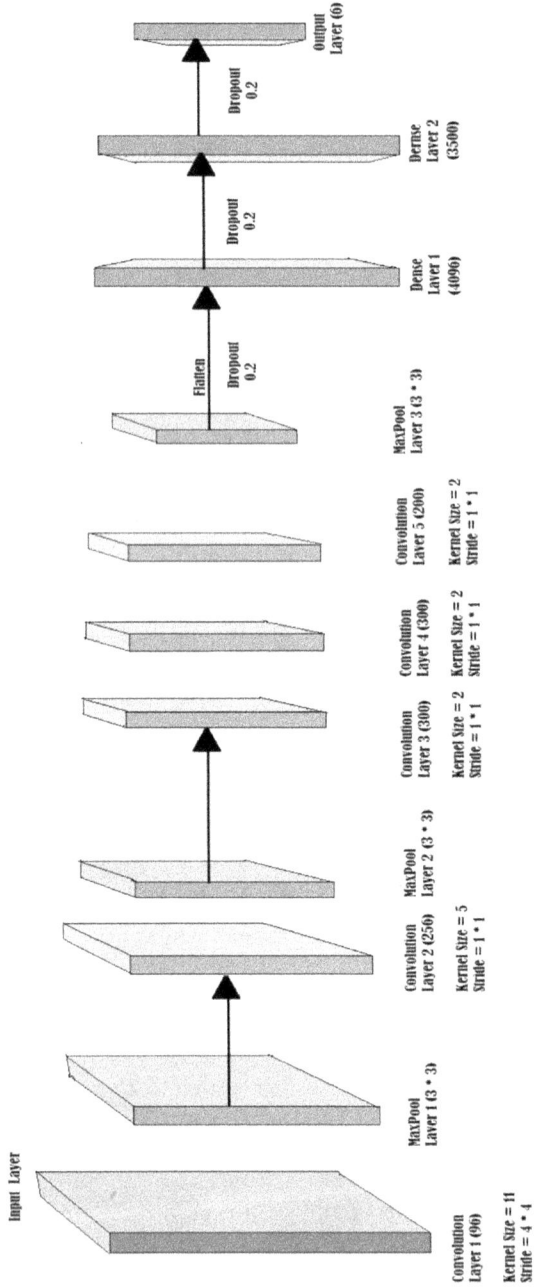

FIGURE 3.8 Architectural diagram of the two-dimensional CNN used.

3.4 RESULTS ANALYSIS AND DISCUSSION

The information gathered through Kinect v2.0 sensors undergoes a lot of processing and test stages for feature reliability-testing and analysis. The data of 10 subjects acquired are properly analyzed through a series of tests. The outcomes thus obtained are hereby discussed. Our 2D CNN architecture consists of nine layers and gives us an aggregate of 96 features for each layer. An outline of the various filters attempted in the various layers and corresponding models is given in Table 3.1. The accuracies obtained by implementing the various models are also shown in Table 3.1. We select the maximum accuracy for further analysis. The accuracy versus epoch curve (Figure 3.9) for the chosen model with the maximum accuracy gives the training and the validation accuracies for the same. The training versus validation graph converges well in Figure 3.9. Thus, a maximum accuracy of 95.1% is attained, which further draws a significant conclusion that the gait features extracted after the application of the 2D CNN model are informative enough for clinical gait analysis. T-Test, KS test, Pearson R, and energy distance are the statistical tests performed for gait feature analysis which also aid in assessing the reliability of features for gait analysis in the future. This section provides an explicit explanation of the obtained results. Tables 3.2 and 3.3 depict the same. The features used are the hip angles obtained from color depth videos and the features extracted automatically from all the layers of our 2D-CNN model in the form of feature maps. Table 3.2 represents tests performed on features obtained from CNN for subjects 1 and 2 walking at speeds of 3 and 5 km/h, respectively, with respect to subject 1 walking at 3 km/h. We use four tests, namely, T-test, KS-test, Pearson-r, and Energy Distance test to validate how informative our results are. Table 3.3 provides similar information for the tests performed on hip angles obtained from depth videos for subjects 1 and 2 walking at different speeds with respect to subject 1 walking at 3 km/h. The statistical tests are performed for all the 10 subjects running at 3 and 5 km/h. For convenience, the test results for only 2 subjects are provided. The 2-sample t-test takes sample data from two groups and boils it down to the t-value. The t-test is any statistical hypothesis test in which the test statistic follows a t-distribution under the null hypothesis. The t-value measures the size of the difference relative to the variation in the sample

TABLE 3.1
Various Models Tested and Their Corresponding Accuracies

Filters in	Model No. 1	Model No. 2	Model No. 3
1st convolution layer	96	45	96
2nd convolution layer	256	284	256
3rd convolution layer	300	440	360
4th convolution layer	300	440	360
5th convolution layer	200	256	300
1st dense layer	3,500	4,096	4,400
2nd dense layer	3,500	4,096	4,400
Accuracy (in %)	92.1%	93.33%	95.1%

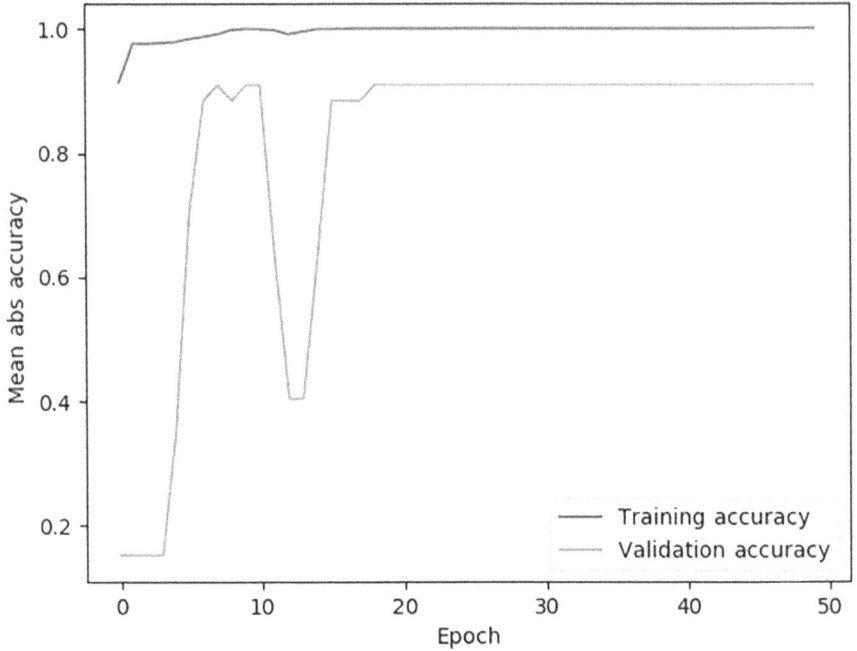

FIGURE 3.9   Accuracy versus epoch curve for the CNN model used.

TABLE 3.2
Statistical Analysis Outcomes for CNN Features

Tests	Subject1_5 km/h	Subject2_3 km/h	Subject2_5 km/h
T-test(t-statistic, p-value)	(1.089, 2.76e$-$1)	(1.46, 1.38e$-$1)	(1.08, 7.113e$-$2)
KS-test (ks-statistic, p-value)	(1.033e$-$1, 1.45e$-$1)	(1.027e$-$1, 1.39e$-$1)	(1.0297e-1, 1.345e$-$1)
Pearson-r	9.99e$-$1	9.789e$-$1	9.48e$-$1
Energy distance	7.89e$-$4	9.24e$-$3	1.87e$-$2

TABLE 3.3
Statistical Analysis Outcomes for Hip Angles Obtained from Depth Videos

Tests	Subject1_5 km/h	Subject2_3 km/h	Subject2_5 km/h
T-test (t-statistic, p-value)	(9.19e$-$2, 9.27e$-$1)	(1.04, 2.52e$-$1)	(1.032, 7.7e$-$2)
KS-test (ks-statistic, p-value)	(1.157e$-$1, 1.779e$-$1)	(1.105e$-$1, 1.73e$-$1)	(1.134e$-$1, 1.76e$-$1)
Pearson's r	9.99e$-$1	9.483e$-$1	7.086e$-$1
Energy distance	9.42e$-$4	1.252	2.0052

data. From Table 3.2, it is realized that when the features from CNN corresponding to subject 1 running at 5 km/h are used in a 2 sample *t*-test with those of the same subject running at 3 km/h, it leads to a *t*-value of 1.089 and p-value of 2.76^{e-1}. Thus, it is concluded that two samples are coming from the same population mean and have very similar distributions since p-value is greater than our confidence interval, i.e., 0.05 [as is evident from the plot for T-distribution (Figure 3.10)]. *p*-value > 0.05 denotes that the feature points follow a specific type of distribution and our null hypothesis is that samples come from a population with the same mean. Only if the *p*-value is < 0.05, the null hypothesis is safely rejected otherwise accepted. Similarly, when CNN features of subject 2 running at 3 km/h and the same subject running at 5 km/h are used in a 2 sample *t*-test with those of subject 1 walking at 3 km/h, the *p*-values obtained are greater than 0.05 and hence null hypothesis cannot be rejected which again infers that the two distributions are coming from the same population mean and have very similar characteristics.

Similarly, in Table 3.3 above, it is seen that t-test between hip angles obtained from the depth videos corresponding to subject 1 walking at 3 km/h is compared with those of the same subject running at 5 km/h, a *t*-value of $9.19e-2$ and a *p*-value of $9.27e-1$ are obtained. This indicates that though the two samples have different sample means and the null hypothesis cannot be rejected, i.e., the two samples have similar distributions and come from the same population. Comparing the values obtained for hip angles from depth videos corresponding to subject 2 moving at 3 km/h and the same subject running at 5 km/h, it is again concluded that *p*-values are

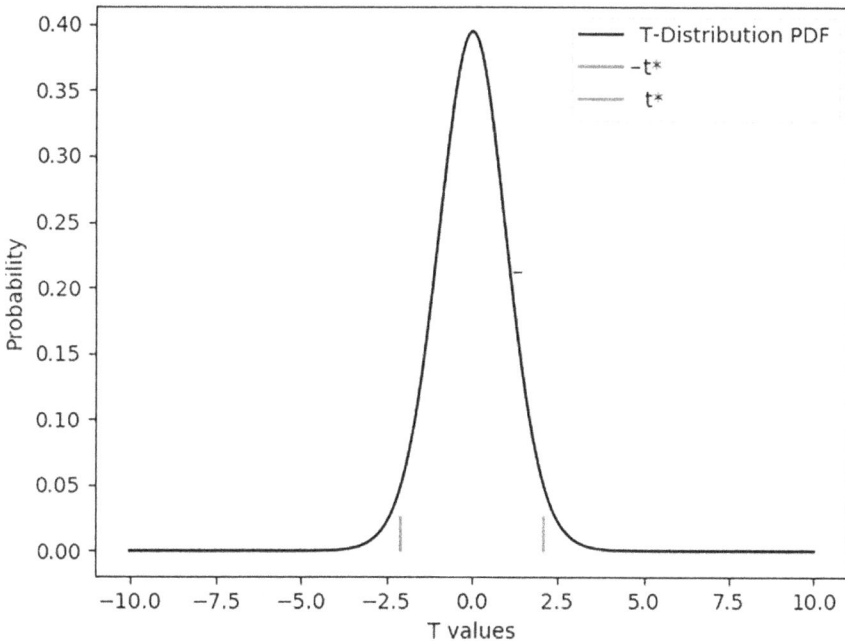

FIGURE 3.10   T distribution plot for extracted CNN features.

greater than 0.05 and hence the null hypothesis cannot be rejected. Thus, the two distributions come from the same population mean. Therefore, the hip angles follow similar patterns and are quite informative for clinical gait analysis.

The Kolmogorov-Smirnov (KS) test verifies and validates whether two samples are drawn from similar distribution. The test uses the two-sided asymptotic KS distribution. If the K-S statistic is small or the p-value is high, then the hypothesis that the distributions of the two samples are same cannot be rejected. From Tables 3.2 and 3.3, the observed values for both the CNN features and the hip angles suggest that the null hypothesis cannot be ignored in all three cases. Hence, the data from multiple samples come from populations of more or less similar means. The plots of cumulative probability distributions for KS test for all the tested features are illustrated below in Figures 3.11 and 3.12.

Energy distance test gives statistical separation between likelihood conveyances. All the axioms of a metric are satisfied by it, which further aids in characterizing the equality of distributions as well. On the other hand, Pearson's r test is a statistical test which quantifies the association between two continuous variables. It gives two values namely Pearson's correlation coefficient and 2-tailed p-value. The 2-tailed p-value is useful for data sets which have sizes of more than 500. In our case, length of the test data set is 90–100. So, only the first parameter, i.e., the Pearson correlation coefficient is used for analysis in our work. This statistical technique is based on the method of covariance and hence is considered one of the best methods for measuring the relationship between variables. Using Pearson's r test and energy distance metrics

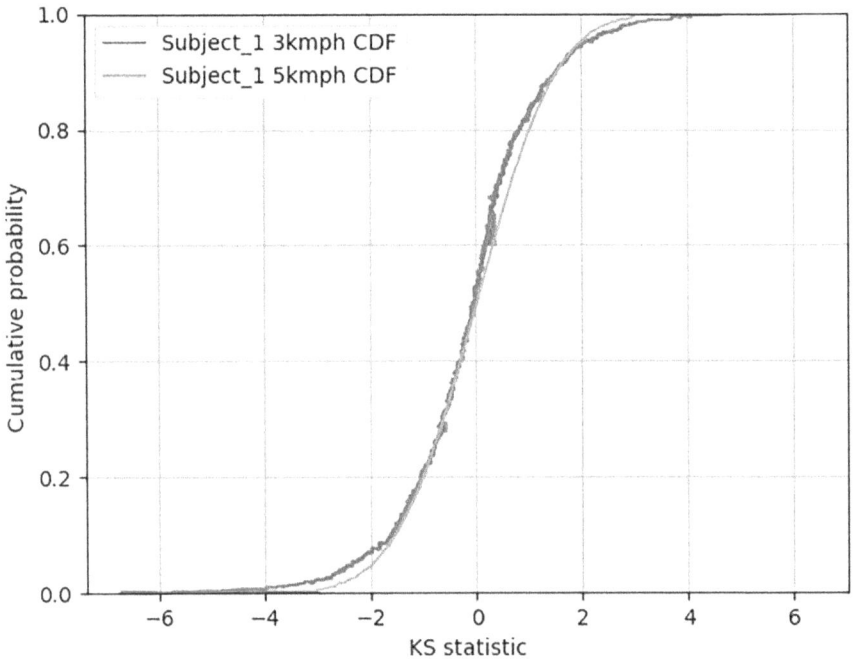

FIGURE 3.11 KS cumulative frequency distribution for CNN features corresponding to Subject 1 at 3 km/h and Subject 2 at 5 km/h.

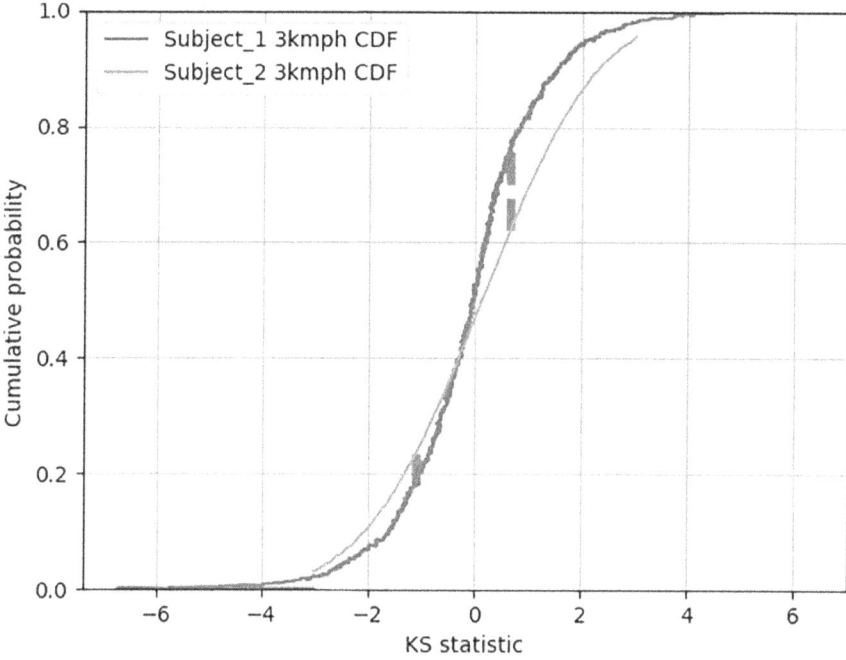

FIGURE 3.12 KS cumulative frequency distribution for hip angles from depth video corresponding to Subject 1 at 3 km/h and Subject 2 at 5 km/h.

as shown in Tables 3.2 and 3.3, it can be concluded that a subject walking at 3 km/h and the same subject running at 5 km/h are statistically of a very similar distribution and have similar statistical properties. All other test results indicate that null hypothesis cannot be rejected. Hence, the effect of speed and subjects on the statistical distributions of CNN features and the hip angles obtained from depth videos are negligible. This study also implies that the hip angles obtained from depth videos are more informative in comparing distributions than features obtained from CNN since they give more discernible test results.

3.5 CONCLUSION AND FUTURE WORK

Color depth videos of subjects are captured using Kinect v2.0 sensors. The videos undergo further processing for extraction of features and hence information is elicited. In one approach, hip joint angles of the subjects are obtained as features. From their plots, the patterns of the hip angles as to how they vary in a gait cycle are observed. The other approach involves feeding the GEIs to CNN for feature extraction. All the extracted features undergo statistical analysis. The hip angle graphs do possess some steep edges. This is due to the fact that every frame contributes to the data and the leg does not undergo similar movement in every frame. Thus a little bit of irregularity is always observed. Interpolation is carried out on the used data and the intermediate points are found to form a smooth cubic graph. As observed from statistical tests, the samples obtained from the subjects tested are almost consistent and null hypothesis cannot be rejected. With all the factors taken into consideration, it is inferred that the hip angles obtained from depth videos prove to be the most promising feature of all the features obtained from depth videos. Features extracted after the application of 2D CNN model on the GEI images provide adequate information for gait analysis. Though it is comparatively less as compared to the information obtained from the hip angles, the calculation of the angles from the depth image has a limitation pertaining to the elevation of the centroid when in motion. The reason being the joints do not always have a translational motion. Hence, measuring the knee angles remains a future work. Also ankle angle detection from both the color depth and RGB images will be worked upon as a part of future analysis. These analyses thus provide sufficient information for recommending the use of deep learning and machine learning techniques in the domain of gait analysis for various medical applications such as in detection and cure of pediatric orthopedics, musculoskeletal problems, mental health issues such as depression and so on.

3.6 EFFECTS OF THIS RESEARCH IN BIOMEDICAL DOMAIN

Existing systems and architectures for gait analysis are either expensive or intrusive in nature. These factors act as restrictions pertaining to the explicit and smooth analysis of human motion signatures having medical implications. Recently, Kinect-based gait analysis is an exciting area of research which has so far explored the solution of human recognition problems. Kinect being a low-cost vision-based sensor offers an user-friendly alternative to the existing costly systems. Gait analysis is performed through the collection of spatio-temporal gait parameters such as lower limb joint angles and GEI-fed CNN features in this work for human activity recognition. This research involves a stringent analysis on the complex process of human walking that involves much balance and coordination. The systematic motion of limbs resulting in bipedal locomotion called gait is considered to be a significant biometric trait with applications on a large scale in the healthcare domain. As gait biometrics can be obtained without much requirement of a person's attention unlike finger scans, DNA or other biometric traits, the data acquisition through Kinect when processed and passed through machine learning and deep learning techniques as explained in this work generates promising outcomes. The portion of our work justifying the extraction of ROI lays emphasis on the techniques available for processing the data acquired and removing the unwanted disturbances present, which otherwise lead to inaccurate and inexact estimations. Gait features are discriminating components which follow certain patterns and distributions. Thus, the reliability testing and the observational assessments of the various features of gait extracted from the depth videos of human subjects in this work introduce the readers to an advanced understanding of extensive gait analysis. The quantitative validations and the statistical analyses carried out in this chapter demonstrate the significance of the parameters contributing to rectified gait analysis for multi-scenario tasks. Also, this work rightfully justifies both the real-time importance and relevance of deep learning strategies in the biomedical field of research. Since many years now, stride assessment has had a long history of being restricted to theoretical disciplines with rare practical applications; this work in its current state addresses the problem of minimal viable application while pondering on rehabilitation alternatives or during clinical decision-making. This chapter provides lot of insights for applications in the biomedical domain. Certain immediate effects are to assist in increasing a more prominent comprehension of stride, survey irregularities of walk in pediatrics field and acquaint the researcher with an essential comprehension of step investigations. Healthcare has become progressively proof-based. Due to which the clinicians nowadays need a consciousness of what instruments are accessible for their patients. Modernized step examinations provision a target and quantitative assessment, which improves the comprehension of reasons for stride irregularities and aids treatment. As the motion of the human joints is not always consistent, measurements of knee and ankle angles remain a future work. These if solved would further encompass a broader spectrum of gait diagnoses and intervention strategies besides permitting future developments in rehabilitation engineering.

ACKNOWLEDGMENTS

We are extremely thankful to Science and Engineering Research Board (SERB), DST, Govt. of India to support this research work. The Kinect v2.0 sensors used in our research experiment are purchased from the project funded by SERB with FILE NO: ECR/2017/000408. We would also like to extend our sincere thanks to the students of Department of Computer Science and Engineering, NIT Rourkela, for their uninterrupted co-operation and participation catering to the data collection.

REFERENCES

Andriluka, Mykhaylo, Stefan Roth, and Bernt Schiele. "Monocular 3d pose estimation and tracking by detection." In *2010 IEEE Computer Society Conference on Computer Vision and Pattern Recognition*, pp. 623–630. IEEE, 2010, San Francisco, CA.

Andriluka, Mykhaylo, Stefan Roth, and Bernt Schiele. "Pictorial structures revisited: People detection and articulated pose estimation." In *2009 IEEE Conference on Computer Vision and Pattern Recognition*, pp. 1014–1021. IEEE, 2009.

Bashir, Khalid, Tao Xiang, and Shaogang Gong. "Feature selection on gait energy image for human identification." In *2008 IEEE International Conference on Acoustics, Speech and Signal Processing*, pp. 985–988. IEEE, 2008, Las Vegas, NV.

Belagiannis, Vasileios, and Andrew Zisserman. "Recurrent human pose estimation." In *2017 12th IEEE International Conference on Automatic Face & Gesture Recognition (FG 2017)*, pp. 468–475. IEEE, 2017, Washington, DC.

Chu, Xiao, Wei Yang, Wanli Ouyang, Cheng Ma, Alan L. Yuille, and Xiaogang Wang. "Multi-context attention for human pose estimation." In *Proceedings of the IEEE Conference on Computer Vision and Pattern Recognition*, pp. 1831–1840. 2017, Honolulu, HI.

Correa, Mauricio, Gabriel Hermosilla, Rodrigo Verschae, and Javier Ruiz-del-Solar. "Human detection and identification by robots using thermal and visual information in domestic environments." *Journal of Intelligent & Robotic Systems* 66, no. 1–2 (2012): 223–243.

Dadashi, Farzin, Babak N. Araabi, and Hamid Soltanian-Zadeh. "Gait recognition using wavelet packet silhouette representation and transductive support vector machines." In *2009 2nd International Congress on Image and Signal Processing*, pp. 1–5. IEEE, 2009, Tianjin.

Dantone, Matthias, Juergen Gall, Christian Leistner, and Luc Van Gool. "Human pose estimation using body parts dependent joint regressors." In *Proceedings of the IEEE Conference on Computer Vision and Pattern Recognition*, pp. 3041–3048. 2013, Portland, OR.

Davis, James W., and Mark A. Keck. "A two-stage template approach to person detection in thermal imagery." In *2005 Seventh IEEE Workshops on Applications of Computer Vision (WACV/MOTION'05)-Volume 1*, 1, pp. 364–369. IEEE, 2005, Washington DC.

Felzenszwalb, Pedro F., and Daniel P. Huttenlocher. "Pictorial structures for object recognition." *International Journal of Computer Vision* 61, no. 1 (2005): 55–79.

Foresti, Gian Luca, Lucio Marcenaro, and Carlo S. Regazzoni. "Automatic detection and indexing of video-event shots for surveillance applications." *IEEE Transactions on Multimedia* 4, no. 4 (2002): 459–471.

Guan, Feng, L. Y. Li, Shuzhi Sam Ge, and Ai Poh Loh. "Robust human detection and identification by using stereo and thermal images in human robot interaction." *International Journal of Information Acquisition* 4, no. 02 (2007): 161–183.

Han, Ju, and Bir Bhanu. "Individual recognition using gait energy image." *IEEE Transactions on Pattern Analysis and Machine Intelligence* 28, no. 2 (2005): 316–322.

Haritaoglu, Ismail, David Harwood, and Larry S. Davis. "W/sup 4: Real-time surveillance of people and their activities." *IEEE Transactions on Pattern Analysis and Machine Intelligence* 22, no. 8 (2000): 809–830.

Ikemura, Sho, and Hironobu Fujiyoshi. "Real-time human detection using relational depth similarity features." In *Asian Conference on Computer Vision*, pp. 25–38. Springer, Berlin, Heidelberg, 2010, Springer, Heidelberg.

Johnson, Sam, and Mark Everingham. "Clustered pose and nonlinear appearance models for human pose estimation." In *bmvc*, 2, no. 4 (2010): 5.

Karlinsky, Leonid, and Shimon Ullman. "Using linking features in learning non-parametric part models." In *European Conference on Computer Vision*, pp. 326–339. Springer, Berlin, Heidelberg, 2012, Springer, Heidelberg.

Ke, Lipeng, Ming-Ching Chang, Honggang Qi, and Siwei Lyu. "Multi-scale structure-aware network for human pose estimation." In *Proceedings of the European Conference on Computer Vision (ECCV)*, pp. 713–728. 2018, Science+Business Media, Berlin.

Krishnamurthy, Sundar Narayan. *"Human Detection and Extraction Using Kinect Depth Images."*, MSc. Thesis, Bournemouth University, 2011, Bournemouth University.

Lan, Xiangyang, and Daniel P. Huttenlocher. "Beyond trees: Common-factor models for 2d human pose recovery." In *10th IEEE International Conference on Computer Vision (ICCV'05) 1*, vol. 1, pp. 470–477. IEEE, 2005, Beijing.

Newell, Alejandro, Kaiyu Yang, and Jia Deng. "Stacked hourglass networks for human pose estimation." In *European Conference on Computer Vision*, pp. 483–499. Springer, Cham, 2016, Springer, Heidelberg.

Pfister, Tomas, James Charles, and Andrew Zisserman. "Flowing convnets for human pose estimation in videos." In *Proceedings of the IEEE International Conference on Computer Vision*, pp. 1913–1921. 2015, Santiago.

Pishchulin, Leonid, Mykhaylo Andriluka, Peter Gehler, and Bernt Schiele. "Poselet conditioned pictorial structures." In *Proceedings of the IEEE Conference on Computer Vision and Pattern Recognition*, pp. 588–595. 2013, Portland, OR.

Ramanan, Deva, David A. Forsyth, and Andrew Zisserman. "Strike a pose: Tracking people by finding stylized poses." In *2005 IEEE Computer Society Conference on Computer Vision and Pattern Recognition (CVPR'05)*, vol. 1, pp. 271–278. IEEE, 2005, San Diego, CA.

Spinello, Luciano, and Kai O. Arras. "People detection in RGB-D data." In *2011 IEEE/RSJ International Conference on Intelligent Robots and Systems*, pp. 3838–3843. IEEE, 2011, San Francisco, CA.

Tang, Wei, Pei Yu, and Ying Wu. "Deeply learned compositional models for human pose estimation." In *Proceedings of the European Conference on Computer Vision (ECCV)*, pp. 190–206. 2018, Science+Business Media, Berlin.

Tompson, Jonathan J., Arjun Jain, Yann LeCun, and Christoph Bregler. "Joint training of a convolutional network and a graphical model for human pose estimation." In *Advances in Neural Information Processing Systems*, pp. 1799–1807. 2014, Montreal.

Wei, Shih-En, Varun Ramakrishna, Takeo Kanade, and Yaser Sheikh. "Convolutional pose machines." In *Proceedings of the IEEE conference on Computer Vision and Pattern Recognition*, pp. 4724–4732. 2016, Las Vegas, NV.

Winter, David A. *Biomechanics and Motor Control of Human Movement*. John Wiley & Sons, 2009, New York.

Xia, Lu, Chia-Chih Chen, and Jake K. Aggarwal. "Human detection using depth information by kinect." In *CVPR 2011 Workshops*, pp. 15–22. IEEE, 2011, Colorado Springs, CO.

Yang, Wei, Shuang Li, Wanli Ouyang, Hongsheng Li, and Xiaogang Wang. "Learning feature pyramids for human pose estimation." In *Proceedings of the IEEE International Conference on Computer Vision*, pp. 1281–1290. 2017, Venice.

Yang, Yi, and Deva Ramanan. "Articulated human detection with flexible mixtures of parts." *IEEE Transactions on Pattern Analysis and Machine Intelligence* 35, no. 12 (2012): 2878–2890.

4 Segmentation of Magnetic Resonance Brain Images Using 3D Convolution Neural Network

S. N. Kumar and Jins Sebastin
Amal Jyothi College of Engineering

H. Ajay Kumar
Mar Ephraem College of Engineering and Technology

CONTENTS

4.1 INTRODUCTION

Image processing refers to the usage of computer-aided algorithms for the analysis of images. Medical image processing uses computerized algorithms for the analysis of CT, MR or ultrasound images for disease diagnosis and for therapeutic applications. A wide number of segmentation algorithms are there in medical image processing and neural networks-based algorithms are gaining much importance nowadays for clinical diagnosis and treatment planning. Magnetic resonance imaging generates high-resolution images and it focuses on the soft tissues. Brain magnetic resonance image (MRI) is used for the analysis of tumors and neuron degenerative diseases like Alzheimer's and Parkinson's disease. The efficient delineation of white matter (WM), gray matter (GM) and cerebrospinal fluid (CSF) is a challenging one in MR brain images due to the Rician noise and artifacts (Wang et al., 2018). The neural network approaches are found to be efficient for large data sets, since automatic segmentation and classification aid the physician for clinical studies. The robustness of neural network algorithm relies on the training and feature extraction also plays an important role. The main advantage of convolution neural network (CNN) over classical neural network architecture is that it does not require any feature extraction technique and hence minimize the computational complexity (Moeskops, Viergever, et al., 2016).

In Milletari et al. (2017), a deep learning algorithm based on the Hough CNN was proposed for the automatic extraction of region of interest (ROI) on MR brain images. The proposed Hough CNN with patch-wise multi-atlas yields efficient results, when compared with the six different architecture models. For the segmentation of 3D MR brain images, Deep Voxel wise Residual Networks that initially extract ROI from 2D MR slices generates the volumetric data. VoxRes Net integrates the low-level image features, shape information and high-level features together for efficient segmentation of the brain volume in the 3D MR brain images (Chen et al., 2016). The CNN with three-dimensional kernels is used for the segmentation of the ROI in the brain MRI of BRATS data sets. The modified U-Net CNN architecture performs better with less number of labeled medical images (Kayalibay et al., 2017). The segmentation of six types of tissues in the brain was done by the single CNN architecture, which also performs multiple segmentation tasks in the breast and cardiac computed tomography angiography (CTA) images. The architecture was trained with tri-planar orthogonal patches for deep learning. The brain segmentation results were found to be comparable with previously published results (Moeskops, Wolterink, et al., 2016). In Ker et al., (2017), a detailed analysis has been done on the deep learning with different types of neural network architecture on various applications like classification, localization, detection, segmentation and registration in medical images. A patch-based CNN was implemented for the automatic ROI extraction on brain images. The neural network was trained using subdivided patches from the CANDI MRI data sets and obtained the training accuracy of 76.86%. The segmentation accuracy was determined by dice ratio that results in a value of 95.19% (Cui et al., 2016).

The automatic segmentation of WM hyper-intensities and the brain tissue in Moeskops et al. (2018) uses T1-weighted, T2-weighted FLAIR and T1-weighted infra-red MRI images. The 2D patches of three different sizes were used for training the fully convolutional neural network from the MRBrainS13 challenge data set. The proposed network model segments accurately the brain tissues and WM hyper-intensities with promising results when evaluated with dice coefficient. The hybrid model was implemented using Gaussian mixture model and deep CNN, trained using the uncertain voxels for the segmentation of the brain tissues in 3D brain MRI images. The implemented model is validated in ISBR18 data set with dice coefficient that outperforms when compared with several other segmentation algorithms (Nguyen et al., 2017). In Bui et al. (2017), the volumetric segmentation of MRI images of the infant brain was efficiently done with greater accuracy using the 3D densely convolutional neural network. The results were comparable with the results of iSeg-2017 challenge. The 3D CNN with RP-Net architecture was proposed for the segmentation of brain tissues from the MR brain images. The classification of voxels acquires the information about local and global features. The proposed network architecture was validated in CANDI, IBSR18 and IBSR20 data sets, which achieves dice coefficient of 90.7%, 90.49% and 84.96%, respectively (Wang, Xie et al., 2019).

A detailed survey was done on the different types of the deep learning algorithms for the ROI extraction on MR brain images. The survey was carried out based on their architecture, segmentation performance, speed, learning efficiency and the quality metrics used for the evaluation of segmentation performance (Akkus et al., 2017). The segmentation of Hippocampus in 7.0 Tesla MR brain image was done using unsupervised deep learning stacked convolutional Independent Subspace Analysis network. In this network image patches with the lower level features were processed by lower layer and higher layer features were processed by higher layer; this hierarchical patch feature representation improves the segmentation in terms of precision, relative overlap and similarity index, when compared with hand-crafted features (Kim et al., 2013). An M-Net-based CNN was used for the segmentation of deep brain structures like Thalamus, Putamen, Pallidum, Hippocampus, Amygdala, Caudate and Accumbens from the ISBR and Diencephalon data set of MICCAI 2013 SATA challenge. The dice coefficient metrics values show that the M-Net outperforms with 2D convolution filter in segmentation of 3D MRI data sets (Mehta & Sivaswamy, 2017). The multi-layer perceptron neural network associated with volumetric shape model was used for extraction of brain tissues. The network uses signed distance maps and intensity-based shape features for training from MRBrainS13 data sets. The evaluation of the proposed algorithm shows that the training time is much low when compared with SVM, MLP, LVQ and RBF techniques (Mahbod et al., 2018). The synthetic MR image and the noncontrast CT image were co-registered for training the fully convolutional modified U-Net and it segments the MR images. The labelling of the synthetic MR images was done using MALP-EM labels and atlases (Zhao et al., 2017). The evaluation by dice coefficient shows contrast-enhanced 4D CT performs better than proposed method, but synthetic MR image segmentation is better than CT image directly.

The CNN was found to be proficient in the segmentation of tumors from the 3D MR data sets of brain; preprocessing was done by median filter and the water cycle optimization algorithm was coupled with CNN model for the accurate identification of tumor regions (Jijja & Rai, 2019). The 2D ensemble model based on 2D pre-trained model was found to be attractive, when compared with the 3D segmentation. Two ensemble models are proposed in this work; the ensemble A employs three 2D models simultaneously for validation and generates a prediction output and the ensemble B employs three 2D models separately for validation and generates a prediction output. The 2D ensemble model segmentation results were found to be proficient, when compared with the 3D scratch segmentation model (Ahn et al., 2019). The semi-dense fully convolutional neural network was found to be robust in the segmentation of infant brain MR images segmentation. The local and global contextual information was utilized in the segmentation and the algorithm was validated by performance metrics and tested on MICCAI iSEG-2017 Grand Challenge database comprising MR images of 6-months-old infant (Dolz et al., 2020).

The 2D CNN features extracted from axial, coronal and sagittal slices images are used as additional inputs for the 3D CNN model and the novel 2D-3D hybrid approach yields efficient results than the 3D and 2D segmentation CNN models (Mlynarski et al., 2019). The spatially localized atlas network tiles (SLANT) technique comprises multiple independent 3D FCNN for MR brain image segmentation. The SLANT-27 architecture was found to be proficient, when compared with the SLANT-8 architecture (Huo et al., 2019). For the segmentation of gliomas in MR images, 3D deep learning approach was used, and for the prediction of tumor stages, random forest classifier was employed. In the 3D deep learning-based segmentation, two CNN architectures are used; one for the extraction of local features and the other one for the extraction of global features (Amian & Soltaninejad, 2020). The CNN architecture was coupled with the distributed dense connection for the accurate segmentation of brain tissues. Three different models of distributed dense architectures cross-skip, skip-1 and skip-2 are proposed in this work. The post-processing stage minimizes the false positives and was tested on BraTS 2019 data set (Zhang et al., 2020).

A hybrid segmentation model comprising multi-cascaded CNN and conditional random field was proposed for the MR brain tumor segmentation. The results obtained from the CNN architecture were refined by the Markov random fields. Prior to segmentation, the pre-procesisng was performed by N4ITK method (Hu et al., 2019). The 3D CNN employed in Ramzan et al. (2020) uses residual learning and dilated convolution operations for the segmentation of brain tissues from MR brain images and yields efficient segmentation results, when compared with the techniques in Luna and Park (2019), Moeskops et al. (2018) and Ahn et al. (2019). The average values of dice coefficient for the WM, GM and CSF are 0.872, 0.872 and 0.896. In Malathi and Sinthia (2019), an automatic segmentation framework based on CNN was proposed for the segmentation of brain tumor from BRATS 2015 database and bias field correction was done by n41TK and both local and global features were taken into account for ROI extraction. For the extraction of the breast tumor from dynamic contrast-enhanced magnetic resonance images, two deep learning architectures; SegNet and U-Net, were proposed. The overall segmentation accuracy of SegNet was 68.88% and U-Net was 78.14% (El Adoui et al., 2019). The cascaded CNN (2.5D CNN) with uncertainty estimation was proposed for the automatic segmentation of the brain tumor from MR images (Wang, Li et al., 2019). The 3D U-net architecture was proposed for the segmentation of brain tumor in MR images and multi-variate linear regression model was proposed for the prediction of survival (Feng et al., 2020). A hybrid CNN architecture comprising 3D U-Net and DeepMedic was proposed for the segmentation of brain tumor in MR images (Kao et al., 2020). The two-stage fusion minimizes the uncertainty in the prediction. A variant of 3D U-Net which comprises three stages was proposed for the infant brain segmentation and validated on iSEG-2017 data set (Qamar et al., 2020).

The chapter framework is as follows: Section 4.1 highlights the MR brain image segmentation characterizing the pros and cons of classical approaches. Section 4.2 describes the pre-processing and the 3D CNN architecture. Section 4.3 depicts the segmentation results of 3D CNN on 3D data sets, and finally, Section 4.4 highlights the conclusion.

4.2 MATERIALS AND METHODS

The 3D CNN architecture is proposed in this chapter for the segmentation of WM, GM and CSF from 3D input MR data set. Prior to segmentation, the pre-processing stage was employed that comprises normalization and contrast adaptive histogram equalization. The flow diagram of the proposed 3D CNN architecture is depicted in Figure 4.1.

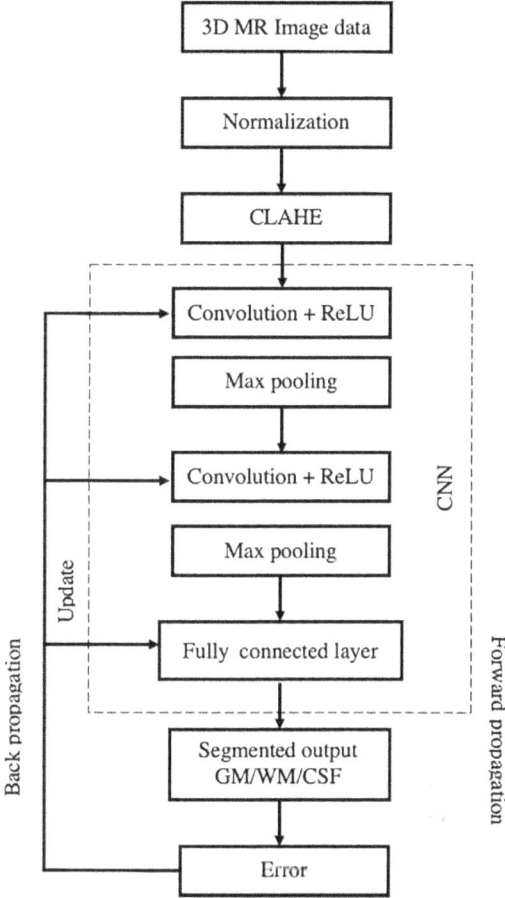

FIGURE 4.1   3D CNN architecture for the segmentation of brain tissues.

4.2.1 PRE-PROCESSING

The pre-processing stage comprises normalization and contrast local adaptive histogram equalization. The normalization is a technique that changes the range of pixel intensity values. The min-max normalization is employed in this work and the expression for normalized voxel values is as follows:

$$imV = (imV - mn)./(mx - mn) \qquad (4.1)$$

where $mx = \max(imV(:))$ and $mn = \min(imV(:))$.

The mx represents the maximum gray value in the data set and mn represents the minimum gray value in the data set. The normalized 3D data are subjected to contrast local adaptive histogram equalization. The CLAHE generates better results than adaptive histogram equalization, since it operates on the smaller regions of image called tiles or blocks rather than on the entire image. The parameter num tiles in CLAHE is set to [4, 4] and it represents the number of regions into which adaptive histogram equalization divides an image. The default value of num tiles is [2, 2] and is chosen based on the nature of the image. The Clip Limit value is set to 0.08 and its default value is 0.01. The Clip Limit, contrast enhanced limit is also termed as contrast factor that eliminates the over-saturation of the image.

4.2.2   3D CNN Architecture

The CNN differs from regular neural network in such a manner that the inputs are images. The neurons in 3D CNN are arranged in 3D pattern; width, height and depth. The CNN architecture comprises the following: convolution layer (CL), pooling layer and fully connected layer. The 3D CNN architecture proposed in this chapter comprises 2 CL, 2 max pooling layers, a fully connected layer and an output layer. The 3D MR input data are utilized in this work. The pre-processing stage comprises normalization and contrast enhancement by contrast local adaptive histogram equalization. The first CL comprises 6 filters with a kernel size of 5×5 and second CL comprises 12 filters with a kernel size of 5×5. The pooling layer comprises filters with kernel size 2×2 and max pooling is employed. The volumetric context information was fully utilized in CNN architecture and was proven to be an efficient one for handling 3D MR images.

> *Convolution layer*: It is termed as the heart of CNN and does most of the computation. The vital parameter of the CL is the set of filters or kernels. The general template of filter is $m \times m \times 3$, where m represents the size of filter and 3 is for the red-green-blue (RGB) images. The convolution operation is performed by sliding the filter over the entire image. A 2D activation map is produced by the sliding operation of filter on the input images.
> *Pooling layer*: The pooling layers are inserted successively between the CL s in the architecture. The objective of the pooling layer is to minimize the size of representation to reduce the number of parameters and computation in the network. The general form of pooling layer comprises filters of size 2×2 with a stride of 2 down samples.

The types of pooling are average pooling, sum pooling and max pooling. The pooling layer is also called as down sampling layer, since it minimizes the features and max pooling is employed here.

> *Fully connected layer*: The neurons in the fully connected layer have full connections for the activation response functions in the predecessor layer. The activation is determined with a matrix multiplication followed by bias effect. The main feature of the fully connected CNN is the flexibility in the input that can be applied; for example, the input can be images or videos. A fully connected neural network comprises a series of fully connected layers. A fully connected layer is defines as a function F_m to F_n and each output dimension relies on the input dimension. The fully connected layer in a deep neural network is depicted in Figure 4.2.

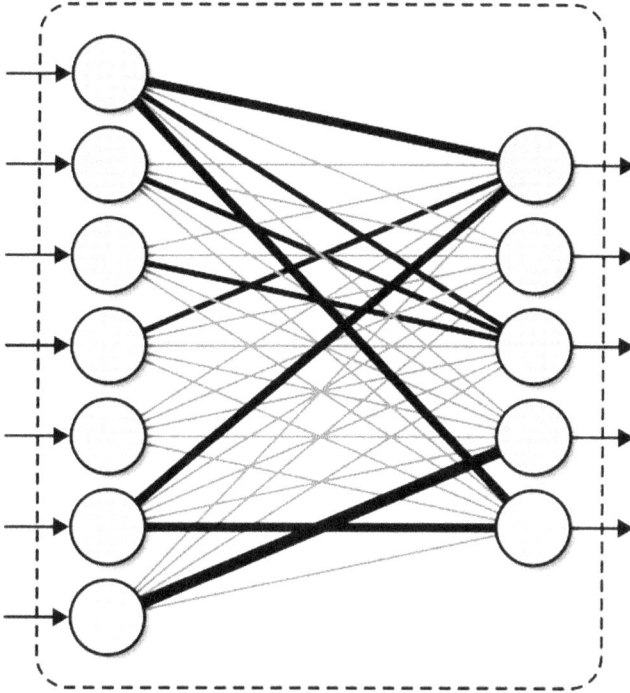

FIGURE 4.2 Fully connected layer in a deep neural network.

The mathematical form of fully connected neural network is expressed as follows. Let $p \in F_m$ depicts the input to the fully connected layer and $q_i \in F$ is the ith output from the fully connected layer.

The $q_i \in F$ is expressed as follows:

$$q_i = \sigma \left(w_1 p_1 + \cdots + w_m p_m \right) \qquad (4.2)$$

The σ is a nonlinear sigmoid function and w_1 represents the learnable parameters in the network.

The entire output q is expressed as follows:

$$q = \sigma \left(w_1, 1 p_1 + \cdots + w_1, m p_m \right) \vdots \, \sigma \left(w_n, 1 p_1 + \cdots + w_m, m p_m \right) \qquad (4.3)$$

The number of epochs used in this architecture for the segmentation is 100. The data organization in 3D CNN architecture is depicted in Figure 4.3.

The 3D volumetric data available are categorized into three groups: training set, testing set and validation test. The training data are employed to train a network; the loss values are determined and propagated. Based on the forward propagation of loss values, parameters are updated through back propagation. The validation data are used to analyze the behavior of the model during the training phase. The test data are employed once at the end to verify the efficiency of the proposed model.

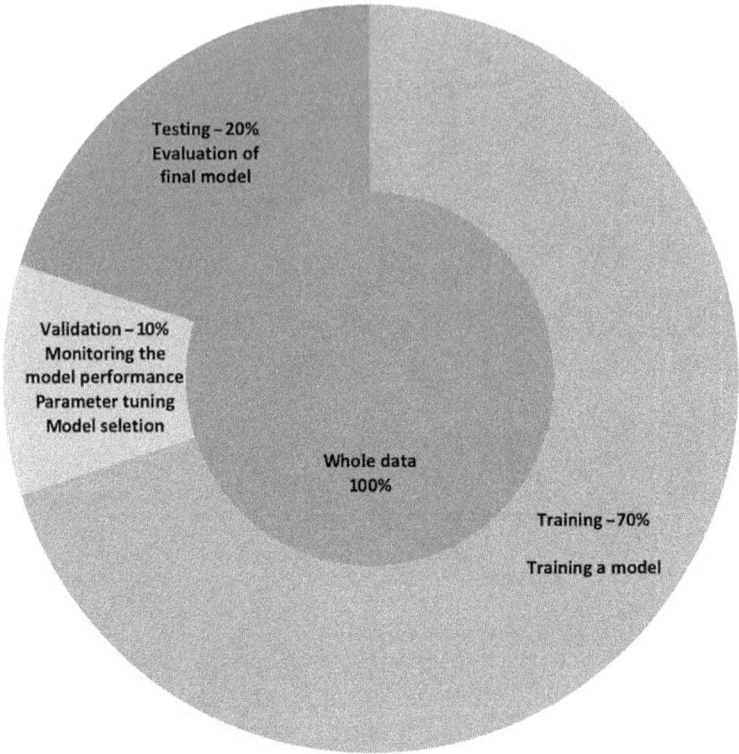

FIGURE 4.3 Data organization in 3D CNN architecture.

4.3 RESULTS AND DISCUSSION

The 3D volumetric input is taken and the GM, WM and CSF threshold values are initialized in the training stage. Prior to segmentation, normalization was done and min max normalization is employed in this work. The two phases of neural network architecture are training and testing. The training phase comprises making the fully connected CNN architecture to recognize the WM, GM and CSF. The gray value features are extracted from the images corresponding to WM, GM and CSF. The threshold values of 192,254 and 128 are set for GM, WM and CSF as prescribed by the database (www.bic.mni.mcgill.ca/brainweb). For performance validation, metrics are used. The metrics in terms of true positive, true negative, false negative and false positive are as follows. The 3D CNN architecture comprises two CL s, two pooling layers and a fully connected layer. The number of samples is arbitrary and ranges from 50, 100,150 and 200 from 3D data set. For analysis 20 3D data sets are used. For training 12 data sets are used and for testing 8 data sets are used. The 20 normal MR brain data sets and the ground truth segmentation results were provided by the center for Morphometric Analysis at Massachusetts General Hospital and are available at "http://www.cma.mgh.harvard.edu/ibsr/." In the training phase, cross-validation testing is also done. Table 4.1 depicts the training phase metrics with cross-validation testing is also done. From Table 4.1, it is evident that with increase in the number of samples, the efficiency of fully connected CNN increases.

The expressions for dice coefficient, Jaccard coefficient, false positive rate, false negative rate and true negative rate are as follows:

$$Dice = \frac{2\,|TP|}{2|TP|+|FN|+|FP|} \tag{4.4}$$

$$Jaccard = \frac{|TP|}{|TP|+|FN|+|FP|} \tag{4.5}$$

Figures 4.4 and 4.5 depict the input data sets in the testing phase. In Figures 4.4 and 4.5, the first column represents the 3D input MRI brain data, second column depicts the representative slice from each data set and third column depicts the contrast limited adaptive histogram equalization (CLAHE) output of second column.

TABLE 4.1
Performance Metrics in the Training Phase of 3D CNN

No. of Samples	Neural Network Phase	Brain Tissue	Jaccard	Dice	RFP	RFN	RTP
50	Training	WM	0.5628	0.7203	0.4175	0.2022	0.7978
		GM	0.5789	0.7333	0.2023	0.3040	0.6960
		CSF	0.7258	0.8411	0.0900	0.2089	0.7911
	Testing	WM	0.5755	0.7306	0.3627	0.2157	0.7843
		GM	0.5750	0.7302	0.2245	0.2959	0.7041
		CSF	0.7297	0.8438	0.1100	0.1900	0.8100
100	Training	WM	0.5725	0.7281	0.3573	0.2230	0.7770
		GM	0.6409	0.7811	0.1650	0.2534	0.7466
		CSF	0.7437	0.8530	0.1190	0.1679	0.8321
	Testing	WM	0.5485	0.7084	0.3267	0.2723	0.7277
		GM	0.6652	0.7989	0.1523	0.2335	0.7665
		CSF	0.7029	0.8256	0.1892	0.1642	0.8358
150	Training	WM	0.6043	0.7533	0.1972	0.2766	0.7234
		GM	0.6791	0.8089	0.2236	0.1691	0.8309
		CSF	0.8123	0.8964	0.1185	0.0915	0.9085
	Testing	WM	0.6005	0.7504	0.2066	0.2754	0.7246
		GM	0.6797	0.8093	0.2169	0.1729	0.8271
		CSF	0.7882	0.8816	0.1333	0.1067	0.8933
200	Training	WM	0.6136	0.7605	0.2150	0.2545	0.7455
		GM	0.7080	0.8290	0.1845	0.1614	0.8386
		CSF	0.8064	0.8928	0.1167	0.0995	0.9005
	Testing	WM	0.5859	0.7389	0.2642	0.2593	0.7407
		GM	0.7045	0.8266	0.1853	0.1650	0.8350
		CSF	0.7407	0.8510	0.1347	0.1596	0.8404

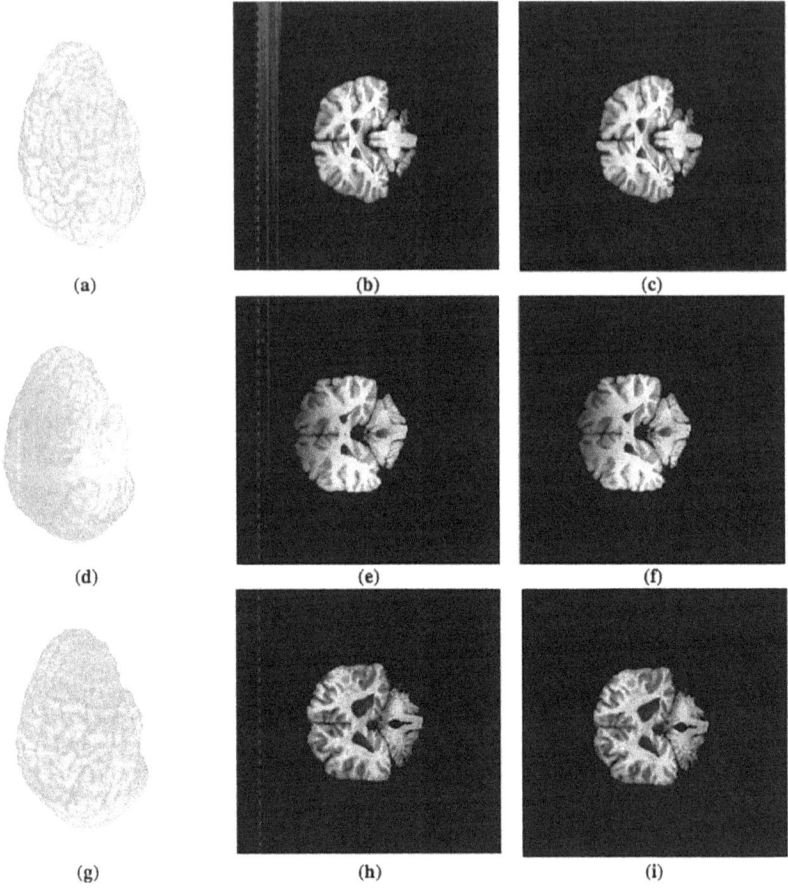

FIGURE 4.4   (a, d, g) 3D input data set (ID1-ID3); (b, e, h) representative slice from each data set; (c, f, i) CLAHE output of (b, e, h).

The ideal value of Dice coefficient and Jaccard coefficient is 1. The values of Dice coefficient and Jaccard coefficient are determined for training phase and testing phase. The FP, FN and TN rates are also determined for training and testing phase.

$$FP \text{ rate} = \frac{|FP|}{|TN| + |FP|} \tag{4.6}$$

$$FN \text{ rate} = \frac{|FN|}{|TP| + |FN|} \tag{4.7}$$

$$TN \text{ rate} = a \frac{|TN|}{|FN| + |TN|} \tag{4.8}$$

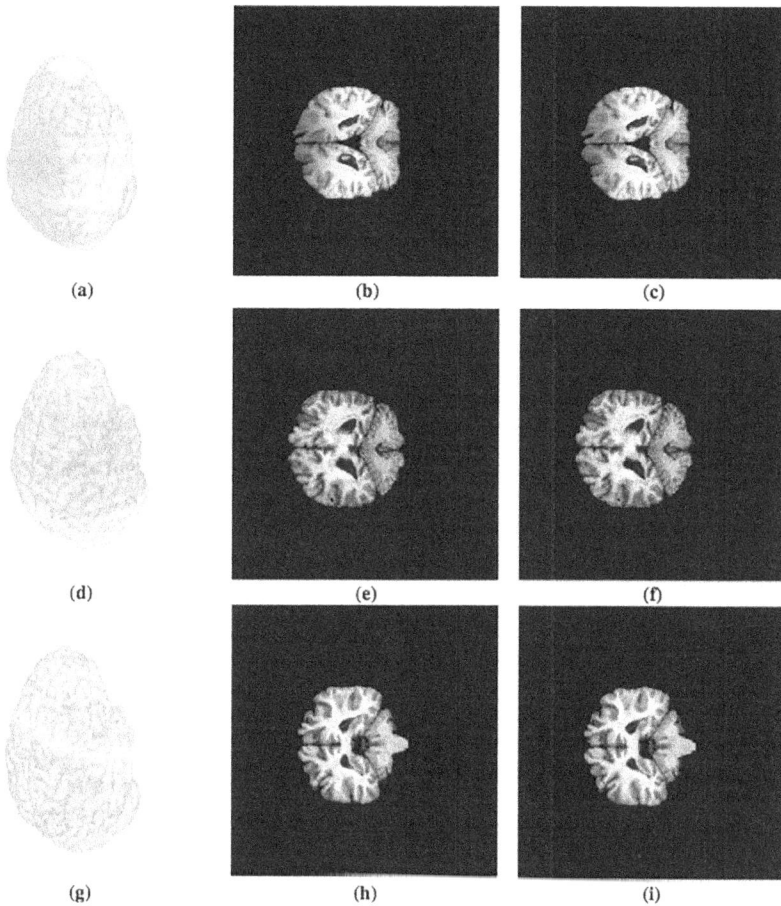

FIGURE 4.5 (a, d, g) 3D input data set (ID4-ID6); (b, e, h) representative slice from each data set; (c, f, i) CLAHE output of (b, e, h).

Figure 4.6 depicts the WM, GM and CSF region extraction corresponding to 3D brain MRI data set (ID1). Figures 4.7–4.9 depict the YZ, XZ, YX and 3D segmentation output of ID1. The WM, GM and CSF region extractions corresponding to 3D brain MRI data set (ID2-ID6) are depicted in Figure 4.10. Table 4.2 depicts the testing phase metrics of the fully connected CNN in the brain tissue segmentation.

The mean values of the performance metrics in the segmentation of brain tissues by the 3D CNN are depicted in Table 4.3. The false positive rate and false negative rate should be low and true negative rate should be high for an efficient algorithm.

4.4   INFERENCES AND FUTURE WORKS

The algorithms are executed in the 8-Core AMD Ryzen7 3800X 3.90GHz processor, 16 GB of RAM and NVIDIA GeForce RTX 3080 graphical processing unit. In the training phase, the 3D CNN architecture proposed in this chapter yields efficient

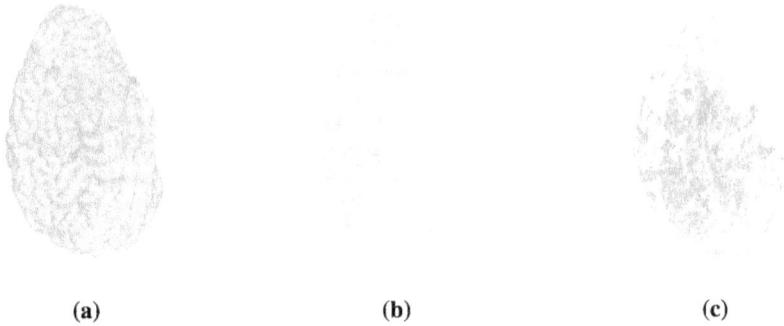

(a)   (b)   (c)

FIGURE 4.6   WM, GM and CSF region exraction corresponding to 3D brain MRI data set ID1.

results for the segmentation of the brain tissues. The cross-validation testing was also done as a part of the training phase and performance metrics values were found to be satisfactory. The final testing results reveal that the 3D CNN architecture proposed in this chapter was found to be efficient in the segmentation of WM and GM; however in the extraction of CSF, the performance was found to be little poor. The threshold values of 192,254 and 128 are set for GM, WM and CSF as prescribed by the database (www.bic.mni.mcgill.ca/brainweb) in the training phase for the extraction of brain tissue. The difference between the threshold values of GM and CSF is 64. The difference between the threshold values of WM and CSF is 126. The difference in gray value difference of GM and CSF is 64, that is, a low value and hence the segmentation of CSF is a crucial one in this work. The segmentation of brain tissues will be efficient, when the difference values $GM_{gray\ value} - CSF_{gray\ value}$ and $WM_{gray\ value} - CSF_{gray\ value}$ are high. Table 4.3 depicts the mean values of performance metrics in the segmentation of brain tissues by the 3D CNN. The results reveal that the proposed 3D CNN architecture is proficient in the extraction of WM and GM, a little difficulty in the proper extraction of CSF. The mean values of false positive and false negative rate of CSF extraction are 0.2919 and 0.2054, and are high when compared with the mean values of WM and GM. The mean value of true negative rate in the extraction of CSF is 0.7946 and is low, when compared with the mean values of WM and GM. The performance of 3D CNN architecture was improved by the utilization of residual learning and dilated convolution operations (Yamashita et al., 2018). The 19 CLs are used here and the first five CL uses 16 kernels, next four CL uses 32 kernels, next four CL uses 64 kernels, next four uses 128 kernels and the last CL uses 80 kernels and prior to that uses 64 kernels. In future work, more training data have to be incorporated and the number of CL can also be increased to improve the efficiency of architecture.

4.5   CONCLUSION

The fully connected CNN architecture is proposed in this work for the segmentation of brain tissues in MR images. Prior to segmentation, normalization is done and the 3D MR brain data sets are used. The fully connected CNN architecture generates efficient segmentation results, when compared with the classical neural

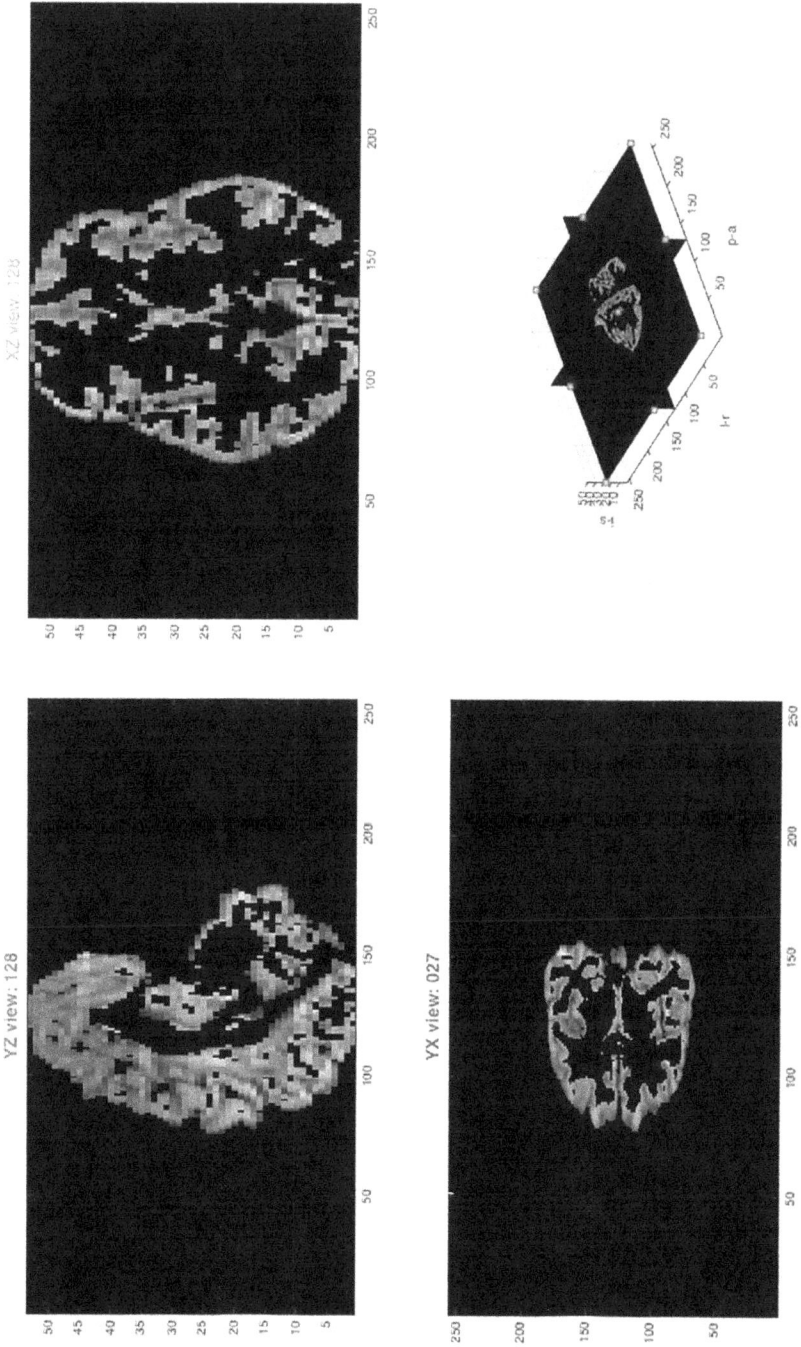

FIGURE 4.7 YZ, XZ, YX and 3D view of GM segmentation output of ID1.

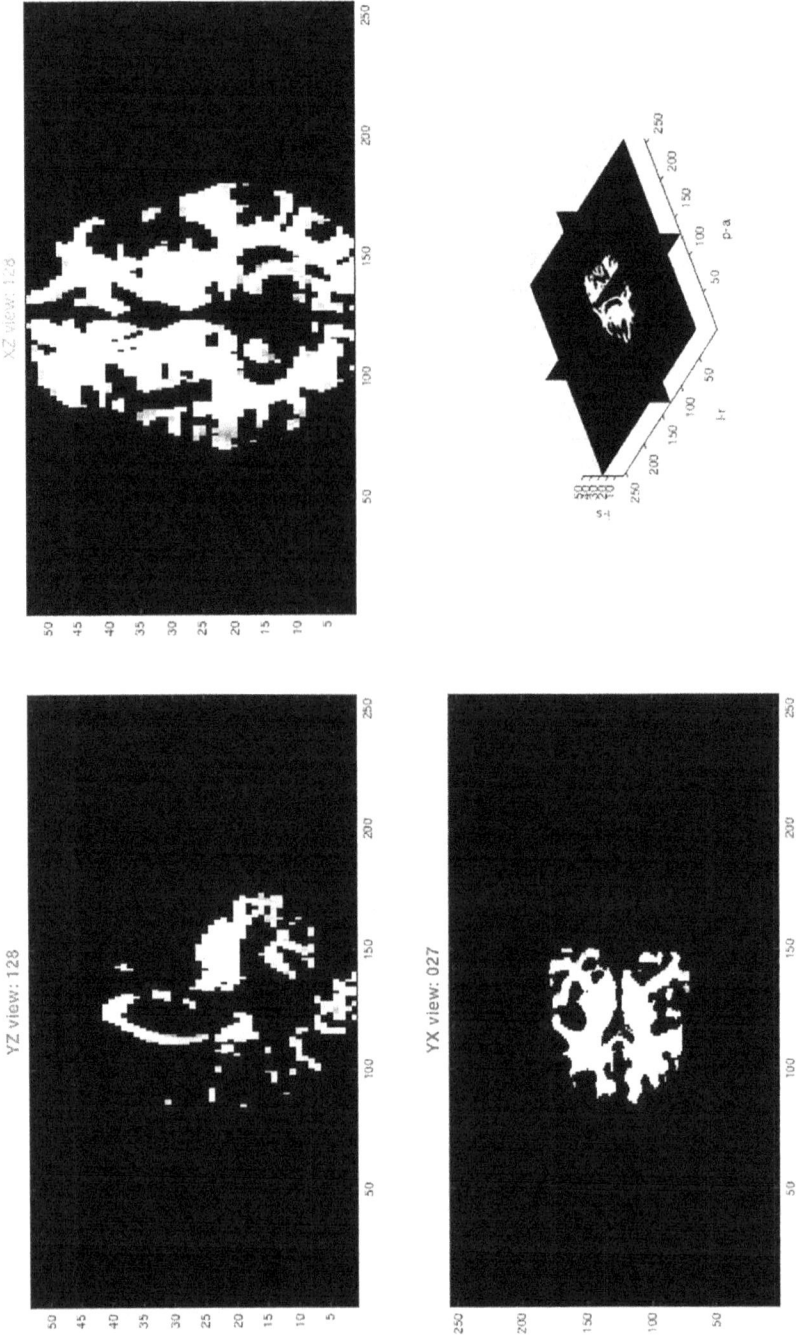

FIGURE 4.8   YZ, XZ, YX and 3D view of WM segmentation output of ID1.

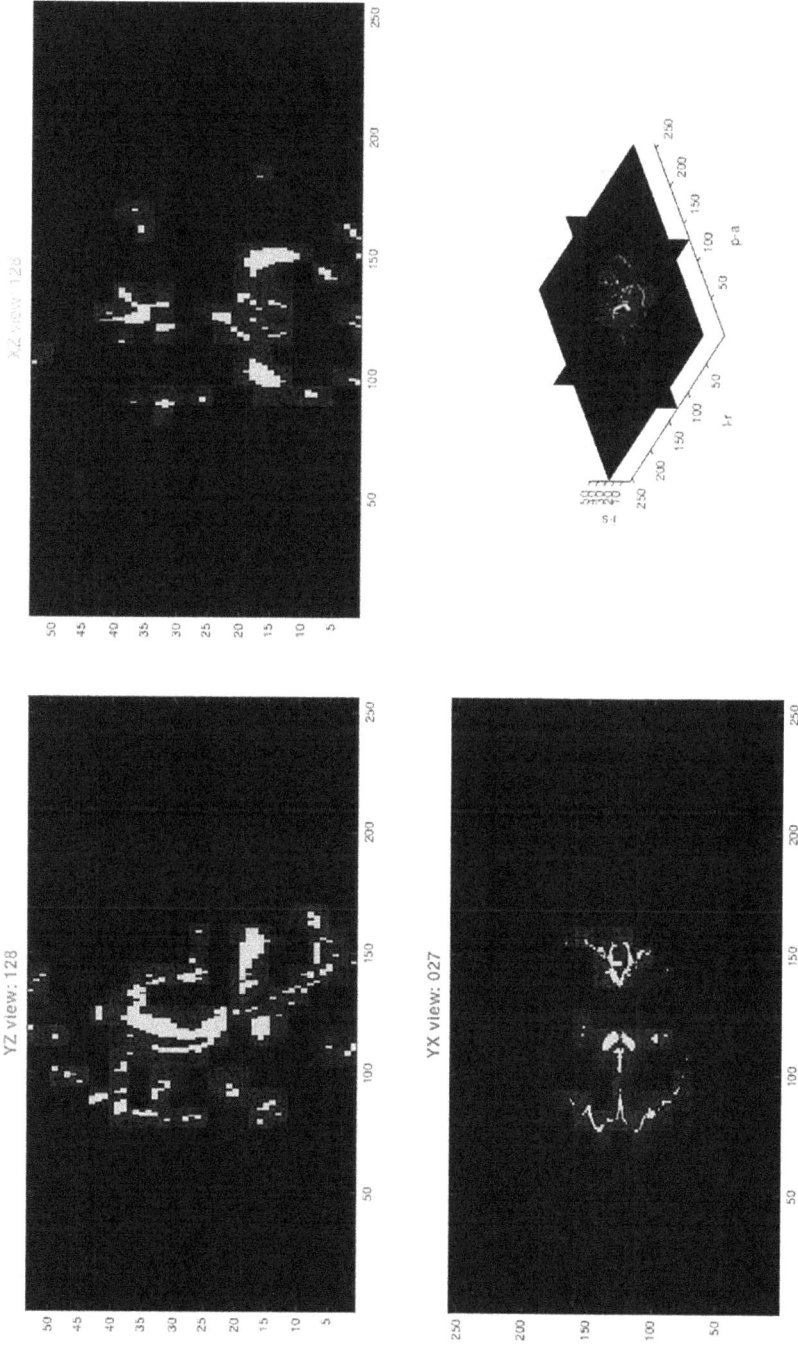

FIGURE 4.9 YZ, XZ, YX and 3D view of CSF output of ID1.

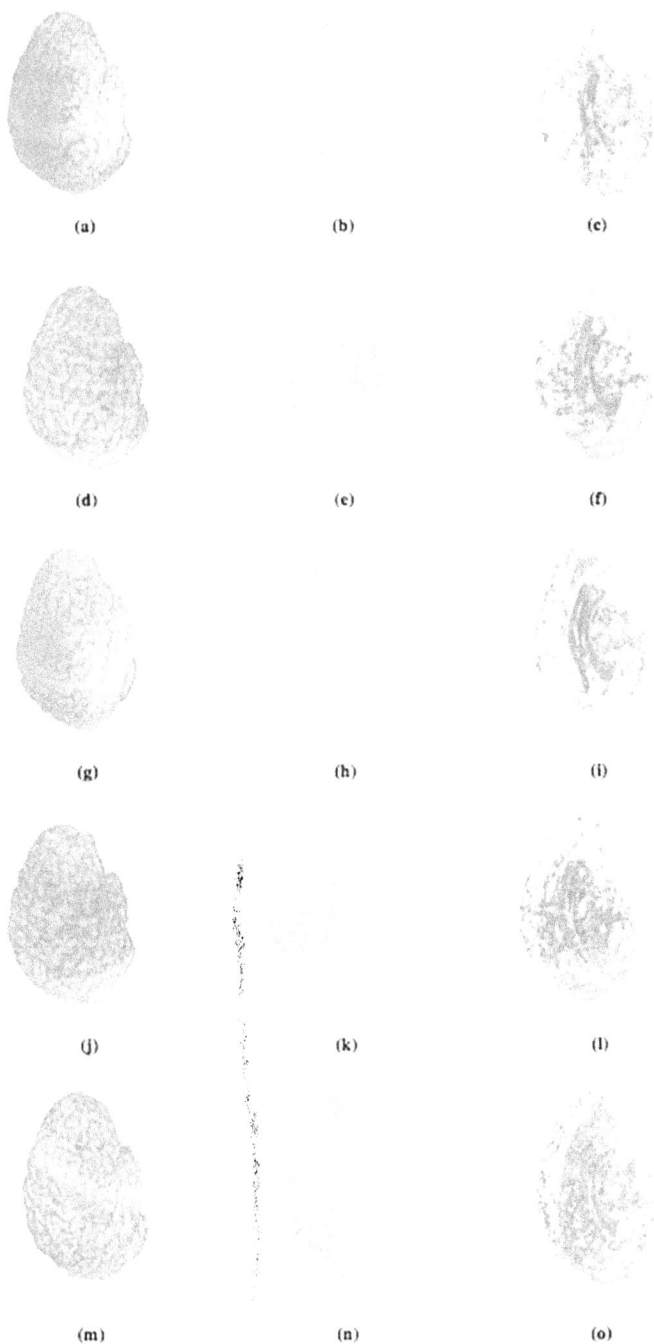

(a)   (b)   (c)

(d)   (e)   (f)

(g)   (h)   (i)

(j)   (k)   (l)

(m)   (n)   (o)

FIGURE 4.10   WM, GM and CSF region exraction corresponding to 3D brain MRI data set ID2-ID6.

TABLE 4.2

Performance Metrics in the Testing Phase of 3D CNN

3D data set	Brain Tissue	Jaccard	Dice	RFP	RFN	RTN
ID 1	GM	0.6932	0.8188	0.0561	0.2679	0.7321
ID 1	WM	0.6487	0.7869	0.3702	0.1112	0.8888
ID 1	CSF	0.2212	0.3622	2.8179	0.1557	0.8443
ID 2	GM	0.6971	0.8215	0.1751	0.1808	0.8192
ID 1	WM	0.5723	0.7280	0.2499	0.2847	0.7153
ID 1	CSF	0.2349	0.3804	1.9990	0.2955	0.7045
ID 3	GM	0.7119	0.8317	0.1719	0.1657	0.8343
ID 1	WM	0.5605	0.7184	0.2281	0.3117	0.6883
ID 1	CSF	0.3256	0.4913	1.6331	0.1427	0.8573
ID 4	GM	0.7039	0.8263	0.1646	0.1802	0.8198
ID 1	WM	0.5723	0.7280	0.2526	0.2831	0.7169
ID 1	CSF	0.4103	0.5819	1.1049	0.1363	0.8637
ID 5	GM	0.7130	0.8324	0.1567	0.1753	0.8247
ID 1	WM	0.6100	0.7578	0.2020	0.2668	0.7332
ID 1	CSF	0.3150	0.4791	1.8529	0.1013	0.8987
ID 6	GM	0.6891	0.8159	0.0559	0.2724	0.7276
	WM	0.6437	0.7832	0.3724	0.1165	0.8835
	CSF	0.2013	0.3352	3.3082	0.1327	0.8673

TABLE 4.3

Mean Values of Performance Metrics in the Segmentation of Brain Tissues by the 3D CNN

Brain Tissue	Jaccard	Dice	RFP	RFN	RTN
GM	0.6183	0.7638	0.2845	0.2041	0.7959
WM	0.6211	0.7658	0.3120	0.1832	0.8168
CSF	0.6136	0.7600	0.2919	0.2054	0.7946

network architecture. For the evaluation of segmentation results, performance metrics are used. The manual segmentation is time-consuming and requires much effort; however, the accuracy plays pivotal role in automated approaches. The segmentation accuracy was evaluated by Dice coefficient, Jaccard coefficient, FP, FN and TN rate. The results reveal that 3D CNN was employed for MR brain images and the results outperform the classical approaches.

ACKNOWLEDGMENTS

The author S.N. Kumar and Jins Sebastin would also like to acknowledge the support provided by Schmitt Centre for Biomedical Instrumentation (SCBMI) of Amal Jyothi College of Engineering.

REFERENCES

Ahn, S., Bui, T. D., Hwang, H., & Shin, J. (2019). Performance of ensemble methods with 2D pre-trained deep learning networks for 3D MRI brain segmentation. *International Journal of Information and Electronics Engineering*, *9*(2), 50–53. Doi: 10.18178/ijiee.2019.9.2.704.

Akkus, Z., Galimzianova, A., Hoogi, A., Rubin, D. L., & Erickson, B. J. (2017). Deep learning for brain MRI segmentation: State of the art and future directions. *Journal of Digital Imaging*, *30*(4), 449–459. Doi: 10.1007/s10278-017-9983-4.

Amian, M., & Soltaninejad, M. (2020). Multi-resolution 3d cnn for mri brain tumor segmentation and survival prediction. *Lecture Notes in Computer Science (Including Subseries Lecture Notes in Artificial Intelligence and Lecture Notes in Bioinformatics)*, *11992 LNCS*, 221–230. Doi: 10.1007/978-3-030-46640-4_21. Bui, T. D., Shin, J., & Moon, T. (2017). *3D Densely Convolutional Networks for Volumetric Segmentation*. http://arxiv.org/abs/1709.03199.

Chen, H., Dou, Q., Yu, L., & Heng, P.-A. (2016). *VoxResNet: Deep Voxelwise Residual Networks for Volumetric Brain Segmentation*. 1–9. http://arxiv.org/abs/1608.05895.

Cui, Z., Yang, J., & Qiao, Y. (2016). Brain MRI segmentation with patch-based CNN approach. *Chinese Control Conference, CCC*, *2016-August*(July), 7026–7031. Doi: 10.1109/ChiCC.2016.7554465.

Dolz, J., Desrosiers, C., Wang, L., Yuan, J., Shen, D., & Ben Ayed, I. (2020). Deep CNN ensembles and suggestive annotations for infant brain MRI segmentation. *Computerized Medical Imaging and Graphics*, *79*, 1–20. Doi: 10.1016/j.compmedimag.2019.101660.

El Adoui, M., Mahmoudi, S. A., Larhmam, M. A., & Benjelloun, M. (2019). MRI breast tumor segmentation using different encoder and decoder CNN architectures. *Computers*, *8*(3). Doi: 10.3390/computers8030052.

Feng, X., Tustison, N. J., Patel, S. H., & Meyer, C. H. (2020). Brain tumor segmentation using an ensemble of 3D U-nets and overall survival prediction using radiomic features. *Frontiers in Computational Neuroscience*, *14*(April), 1–12. Doi: 10.3389/fncom.2020.00025.

Hu, K., Gan, Q., Zhang, Y., Deng, S., Xiao, F., Huang, W., Cao, C., & Gao, X. (2019). Brain tumor segmentation using multi-cascaded convolutional neural networks and conditional random field. *IEEE Access*, *7*, 92615–92629. Doi: 10.1109/ACCESS.2019.2927433.

Huo, Y., Xu, Z., Xiong, Y., Aboud, K., Parvathaneni, P., Bao, S., Bermudez, C., Resnick, S. M., Cutting, L. E., & Landman, B. A. (2019). 3D whole brain segmentation using spatially localized atlas network tiles. *NeuroImage*, *194*(November 2018), 105–119. Doi: 10.1016/j.neuroimage.2019.03.041.

Jijja, A., & Rai, D. (2019). Efficient MRI segmentation and detection of brain tumor using convolutional neural network. *International Journal of Advanced Computer Science and Applications*, *10*(4), 536–541. Doi: 10.14569/ijacsa.2019.0100466.

Kao, P. Y., Shailja, F., Jiang, J., Zhang, A., Khan, A., Chen, J. W., & Manjunath, B. S. (2020). Improving patch-based convolutional neural networks for MRI brain tumor segmentation by leveraging location information. *Frontiers in Neuroscience*, *13*(January), 1–14. Doi: 10.3389/fnins.2019.01449.

Kayalibay, B., Jensen, G., & van der Smagt, P. (2017). *CNN-based Segmentation of Medical Imaging Data*. http://arxiv.org/abs/1701.03056.

Ker, J., Wang, L., Rao, J., & Lim, T. (2017). Deep learning applications in medical image analysis. *IEEE Access*, *6*, 9375–9379. Doi: 10.1109/ACCESS.2017.2788044.

Kim, M., Wu, G., & Shen, D. (2013). Unsupervised deep learning for hippocampus segmentation in 7.0 Tesla MR images. *Lecture Notes in Computer Science (Including Subseries Lecture Notes in Artificial Intelligence and Lecture Notes in Bioinformatics), 8184 LNCS*, 1–8. Doi: 10.1007/978-3-319-02267-3_1.

Mahbod, A., Chowdhury, M., Smedby, Ö., & Wang, C. (2018). Automatic brain segmentation using artificial neural networks with shape context. *Pattern Recognition Letters, 101*, 74–79. Doi: 10.1016/j.patrec.2017.11.016.

Malathi, M., & Sinthia, P. (2019). Brain tumour segmentation using convolutional neural network with tensor flow. *Asian Pacific Journal of Cancer Prevention, 20*(7), 2095–2101. Doi: 10.31557/APJCP.2019.20.7.2095.

Mehta, R., & Sivaswamy, J. (2017). M-net: A convolutional neural network for deep brain structure segmentation. *Proceedings - International Symposium on Biomedical Imaging, April*, 437–440. Doi: 10.1109/ISBI.2017.7950555.

Milletari, F., Ahmadi, S. A., Kroll, C., Plate, A., Rozanski, V., Maiostre, J., Levin, J., Dietrich, O., Ertl-Wagner, B., Bötzel, K., & Navab, N. (2017). Hough-CNN: Deep learning for segmentation of deep brain regions in MRI and ultrasound. *Computer Vision and Image Understanding, 164*, 92–102. Doi: 10.1016/j.cviu.2017.04.002.

Mlynarski, P., Delingette, H., Criminisi, A., & Ayache, N. (2019). 3D convolutional neural networks for tumor segmentation using long-range 2D context. *Computerized Medical Imaging and Graphics, 73*, 60–72. Doi: 10.1016/j.compmedimag.2019.02.001.

Moeskops, P., de Bresser, J., Kuijf, H. J., Mendrik, A. M., Biessels, G. J., Pluim, J. P. W., & Išgum, I. (2018). Evaluation of a deep learning approach for the segmentation of brain tissues and white matter hyperintensities of presumed vascular origin in MRI. *NeuroImage: Clinical, 17*(April 2017), 251–262. Doi: 10.1016/j.nicl.2017.10.007.

Moeskops, P., Viergever, M. A., Mendrik, A. M., De Vries, L. S., Benders, M. J. N. L., & Isgum, I. (2016). Automatic segmentation of MR brain images with a convolutional neural network. *IEEE Transactions on Medical Imaging, 35*(5), 1252–1261. Doi: 10.1109/TMI.2016.2548501.

Moeskops, P., Wolterink, J. M., van der Velden, B. H. M., Gilhuijs, K. G. A., Leiner, T., Viergever, M. A., & Išgum, I. (2016). Deep learning for multi-task medical image segmentation in multiple modalities. *Lecture Notes in Computer Science (Including Subseries Lecture Notes in Artificial Intelligence and Lecture Notes in Bioinformatics), 9901 LNCS*(October), 478–486. Doi: 10.1007/978-3-319-46723-8_55.

Nguyen, D. M. H., Vu, H. T., Ung, H. Q., & Nguyen, B. T. (2017). 3D-Brain segmentation using deep neural network & Gaussian mixture model. *Proceedings -2017 IEEE Winter Conference on Applications of Computer Vision, WACV 2017*, 815–824. Doi: 10.1109/WACV.2017.96.

Qamar, S., Jin, H., Zheng, R., Ahmad, P., & Usama, M. (2020). A variant form of 3D-UNet for infant brain segmentation. *Future Generation Computer Systems, 108*, 613–623. Doi: 10.1016/j.future.2019.11.021.

Ramzan, F., Khan, M. U. G., Iqbal, S., Saba, T., & Rehman, A. (2020). Volumetric segmentation of brain regions from MRI scans using 3d convolutional neural networks. *IEEE Access, 8*, 103697–103709. Doi: 10.1109/ACCESS.2020.2998901.

Wang, G., Li, W., Ourselin, S., & Vercauteren, T. (2019). Automatic brain tumor segmentation based on cascaded convolutional neural networks with uncertainty estimation. *Frontiers in Computational Neuroscience, 13*(August), 1–13. Doi: 10.3389/fncom.2019.00056.

Wang, L., Xie, C., & Zeng, N. (2019). RP-net: A 3D convolutional neural network for brain segmentation from magnetic resonance imaging. *IEEE Access, 7*, 39670–39679. Doi: 10.1109/ACCESS.2019.2906890.

Wang, Y., Wang, Y., Zhang, Z., Xiong, Y., Zhang, Q., Yuan, C., & Guo, H. (2018). Segmentation of gray matter, white matter, and CSF with fluid and white matter suppression using MP2RAGE. *Journal of Magnetic Resonance Imaging, 48*(6), 1540–1550. Doi: 10.1002/jmri.26014.

Yamashita, R., Nishio, M., Do, R. K. G., & Togashi, K. (2018). Convolutional neural networks: An overview and application in radiology. *Insights into Imaging, 9*(4), 611–629. Doi: 10.1007/s13244-018-0639-9.

Zhao, C., Carass, A., Lee, J., He, Y., & Prince, J.L. (2017). Whole brain segmentation and labeling from CT using synthetic MR images. In Q. Wang, Y., Shi, H.-Il Suk, & K. Suzuki. (Eds.), *Machine Learning in Medical Imaging. MLMI 2017* (Vol. 10541, Issue November, pp. 291–298,). Springer, Cham. Doi: 10.1007/978-3-319-67389-9_34.

Zhang, H., Li, J., Shen, M., Wang, Y., & Yang, G. Z. (2020). DDU-Nets: Distributed dense model for 3D MRI brain tumor segmentation. *Lecture Notes in Computer Science (Including Subseries Lecture Notes in Artificial Intelligence and Lecture Notes in Bioinformatics), 11993 LNCS,* 208–217. Doi: 10.1007/978-3-030-46643-5_20.

5 Performance Analysis of Deep Learning Models for Biomedical Image Segmentation

T. K. Saj Sachin, V. Sowmya, and K. P. Soman
Amrita School of Engineering

CONTENTS

5.1   INTRODUCTION

In the recent years, deep convolutional neural networks have outperformed the state-of-art-architecture in many visual recognition tasks (Ronneberger, Fischer, & Brox, 2015; Shin et al., 2016) such as object detection, classification, biomedical image segmentation, etc. (Khan, Sohail, Zahoora, & Qureshi, 2020). In the present scenarios, automatic as well as an accurate segmentation of lesions is very much essential as the rates of cancer are increasing all over the world. Through automatic lesion segmentation, we can study/detect the progress of a particular disease, diagnose, monitor, and assess clinical trials for new treatments (Lameski, Jovanov, Zdravevski, Lameski, & Gievska, 2019; Yuan, Chao, & Lo, 2017). One of the most common as well dangerous skin cancers is melanoma, which is the rapidly increasing cancer all over the world. Although we have advanced treatments such as immunotherapy and radiation therapy, etc., still the survival rate of the advanced stage of this cancer for 5 years is still less than 15%, whereas if this is detected during the earlier stages the 5-year survival rate is over 95% (Wu et al., 2019). This big difference in survival rate in earlier detection gives the importance of detecting these types of diseases (Wu et al., 2019). Similarly, brain cancer is also increasing in all over the world, which is also termed as one of the most dangerous cancer in the world. Since manual annotation by the doctor for these two cancer types is highly time-consuming and prone to have human error because of tumor being in different shape, size, contrast, and many other factors. Thus, we require an automatic and accurate image segmentation technique to accomplish this task, which can be used for both clinical as well as research purpose (Xue, Xu, Zhang, Long, & Huang, 2018). These factors motivated us to use deep learning technique, since it is successful in giving best results in most of the areas (Saj et al., 2019; Saj, Mohan, Kumar, & Soman, 2019; Zhou, 2020).

The authors have used deep learning architectures for skin lesion image segmentation such as TernausNet and DeepLabV3+ with International Skin Imaging Collaboration (ISIC) 2018 skin lesion data set and achieved a maximum Jaccard index of 87.6% by DeepabV3+ (Lameski et al., 2019). In Ronneberger et al. (2015), the authors proposed the architecture named as U-Net for biomedical image segmentation. The architecture was exclusively designed for biomedical community. Because of this, the architecture was able to give better performance with very less number of biomedical images; as the availability of the medical images is less in the current scenario, the architecture learns with the power of data augmentations with lesser number of images given for training. The architecture was able to outperform all the architectures available at that time for the task of biomedical image segmentation. Whereas in Wu et al. (2019), the authors have used C-UNet architecture with ISIC 2018 skin lesion data set; C-UNet architecture incorporates the inception like convolutional block, the recurrent convolutional block, and dilated convolutional layers. The authors have trained different types of models to study the contribution of each components of C-UNet such as (a) C-UNet (Inception + Recurrent convolutional layers), (b) C-UNet (Dilated), (c) C-UNet (Conditional Random Fields), and C-UNet (Dice fine-tune). Among this C-UNet with Dice fine tune gave the best results of 77.5% and 86.9% for Jaccard and Dice score, respectively. The C-UNet architecture was able to outperform U-Net architecture in the biomedical segmentation with ISIC 2018 data set. The authors have used deep convolutional neural network (DCNN) model based on U-Net for skin lesion segmentation. When compared with normal U-Net architecture they have used batch normalization layer, which helped in solving the overfitting problem, and dilated convolution layer for increasing the receptive field during the training, this helped in significantly improving their accuracy. The authors have done segmentation with ISIC 2017 skin lesion data set and were able to achieve comparable performance with the existing approaches (Liu, Mou, Zhu, & Mandal, 2019). For brain tumor image segmentation, the authors have used cGAN, which belongs to the GAN family. The data set, which the authors used, was BraTs-2017 challenge data set. In this, the authors have considered three subsections within tumor region named as whole, core, and enhancing tumor in both malignant and nonmalignant tumor cases. The whole tumor is the actual size of the tumor inside the brain; if we remove the fluid part inside the tumor, the resulting tumor is called as core tumor and finally enhancing/active tumor is achieved by removing the nonactive region of tumor from the core tumor. The authors were able to get state-of-the-art accuracy with cGAN (Rezaei et al., 2017). In Xue, Xu, Zhang et al. (2018), the authors proposed segmentor adversarial network (SegAN), where they introduced multiscale loss function which showed a superior performance than single-scale loss function or the conventional pixel-wise softmax loss. The data sets the authors used were BraTs 2013 and 2015 brain tumor data sets. In these data sets, there were three subsections within a tumor named as: (a) whole tumor, (b) core tumor, and (c) enhancing tumor and were able to achieve very good performance in terms of Dice score and outperformed U-Net architecture. In Buda, Saha, and Mazurowski (2019), they proposed a fully automatic brain tumor segmentation by finding relationship between tumor imaging characteristics with tumor genomic subtypes, the data set they used was preprocessed BraTs 2015, where only nonmalignant tumor is considered and only one subsection of tumor is used named as whole tumor and they were able to achieve a mean Dice score of 82%. The authors proposed a deep convolutional network for the task of semantic segmentation. The motivation behind the design of this architecture was to efficiently segment road and indoor scene, and the architecture is also efficient in terms of memory and computational time. This architecture was able to outperform many architectures and author's future work will be to extend the applicability of this architecture in other domains too (Badrinarayanan, Kendall, & Cipolla, 2017). SegNet was used for biomedical image segmentation in Tang, Li, and Xu, (2018). The task was to segment gland structures from colon cancer histology images (colon cancer occurs at the inner lining of large intestine). The data set used was gland segmentation challenge 2015, which consists of both malignant as well nonmalignant patients and the architecture was able to achieve a maximum dice score of 86.3%. Thus it has been proved that the architecture can also be used for biomedical image segmentation. The difference between the SegNet and U-Net (which was proposed for the biomedical community) is that U-Net does not reuse the pooling indices, instead it transfers entire feature maps from the encoder to the corresponding decoder at the cost of memory and concatenates them to up-sampled decoder feature maps, whereas, in SegNet, only pooling indices are transferred from the encoder to the decoder network (Badrinarayanan et al., 2017).

Therefore, in this chapter, we propose to do biomedical image segmentation of skin lesion/tumor as well brain tumor with two data sets named as BraTs 2017/preprocessed BraTs 2015 (Buda et al., 2019) and ISIC 2018. Initially, performance analysis of SegAN, which belongs to generative adversarial network family, is done using these two data sets: (a) BraTs 2017 and (b) ISIC 2018. From Rezaei et al. (2017), it is clear that GAN has received increased attention all over the world for various computer vision tasks such as object detection, video prediction, and biomedical image segmentation (Creswell et al., 2018; Antoniou, Storkey, & Edwards, 2017), so thus motivated us to explore SegAN on this two data sets as there is minimal literature available for SegAN architecture. In addition, along with that two other general deep convolution neural network such as U-Net, SegNet will be also be used for increasing the segmentation accuracy. Both of these architecture were never been applied before for these data sets (ISIC 2018) and preprocessed BraTs 2015 (Buda et al., 2019) according to the literature survey, whereas these architectures U-Net and SegNet were able to give a better performance in the image segmentation task. The rest of the chapter is as follows: (a) methodology, (b) data set description, (c) results discussion, (d) comparison with existing approaches, and (e) conclusion.

5.2 METHODOLOGY

Figure 5.1 shows the flow chart of the chapter. In this chapter, since we use three state-of-the-art architectures named as SegAN, U-Net, and SegNet. Two different types of cancer were considered for image segmentation task: (a) skin cancer (ISIC 2018) and (b) brain tumor (BraTs 2017/preprocessed BraTs 2015); the reason for considering two data sets for brain tumor image segmentation is that architecture with preprocessed BraTs 2015 was able to give much better segmentation accuracy than BraTs 2017. Thus it has motivated us to continue the segmentation task with preprocessed BraTs 2015 data set.

The evaluation parameters considered were Dice score and Jaccard index, which is commonly used evaluation metrics for the image segmentation task that shows the similarity between the segmentation mask produced by the architecture with that of ground truth label. A detailed explanation for each is shown in the following sections.

5.3 DATA SET DESCRIPTION

5.3.1 BraTs 2017 Brain Tumor

In this data set, it consists of both malignant and nonmalignant tumors respectively: (a) high-grade glioma (HGG) and (b) low-grade glioma (LGG). 243 patients were considered in which 135 patients were having HGG and 108 were having LGG. For each patient, four MRI modalities/scans are taken: (a) T1-weighted, (b) T2-weighted,

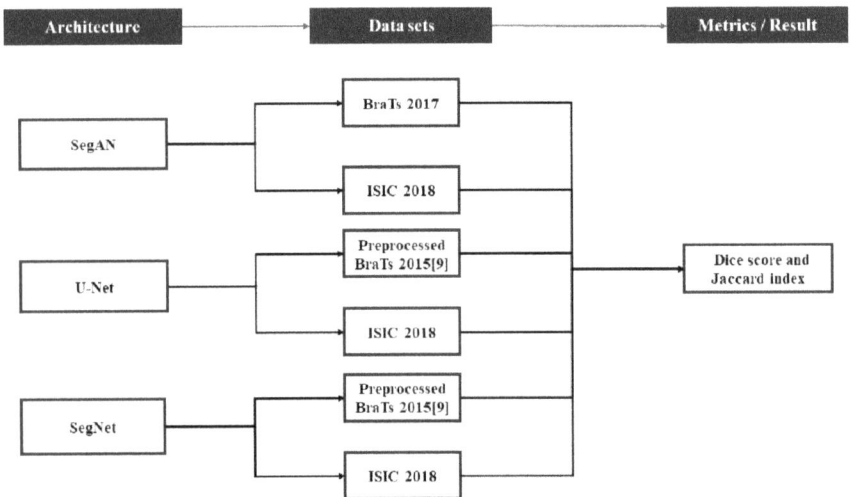

FIGURE 5.1 Flow chart of the chapter.

(c) T1-Gd, and (d) T2-FLAIR (fluid attenuated inversion recovery). Along with two segmentation labels were also available: (a) manually corrected segmentation label and (b) computer-aided segmentation label (Bakas et al., 2017b, c).

The most common MRI sequences (scans) are as follows: (a) T1-weighted and T2-weighted. T1-weighted scan is produced by using short TE and TR (this are settings in the hardware), where TE is defined as the time-to-echo and is the time between the delivery of the radio frequency pulse and the receipt of the echo signal and TR is defined as the repetition time and is the amount of time between successive pulse sequence applied to the same slice. T2-weighted scans are produced using longer TE and TR. T2-FLAIR is similar to T2-weighted imaging except that TE and TR are very long. T1-weighted can also be performed by infusing contrast enhancement agent named as gadolinium. Gad-enhanced images are especially used in detecting tumors (Menze et al., 2014; Bakas et al., 2017a). T2-weighted MRI scan is used to find the core region of the tumor. T2-FLAIR MRI scan is used to find the whole region of tumor. T1-Gd MRI scan is used to find the active region of the tumor. Finally, T1-weighted scan shows the native image of the brain. There are three ground truth labels available in this data set: (a) whole tumor, (b) core tumor, and (c) enhanced tumor. The tumor information can be found out through different scans of MRI. Finally, different MRI scans are used to provide different types of biological information of the brain tissues.

5.3.2 Preprocessed BraTs 2015 Brain Tumor

In this data set, 120 patients were having low-grade glioma cases, which have FLAIR sequence available, out of which only 10 patients were excluded since they did not have genomic cluster information. Therefore, the data set resulted in 110 patients, in which 101 patients consisted of all MRI modalities such as precontrast, postcontrast, and FLAIR sequence. The remaining nine patients were not having either precontrast or postcontrast sequence, so they used FLAIR sequence itself in places where they wanted either precontrast or postcontrast sequence. Finally, each patient has at least 20–88 slice information (images). The data set has undergone different preprocessing before it was available online (Buda et al., 2019). The sample images from the data set are shown in Figure 5.2.

- Scaling of all the images (slice) within every subject to common frame of reference.
- Removal of skull, making to focus on only the brain region (skull stripping process).

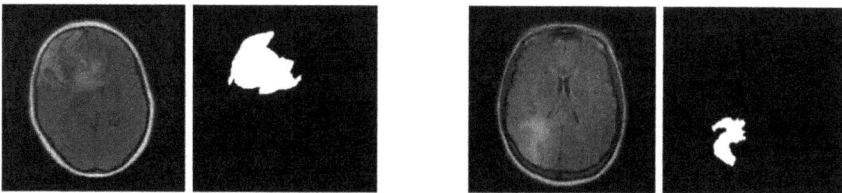

FIGURE 5.2 Sample images from the data set (Buda et al., 2019).

- Adaptive window and level adjustment on the image histogram to normalize intensities.
- Z-score normalization.

5.3.3 ISIC 2018 Skin Tumor

In this data set, there are about 2,594 dermoscopic images and corresponding segmentation masks. Dermoscopy is the process of examination of the skin using skin surface microscopy. This process is mainly used for evaluating the pigmented skin lesions. Among this training data, we divided the data set into training and testing with different data split ratios. There are three different types of skin lesions in this data set, namely, (a) nevus, (b) seborrhoeic keratosis, and (c) melanoma; among this melanoma is the most dangerous as it is malignant tumor and other two are nonmalignant/benign tumor (Tschandl, Rosendahl, & Kittler, 2018; Codella et al., 2019). The sample images from the data set are shown in Figure 5.3.

5.4 ARCHITECTURE

5.4.1 Segmentor Adversarial Network

Generative adversarial network has recently gained lot of attentions in the areas of computer vision. In GANs, there are two parts: (a) generator network and (b) discriminator network (Arjovsky & Bottou, 2017; Wang et al., 2017). The generator network tries to generate fake samples after seeing the distribution of data fed into it such as image, audio, etc., and tries to fool the other part of the architecture, discriminator. This network discriminator tries to distinguish between this fake sample generated by the generator from the original sample in a way that both run in a competition during the training phase (Xue, Xu, & Huang, 2018; Goodfellow, 2016). The architecture is shown in Figure 5.4.

SegAN belongs to this GAN family, which is exclusively used as per now for image segmentation task. Similar to GAN, SegAN also have two parts: (a) segmentor, which act as a generator in this architecture; (b) critic, which act as a discriminator in this architecture. The segmentor consists of encoder-decoder network, which helps in creating the segmentation label corresponding to the input image given. Here, the role of critic is to differentiate between the two different types of inputs given into the network: (a) the original image masked with ground truth label and (b)

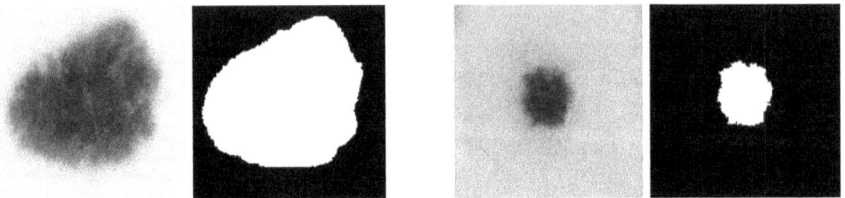

FIGURE 5.3   Sample images from the data set (ISIC 2018) (Tschandl et al., 2018; Codella et al., 2019).

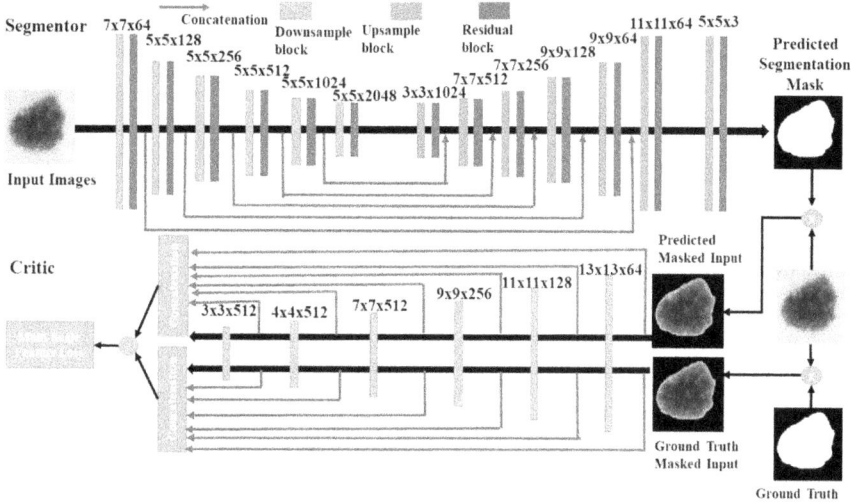

FIGURE 5.4 SegAN (Xue, Xu, & Huang, 2018).

the original image masked with predicted label generated by the segmentor. During the training phase, here the critic tries to maximize the loss function (multiscale loss function) and segmentor tries to minimize this loss function. At the end, both the network will learn to do their task perfectly and the segmentor will be able to predict segmentation label very similar to ground truth label corresponding to the input image given to the architecture (Xue, Xu, Zhang et al., 2018).

Segmentor is encoder-decoder network, where down-sampling of images takes place to extract the features from the input image. In decoder, up-sampling is done where larger receptive field is created using large convolution kernel and incorporates more spatial information for constructing segmentation label from the features extracted from the encoder. Skip connection is used for the concatenation between the encoder and decoder to connect different levels of features. Residual block is also added after each down-sampling and up-sampling block. Last layer of segmentor is adaptive logistic function instead of softmax or sigmoid function (Xue, Xu, Zhang et al., 2018).

Critic network structure is similar to segmentor decoder network with reverse in direction and no residual blocks. Hierarchical features from multiple layers of critic network are extracted from both the images and their values are concatenated to compute multiscale loss function. The formula is give below in Equation (5.1)

$$\min_{\theta_S} \max_{\theta_C} = \frac{1}{N} \sum l_{mae} \left(f_c \left(x_n \circ S(x_n) \right), f_c(x_n \circ y_n) \right) \qquad (5.1)$$

5.4.2 SegNet Architecture

SegNet is an encoder-decoder network, where encoder captures the context of the input image and the decoder is used to enable precise localization. The encoder consists of 13 convolutional layers, which corresponds to pretrained VGG16 network,

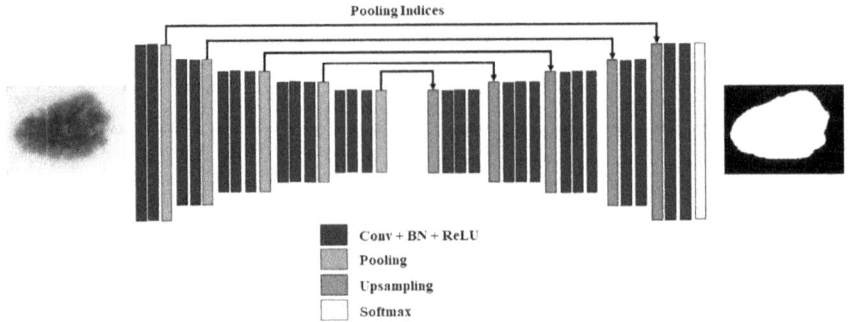

FIGURE 5.5   SegNet architecture (Badrinarayanan et al., 2017).

excluding the last fully connected layer for maintaining the higher resolution feature maps at the encoder output. This also reduced the number of learnable parameters to a very large extent. Each encoder in encoder network consists of convolutional layer with filter bank producing feature maps followed by batch normalization and ReLU activation function because of the loss of spatial information which can result in poor segmentation result. Storing of max-pooling indices, i.e., the location of maximum feature value in the pooling window, is memorized for each encoder feature map. For each encoder layer there are corresponding decoder layers, i.e., 13 layers of convolution layer followed by a softmax classifier. In decoder, up-sampling of input feature map takes places with the help of memorized max-pooling indices from the corresponding encoder feature maps followed by convolution to produce dense feature maps; batch normalization is applied followed by ReLU. The high-dimensional feature map at the end of decoder network is fed to softmax classifier. This softmax classifier classifies each pixel independently. The output of the softmax classifier is K channel image of probabilities where K is the number of classes (Badrinarayanan et al., 2017; Badrinarayanan, Handa, & Cipolla, 2015; Khagi & Kwon, 2018). The architecture is shown in Figure 5.5.

5.4.3 U-Net Architecture

The U-Net architecture consists of two parts: (a) contracting path (encoder) and (b) expansive path (decoder). In U-Net, each blue box represents the multichannel feature map, gray arrow denotes the concatenation of features from encoder to decoder, and finally, white box denotes the copied features from the contracting path. Contracting path (encoder) helps in capturing the context (focusing on the relationship of the nearby pixels) information of the input image and it consists of two 3×3 convolutional layers, each followed with ReLU activation function. For down-sampling 2×2 max-pooling operation is done. Expansive path (decoder) helps in enabling precise localization. It consists of up-sampling of the feature map using transposed convolution, concatenation of features is done at each step of expansive path to the corresponding contracting path, and two 3×3 convolutional layers each followed by ReLU activation function. Since in the up-sampling part we have large number of feature maps, they help the network in propagating context information to higher resolution

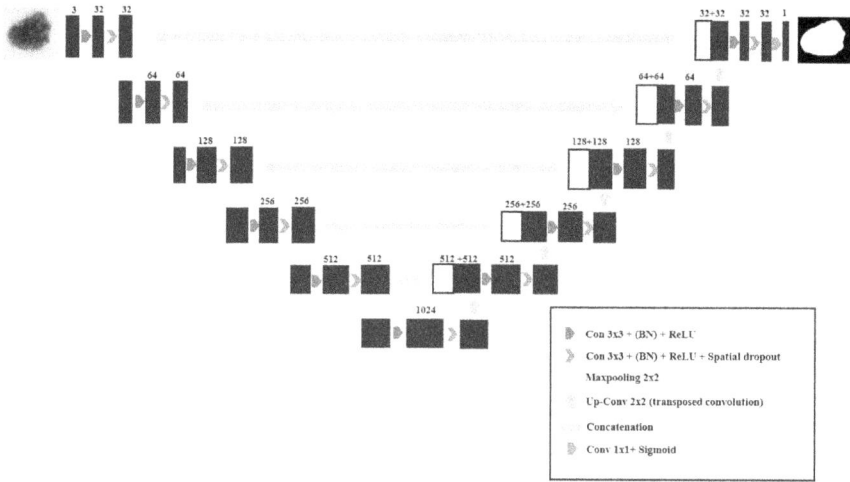

FIGURE 5.6 U-Net architecture (Ronneberger et al., 2015).

layers. Therefore, the expansive path is more or less symmetric to the contracting path (encoder); as a result u-shaped architecture is formed. At the last layer, 1×1 convolution is used to map the feature vector to the desired number of classes. In this architecture, there are about 23 convolution layers (Ronneberger et al., 2015; Liu, Cao, Wang, & Wang, 2019). The architecture is shown in Figure 5.6.

5.5 EVALUATION PARAMETERS

The most commonly used evaluation parameters for image segmentation task are (a) Dice score and (b) Jaccard index. Both the parameters are used in finding the similarity between the image samples: (a) predicted image by the architecture and (b) ground truth image. The formula for Dice score is shown in Equation (5.2)

$$\text{Dice} = \frac{2|P \cap T|}{|P| + |T|} = \frac{2|PT|}{|P|^2 + |T|^2} \qquad (5.2)$$

Dice score is defined as twice the area of overlap of the images (predicted and target image) divided by the total number of pixels in both the images. Since we are having binary output consisting of 0 and 1, the formula can also be written in another way, where area of overlap can be written as element-wise multiplication between the predicted and target image and sum of the total pixels divided by sum of the square of pixels in both the images.

$$\text{Jaccard} = \frac{P \cap T}{P \cup T} = \frac{P \cap T}{|P| + |T| - |P \cap T|} = \frac{|PT|}{|P|^2 + |T|^2 + |P \cdot T|} \qquad (5.3)$$

Jaccard index shown in Equation (5.3) is defined as the area of overlap divided by area of the union. This can also be written in another form as shown in Equation (5.2) and the calculation is similar to Dice score calculation. The relationship between the Jaccard index and Dice is show in Equation (5.4). Both Jaccard index and Dice score range from values 0 to 1, where 0 means the worst similarity between the samples and 1 indicated the prefect similarity between the samples.

$$\text{Jaccard} = \frac{\text{Dice}}{2 - \text{Dice}} \qquad (5.4)$$

5.6   RESULTS AND DISCUSSION

Initially we used BraTs 2017 data set for brain tumor image segmentation. It consists of both LGG and HGG cases; in each patient there are four MRI scans, which is of dimension $240 \times 240 \times 155$. According to Xue, Xu, Zhang et al. (2018) we considered only three scans (T2-weighted, T2-FLAIR, and T1-Gd) among four scans and took five slices among 155 slices in each scan of each subject. All these three scan slices were concatenated to form an image of size $160 \times 160 \times 3$ after central cropping process is done to reduce the dimension of the image. This process can generate five images per patient and there are about 243 patients in total in this data set. Thus, creating 1,215 images, among this approximately 215 images contain no tumor information and thus it is removed to increase the segmentation accuracy.

Since we are using S1-1C SegAN architecture, which means one segmentor and one critic, through this we can predict only one label at a time and the segmentation label available from the data set consists of all three tumor information together (whole tumor, core tumor, enhancing tumor). So all three-label information are extracted and created as separate image for each of them with dimension $160 \times 160 \times 1$. Apart from this, various other data augmentation techniques are also used such as (a) random vertical and horizontal flip, (b) scaling of images, and (c) color jitter including randomly changing brightness, contrast, saturation, and hue values.

Table 5.1 shows the result of SegAN architecture with BraTs 2017 data set. The architecture ran separately for whole, core, and enhancing tumor with total images of 4,000. Data split was in the ratio of 90:10, ran for a maximum epochs of 2,500. The evaluation parameters used for segmentation accuracy by the architecture are Dice score and Jaccard index.

TABLE 5.1
SegAN Results with BraTs 2017 Brain Tumor Data Set

Number of Images	Data Split	Epochs	Whole Dice	Jaccard	Core Dice	Jaccard	Active Dice	Jaccard
		250	16.20	13.20	16.78	13.58	8.25	4.36
4,000	90:10	500	20.94	15.99	20.96	15.92	10.50	5.00
		1,000	24.5	18.30	23.56	17.46	11.52	6.25
		2,000	26.29	19.46	25.12	18.62	13.0	7.5
		2,500	26.29	19.46	25.12	18.62	13.5	7.5

Ground Truth Label   Predicted Label

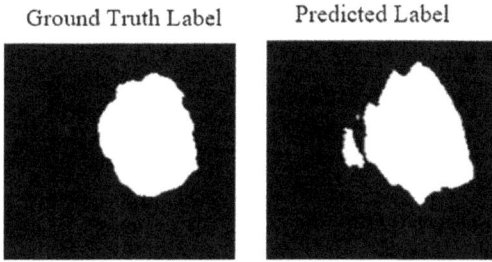

FIGURE 5.7   SegAN segmentation output for brain tumor (best output).

From Figure 5.7, it is clear that the segmentation output (predicted) is not similar to the ground truth label because of less Jaccard index and Dice score value that the model has achieved. We can see that the architecture was predicting noncancerous region also as cancerous one. Since with BraTs 2017 segmentation accuracy achieved was comparatively low. Therefore, we have proposed to continue our experiments with new data set, preprocessed BraTs 2015 data set (Buda et al., 2019). The next architecture chosen for biomedical segmentation was U-Net, because this architecture has a good record in dealing with biomedical images. Table 5.2 shows the results achieved with U-Net architecture with preprocessed BraTs 2015 data.

This data set consists of total 886 images, excluding all the images, which had blank information (images with no tumor information). The image is resized to 160×160, to remove all the blank border information, and to reduce the computational complexity. The architecture was run with three different data split ratio such as: (a) 70:30, (b) 80:20, and (c) 90:10. For all this data-split, the model was trained for 250 epochs and evaluated based on Jaccard index and Dice score. It was found that data spilt ratio of 80:20 achieved maximum segmentation accuracy. Now, for improving the accuracy data augmentation techniques such as (a) horizontal flip, (b) vertical flip, and (c) random rotation are used and increased the number of images to 3,544 images. The model has now trained with 80:20 data-spilt and has achieved a maximum accuracy of 74.23% and 85.01% for Jaccard index and Dice score, respectively, trained for 1,000 epochs. The segmentation outputs are shown in Figure 5.8.

From Figure 5.8 it is clear that compared to BraTs 2017 data set, preprocessed BraTs 2015 data set performed better for brain tumor image segmentation task. For

TABLE 5.2
U-Net Results with Preprocessed BraTs 2015 Brain Tumor Data Set

Data and No. of Images	Data Split	Epochs	Jaccard Index	Dice Score
Without data augmentation 886	70:30	250	70.02	83.81
	80:20	250	70.03	83.80
	90:10	250	67.75	83.80
With data augmentation 3,544	80:20	250	71.26	83.84
		500	73.57	84.84
		1,000	74.23	85.01

Ground Truth Label   Predicted Label   Ground Truth Label   Predicted Label

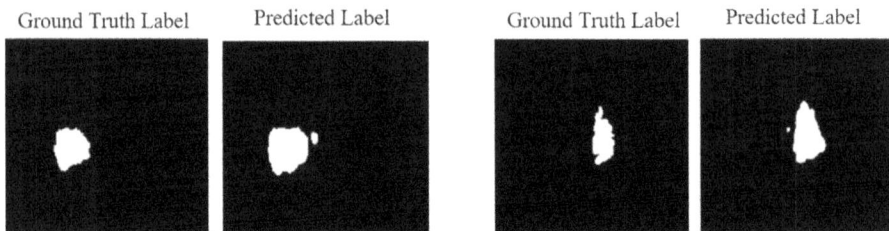

FIGURE 5.8   U-Net segmentation output for brain tumor.

next experiment, SegNet architecture is used for biomedical image segmentation with preprocessed BraTs 2015 data set. SegNet has recently gained popularity for the task of image segmentation and thus motivated us to use this architecture for this task. The results are shown in Table 5.3.

For this experiment also, both cases were considered with and without data augmentation. In without data augmentation, for a data split of 80:20 performed better than 70:30 and 90:10. With data augmentation and 80:20 split, the model was trained for maximum 1,000 epochs and achieved 71.23% and 84.06% for Jaccard index and Dice score, respectively. The segmentation outputs are shown in Figure 5.9. When compared with previous architectures such as SegAN and U-Net, SegNet output is smooth-edged.

For the second data set, skin lesion image segmentation, SegAN architecture is used first, with a data-split ratio of 90:10. The ISIC 2018 data set consists of 2,594 images and corresponding segmentation label along with it. The image is resized to

TABLE 5.3
SegNet Results with Preprocessed BraTs 2015 Brain Tumor Data Set

Data and No. of Images	Data Split	Epochs	Jaccard Index	Dice Score
Without data augmentation 886	70:30	250	66.7	81.01
	80:20	250	70.09	82.0
	90:10	250	67.74	80.01
With data augmentation 3,544	80:20	250	69.77	83.96
		500	71.01	83.96
		1,000	71.23	84.06

Ground Truth Label   Predicted Label   Ground Truth Label   Predicted Label

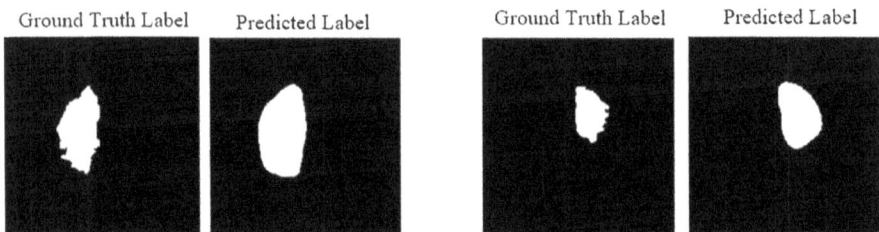

FIGURE 5.9   SegNet segmentation output for brain tumor.

TABLE 5.4

SegAN Results with ISIC 2018 Skin Lesion Data Set

Number of Images	Data Split	Epochs	Jaccard Index	Dice Score
10,376	90:10	250	56.57	67.62
		500	56.89	68.04
		1,000	56.89	68.04
		2,000	58.46	69.45
		2,500	58.46	69.45

a size of 160×160, to remove all blank border information for reducing the computational complexity. The results are shown in Table 5.4. From Table 5.4, it is understood that SegAN was able to achieve comparable segmentation performance with a maximum Jaccard and Dice of 58.46% and 69.45%, respectively, after training for 2,500 epochs. The SegAN showed much better performance with ISIC 2018 data set than Brats 2017 data set. The reason because of loss of quality in brats 2017 images after preprocessing. This was another reason for us to go ahead with a preprocessed data directly such as preprocessed Brats 2015 (Buda et al., 2019). The segmentation output is shown in Figure 5.10. For improving the segmentation accuracy for skin lesion, U-Net and SegNet architectures are also used in this case.

It is clear from Table 5.5 that the U-Net architecture was able to achieve very good performance in terms of Jaccard index and Dice score, respectively, with 10,376

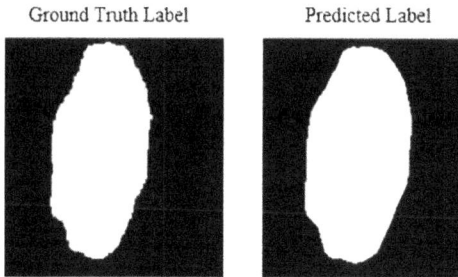

FIGURE 5.10   SegAN segmentation output for skin lesion (best output).

TABLE 5.5

U-Net Results with ISIC 2018 Skin Lesion Data Set

Data and No. of Images	Data Split	Epochs	Jaccard Index	Dice Score
Without data augmentation 2,594	70:30	250	74.34	86.12
	80:20	250	75.01	86.35
	90:10	250	72.67	86.23
With data augmentation 10,376	80:20	250	74.32	86.43
		500	75.67	86.54
		1,000	75.96	87.56

Ground Truth Label   Predicted Label   Ground Truth Label   Predicted Label

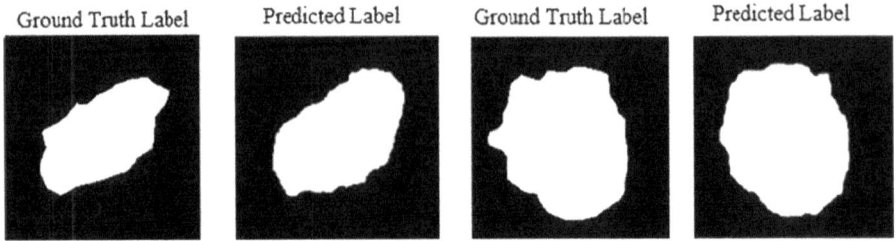

FIGURE 5.11   U-Net segmentation output for skin lesion.

TABLE 5.6
SegNet Results with ISIC 2018 Skin Lesion Data Set

Data and No. of Images	Data Split	Epochs	Jaccard Index	Dice Score
Without data augmentation2,594	70:30	250	70.30	84.67
	80:20	250	71.01	83.21
	90:10	250	66.24	81.32
With data augmentation 10,376	80:20	250	72.56	84.88
		500	72.94	85.88
		1000	73.01	85.98

Ground Truth Label   Predicted Label   Ground Truth Label   Predicted Label

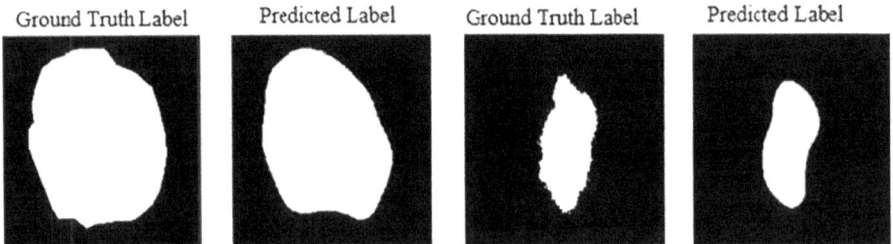

FIGURE 5.12   SegNet segmentation output for skin lesion.

images after data augmentation, data-split of 80:20, ran for 1,000 epochs. The segmentation outputs are shown in Figure 5.11.

Table 5.6 shows that SegNet was also able to achieve comparable results in terms of Jaccard index and Dice score with ISIC 2018. The segmentation outputs are shown in Figure 5.12. From Figure 5.12, it can be noticed that the segmentation output for SegNet is smooth-edged, when compared with other two architectures: (a) SegAN and (b) U-Net.

5.6.1 COMPARISON WITH EXISTING APPROACHES

In this section, we compared SegNet and U-Net with preprocessed BraTs 2015 data set with existing benchmark paper. Table 5.7 shows the comparison.

TABLE 5.7

Comparison of Our Work with Existing Approaches for Brain Tumor Image Segmentation

Architecture (with Preprocessed BraTs 2015)	Jaccard Index	Dice Score
U-Net (Ronneberger et al., 2015)	-	82
SegNet	71.23	84.06
U-Net	74.23	85.01

TABLE 5.8

Comparison of Our Work with Existing Approaches for Skin Lesion Image Segmentation

Architecture (with ISIC 2018)	Jaccard Index	Dice Score
TernausNet (Lameski et al., 2019)	82.1	-
DeepLabV3+ (Lameski et al, 2019)	87.6	-
C-UNet (Wu et al., 2019)	77.5	86.5
SegAN	56.8	68.04
SegNet	73.01	85.98
U-Net	75.96	87.56

This data set as per now is used only by this author (Buda et al., 2019); in this paper for image segmentation U-Net architecture is used and achieved a mean dice score of 82%. Whereas both SegNet and U-Net architectures were able to outperform the benchmark accuracy. The U-Net that we have used had additional two more convolutional layers at encoder and decoder, which helped in improving the segmentation accuracy. Table 5.8 shows the comparison of skin lesion (ISIC 2018) segmentation with our proposed work with existing approaches in the literature.

According to the literature survey, three architectures were used for ISIC 2018 skin lesion segmentation. Our work was able to achieve comparable performance with the existing approaches. In terms of Jaccard index, our method showed comparatively lower performance when compared with existing approaches, in that U-Net outperformed both SegNet and SegAN. In terms of Dice score, U-Net was able to outperform the existing benchmark accuracy achieved by C-UNet (Wu et al., 2019). Table 5.9 shows the number of learnable parameter and the time to train the model for one epoch for each proposed architecture that we have used.

Table 5.9 shows that SegAN model consists of higher number of learnable parameter, since it consists of two networks: (a) segmentor and (b) critic, followed by SegNet and finally U-Net in the number of learnable parameters. Since SegAN consists of approximately 222 billion learnable parameter, it takes approx. 1,200 secs to complete one epochs, and the computational complexity of this architecture is very high. All these models were trained in Kaggle platform, where it has NVIDIA Tesla P100 GPU and consists of 16 GB GPU memory and 12 GB RAM memory. Now, the comparison of segmentation outputs by the three architectures is shown in Figure 5.13.

TABLE 5.9

Comparison of Learnable Parameters among the Proposed Architecture

Architecture	No. of Learnable Parameters	Computation Time (per Epochs)
SegAN (Xue, Xu, Zhang et al., 2018)	222,328,178,100 (222 billion) (approx.)	1,200 s (approx.)
SegNet (Badrinarayanan et al., 2017)	33,393,669 (33 million)	41 s
U-Net (Ronneberger et al., 2015)	31,454,721 (31 million)	30 s

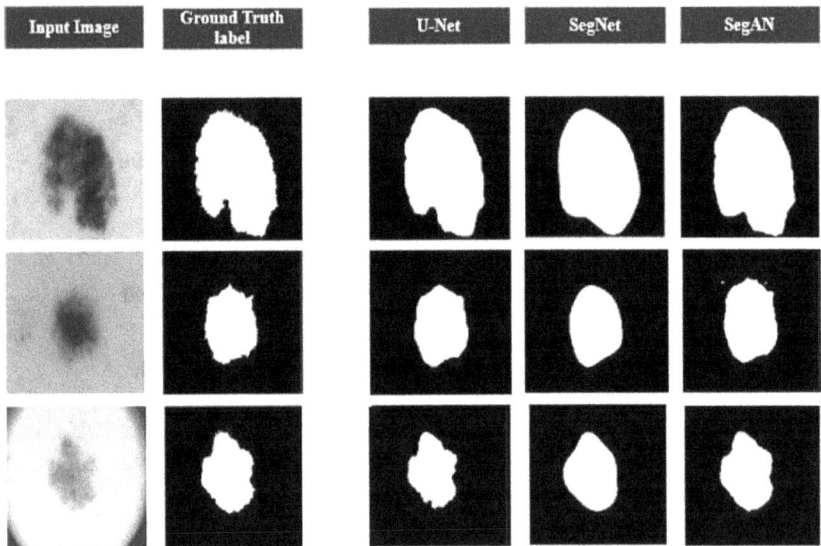

FIGURE 5.13   Comparison of the segmentation output (U-Net, SegNet, and SegAN).

Figure 5.13 shows the comparison of segmentation output by three architectures with ISIC 2018 skin lesion data set. From Figure 5.13, it is understood that U-Net was able to give the best segmentation output when compared with SegNet and SegAN segmentation outputs. When compared, SegNet output is too smooth-edged output when compared with the rest of the proposed method. SegAN segmentation output was able to reach par with U-Net segmentation output.

5.7   DISCUSSION

Although we have achieved comparable results, it can be further improved by utilizing many more preprocessing techniques and using architectures such as DeepLabV3+, MobileNetV2, NasNet because these architectures were able to give good performances in segmentation. Finally, after achieving 90%–95% segmentation accuracy, the model can be deployed and can be used by doctors for detecting tumors, which will avoid human error factor and accurately determine tumor well before and can start the diagnosis as soon as possible.

5.8 CONCLUSION

In this chapter, for automatic biomedical image segmentation, two different types of cancers were used: (a) brain tumor and (b) skin tumor. We proposed to do this task with three different architectures: (a) SegAN, (b) SegNet, and (c) U-Net. In addition, it was understood that U-Net gave the best performance when compared with rest of the proposed architecture, with lesser number of learnable parameters, whereas the SegAN learnable parameters were high. When compared with respect to the segmentation output, U-Net showed the best result, SegAN was able to reach par with U-Net and SegNet segmentation output was smooth-edged. The proposed architecture was compared with the existing approaches and our proposed work was able to achieve comparable performance with skin lesion, and showed better performance than the existing approaches with brain tumor data set. In future, segmentation accuracy can be increased by doing more preprocessing techniques such as haarcascade, in order to improve the performance of the standard architectures such as U-Net, DeepLabV3+, MobileNetV2, NasNet, etc.

REFERENCES

Antoniou, A., Storkey, A., & Edwards, H. (2017). Data augmentation generative adversarial networks. *arXiv Preprint arXiv:1711.04340.*

Arjovsky, M., & Bottou, L. (2017). Towards principled methods for training generative adversarial networks. *arXiv Preprint arXiv:1701.04862.*

Badrinarayanan, V., Handa, A., & Cipolla, R. (2015). Segnet: A deep convolutional encoder-decoder architecture for robust semantic pixel-wise labelling. *arXiv preprint arXiv: 1505.07293.*

Badrinarayanan, V., Kendall, A., & Cipolla, R. (2017). Segnet: A deep convolutional encoder-decoder architecture for image segmentation. *IEEE Transactions on Pattern Analysis and Machine Intelligence, 39*(12), 2481–2495.

Bakas, S., Akbari, H., Sotiras, A., Bilello, M., Rozycki, M., Kirby, J. S., ... Davatzikos, C. (2017a). Advancing the cancer genome atlas glioma mri collections with expert segmentation labels and radiomic features. *Scientific Data, 4*, 170117.

Bakas, S., Akbari, H., Sotiras, A., Bilello, M., Rozycki, M., Kirby, J., ... Davatzikos, C. (2017b). Segmentation labels and radiomic features for the pre-operative scans of the TCGA-GBM collection. *The Cancer Imaging Archive 2017, 286.*

Bakas, S., Akbari, H., Sotiras, A., Bilello, M., Rozycki, M., Kirby, J., ... Davatzikos, C. (2017c). Segmentation labels and radiomic features for the pre-operative scans of the tcga-lgg collection. *The Cancer Imaging Archive, 286.*

Buda, M., Saha, A., & Mazurowski, M. A. (2019). Association of genomic subtypes of lower-grade gliomas with shape features automatically extracted by a deep learning algorithm. *Computers in Biology and Medicine, 109*, 218–225.

Codella, N., Rotemberg, V., Tschandl, P., Celebi, M. E., Dusza, S., Gutman, D., ... Kittler, H. (2019). Skin lesion analysis toward melanoma detection 2018: A challenge hosted by the international skin imaging collaboration (ISIC). *arXiv Preprint arXiv:1902.03368.*

Creswell, A., White, T., Dumoulin, V., Arulkumaran, K., Sengupta, B., & Bharath, A. A. (2018). Generative adversarial networks: An overview. *IEEE Signal Processing Magazine, 35*(1), 53–65.

Goodfellow, I. (2016). Nips 2016 tutorial: Generative adversarial networks. *arXiv Preprint arXiv:1701.00160.*

Khagi, B., & Kwon, G.-R. (2018). Pixel-label-based segmentation of cross-sectional brain mri using simplified segnet architecture-based cnn. *Journal of Healthcare Engineering,* 2018.

Khan, A., Sohail, A., Zahoora, U., & Qureshi, A. S. (2020). A survey of the recent architectures of deep convolutional neural networks. *Artificial Intelligence Review,* 1–62.

Lameski, J., Jovanov, A., Zdravevski, E., Lameski, P., & Gievska, S. (2019). Skin lesion segmentation with deep learning. In *IEEE EUROCON 2019-18th International Conference on Smart Technologies,* (pp. 1–5), Novi Sad.

Liu, L., Mou, L., Zhu, X. X., & Mandal, M. (2019). Skin lesion segmentation based on improved u-net. In *2019 IEEE Canadian Conference of Electrical and Computer Engineering (CCECE),* (pp. 1–4), Edmonton.

Liu, Z., Cao, Y., Wang, Y., & Wang, W. (2019). Computer vision-based concrete crack detection using u-net fully convolutional networks. *Automation in Construction, 104,* 129–139.

Menze, B. H., Jakab, A., Bauer, S., Kalpathy-Cramer, J., Farahani, K., Kirby, J., … Lanczi, L. (2014). The multimodal brain tumor image segmentation benchmark (brats). *IEEE Transactions on Medical Imaging, 34*(10), 1993–2024.

Rezaei, M., Harmuth, K., Gierke, W., Kellermeier, T., Fischer, M., Yang, H., & Meinel, C. (2017). A conditional adversarial network for semantic segmentation of brain tumor. In *International MICCAI Brainlesion Workshop,* (pp. 241–252).

Ronneberger, O., Fischer, P., & Brox, T. (2015). U-net: Convolutional networks for biomedical image segmentation. In *International Conference on Medical Image Computing and Computer-Assisted Intervention,* (pp. 234–241), Springer, Munich.

Saj, T. S., Babu, S., Reddy, V. K., Gopika, P., Sowmya, V., & Soman, K. (2019). Facial emotion recognition using shallow CNN. In *Symposium on Machine Learning and Metaheuristics Algorithms, and Applications,* (pp. 144–150), Springer, Kerala, India.

Saj, T. S., Mohan, N., Kumar, S. S., & Soman, K. (2019). Significance of incorporating cheb-function coefficients for improved machine fault diagnosis. *In IOP Conference Series: Materials Science and Engineering, 561,* p. 012090, IOP Press, Tamil Nadu.

Shin, H.-C., Roth, H. R., Gao, M., Lu, L., Xu, Z., Nogues, I., … Summers, R. M. (2016). Deep convolutional neural networks for computer-aided detection: Cnn architectures, dataset characteristics and transfer learning. *IEEE Transactions on Medical Imaging, 35*(5), 1285–1298.

Tang, J., Li, J., & Xu, X. (2018). Segnet-based gland segmentation from colon cancer histology images. In *2018 33rd Youth Academic Annual Conference of Chinese Association of Automation (YAC),* (pp. 1078–1082), Nanjing.

Tschandl, P., Rosendahl, C., & Kittler, H. (2018). The ham10000 dataset, a large collection of multi-source dermatoscopic images of common pigmented skin lesions. *Scientific data, 5,* 180161.

Wang, K., Gou, C., Duan, Y., Lin, Y., Zheng, X., & Wang, F.-Y. (2017). Generative adversarial networks: Introduction and outlook. *IEEE/CAA Journal of Automatica Sinica, 4*(4), 588–598.

Wu, J., Chen, E. Z., Rong, R., Li, X., Xu, D., & Jiang, H. (2019). Skin lesion segmentation with c-unet. In *2019 41st Annual International Conference of the IEEE Engineering in Medicine and Biology Society (EMBC),* (pp. 2785–2788), Berlin.

Xue, Y., Xu, T., & Huang, X. (2018). Adversarial learning with multi-scale loss for skin lesion segmentation. In *2018 IEEE 15th International Symposium on Biomedical Imaging (ISBI 2018),* (pp. 859–863), Washington DC.

Xue, Y., Xu, T., Zhang, H., Long, L. R., & Huang, X. (2018). Segan: Adversarial network with multi-scale l 1 loss for medical image segmentation. *Neuroinformatics, 16*(3-4), 383–392.

Yuan, Y., Chao, M., & Lo, Y.-C. (2017). Automatic skin lesion segmentation using deep fully convolutional networks with jaccard distance. *IEEE Transactions on Medical Imaging, 36*(9), 1876–1886.

Zhou, D.-X. (2020). Universality of deep convolutional neural networks. *Applied and Computational Harmonic Analysis, 48*(2), 787–794.

6 Deep Learning for Ophthalmological Images

Safiye Pelin Taş, Sezin Barin, and Gür Emre Güraksin
Afyon Kocatepe University

CONTENTS

6.1 INTRODUCTION

The retina is a layer of the eye and contains light-sensitive cells, color-sensitive cells, and nerve fibers for vision. It is directly connected to the brain and transfers perceived visual signals to the brain for interpretation, thereby assisting the completion of a vision action (Kermany et al., 2018). For this reason, disorders that occur in the retina can lead to loss of vision loss and the ensuing diseases can cause blindness. Thus, the early diagnosis and treatment of retinal disorders are very important to prevent or minimize such negative outcomes.

There are many eye diseases caused by retinal disorders. The examples of important retinal diseases include age-related macular degeneration (AMD), diabetic retinopathy (DR), diabetic macular edema (DME), and myopic choroidal neovascularization (CNV). Among these diseases, AMD is a retinal disease that occurs as a result of damage to the macular layer, which is located at the center of the retina and provides visual clarity and acuity. This disease, which frequently occurs in people aged 50 and above, may cause vision loss (Mishra et al., 2019). Macular degeneration is divided into two categories: dry and wet AMD. Dry AMD is the most common type. Here, the aging and thinning of the macular tissues arise as a result of accumulating protein clusters (commonly known as Drusen) or damaged due to both reasons. Wet AMD is a more advanced form of dry AMD, where new abnormal blood vessels form and grow under the retina. These vessels leak blood or fluid which leads to the formation of scars in the macular (Wang et al., 2019). DR, another type of retinal disease, causes damage to the blood vessels in the retina due to diabetes or high blood pressure. The blood vessels grow and leak and the prevention of blood flow may cause edema. In the advanced stage, the formation of new blood vessels in the retina leads to sudden intraocular bleeding. These symptoms become visible in both eyes. Additionally, DR can introduce different ailments to the human eye (Ishtiaq et al., 2019). For example, DME is a retinal disease caused by DR. The leakage present in blood vessels due to DR causes fluid accumulation, edema and result in DME disease (Varma et al., 2014). Finally, myopic CNV is a medical condition that occurs when the blood vessels located behind the eyes fail to grow properly (Wang et al., 2020). As a result of the leak, symptoms such as impaired vision and blurred image may occur.

As mentioned above, there are many eye diseases caused by retinal disorders and early diagnosis is very important for the treatment process. However, the analysis of ophthalmological images is inevitably time-consuming, costly and prone to human error. The emergence of imaging techniques allows the scanning and detection of retinal diseases based on the knowledge and experience of a specialist. But unnoticed symptoms can lead to misdiagnosis by a specialist. Additionally, the symptoms observed by a specialist can be confused with the symptoms of another retinal disease. For example, the symptoms of DR are very similar to the symptoms of vascular rupture or myopic CNV. Thus, during the examination of the retinal images of a patient with a DR disease, a specialist is likely to make a wrong diagnosis which would cause the patient to undergo an incorrect treatment. Based on these narratives, artificial intelligence-based studies had become necessary to minimize the disadvantages mentioned and support physicians in the clinical setting. In this context, it is observed that there has been an increase in deep learning-based studies in the literature, especially in recent years.

This manuscript presents a thorough literature review of the above-mentioned retinal diseases detection using OCT images and CNN-based algorithms between 2019 and 2020. First, detailed information about fundus fluorescein angiography (FFA) and optical coherence tomography (OCT) techniques, which are retinal imaging techniques, is given in Section 6.2 and these two methods are compared. In Section 6.3, neural network architectures of deep learning methods used in determining retinal diseases in literature studies are mentioned. In Section 6.4, studies that conducted deep learning studies with OCT images in determining retinal diseases are mentioned and the statistical results obtained are presented in a table. Finally, in Section 6.5, the importance of the analysis of retinal-borne diseases is mentioned and the importance of study is briefly explained.

6.2 RETINAL IMAGING TECHNIQUES

6.2.1 FUNDUS FLUORESCEIN ANGIOGRAPHY

Recently, FFA and OCT imaging techniques are being used to aid diagnosis of these retinal diseases. Fundus fluorescent angiography is based on the principle of monitoring the movement of a substance in the vessels located in the retina by introducing a dye called fluorescein through the blood vessels present in the hand or arm. Fluorescein dye is administered intravenously and expected to spread throughout the body. After the paint reaches the retina, a fundus camera with special excitation and barrier filters are used to capture images of the retina. To obtain the images for analysis from a camera, there needs to be excitation of the administered fluorescein dye present in the retina. To resolve this, the white light emitted with the camera flash system is passed through a blue filter (Khochtali et al., 2016). The blue light is absorbed by fluorescein dye resulting in the emission of rays with yellow-green wavelength. In this way, the excitation process is completed. Afterward, both the yellow-green fluorescein rays and blue rays from fluorescein-free eye tissues return to the system. At this stage, a yellow-green barrier filter prevents blue light from passing and ensures the imaging of only the fluorescein dye. The image consists of black and white pixels. The parts with the dye are white whereas the other parts are black (Khochtali et al., 2016). This image is examined by a specialist according to the movement of fluorescein in the retinal vessels and a diagnosis is made.

6.2.2 OPTICAL COHERENCE TOMOGRAPHY

OCT, on the other hand, is a non-invasive technique of obtaining high-resolution images by sending infrared rays to the eye (Rawat & Gaikwad, n.d.). Taking the tomographic sections allows the 3D viewing of all layers of the eye. A specialist examines the size, thickness, shape, etc., of these images to make a diagnosis. Thus, retinal diseases can be detected by examining them according to their characteristics (Zhang et al., 2020). The operational logic of an OCT system includes the scanning of the eye with infrared light, the acquisition of the reflected light with the help of a special system, the interpretation of the acquired information with mathematical expressions and the creation of an image. Rays from a low-intensity light source are sent to both the eye and the reference system with the aid of a beam splitter (Akram & Nasim, n.d.). The rays reflected back from the eye and the rays reflected back from the reference system are compared, interpreted and converted into images. The use of OCT-A scanning system allows the acquisition of deep OCT images. In other words, the desired area is scanned by the above-mentioned system. Transverse images are created by the side by side placement of the obtained OCT-A images (Rawat & Gaikwad, n.d.).

6.2.3 COMPARISON OF FUNDUS AND OCT

These two imaging techniques (FFA and OCT) are the most frequently used methods in the diagnosis of retinal diseases. However, these two systems have both positive and negative aspects. FFA is an older, traditional and more reliable system while OCT is a newly developed imaging technique with features that replace FFA. These two technologies are compared using criteria such as image acquisition methods, image characteristics and the success rate of disease diagnosis.

FFA is a slow and invasive method whereas OCT is a faster non-invasive system. In OCT, there is a balance between resolution and field of view, and the image quality decreases as the field of view increases. On the other hand, the FFA method can superficially display the entire macular region without compromising the image quality. The posterior segment of the FFA method produces two-dimensional images showing details of the vascular and superficial retinal capillary plexus. However, this method depicts poor images of the radial peripapillary network, the deep retinal capillary plexus and the choroid vascular system (Spaide et al., n.d.). In contrast, OCT provides 3D detailed and cross-sectional images of flow in the superficial retinal capillary plexus in addition to the medium and deep retinal capillary plexuses, radial peripapillary network and choriocapillaris (Talisa et al., n.d.). Thus, OCT can evaluate a larger capillary structure than FFA, and it provides an anatomically exact location and deep information about all layers of the eye (Moraes et al., n.d.). Since the FFA is based on monitoring the movement of fluorescein dye within the vessels in the retina of a patient, this method provides a detailed view of the blood circulation in the retina and is evaluated according to criteria such as infiltration, obstruction, and accumulation. However, OCT provides a snapshot of the blood flow and gives information about the anatomical structure of the eye (Chhablanı & Sudhalkar, n.d.). Both techniques can be used to diagnose diseases like AMD, DME, DR, and CNV. However, these two technologies have different advantages and disadvantages in the diagnosis of retinal diseases due to their image characteristics.

6.3 DEEP LEARNING

The deep learning concept, which has made received numerous attentions in recent years, is a sub-branch of machine learning. Today, there are continuous developments from the incorporation of deep learning with several applications in almost every field, including military, industry, economy, biomedical, voice recognition, video processing, image analysis, language processing, etc. (Arel et al., n.d.). Deep learning consists of multiple layers and works with large data sets (Boulemtafes et al., n.d.). These layers allow the derivation of representative features for a data set during the training of a model and permit continuous self-improvement of a model during the training stage (Şeker et al., 2017). The layers are also very similar to the neural network structure of the human brain, where the artificial neurons are interconnected. Just like in the human nervous system with a multi-stage processing capability to separate and abstract input data, there is continuous training of a model to learn the characteristics of the input data and make new inferences (Arel et al., n.d.). The extracted features for each layer serve as an input for the consecutive layer, where the transfer of these features is done through artificial neurons (Deng & Yu, 2013). In brief, deep learning architecture consists of an input, an output, and fully connected multi-layered neural networks, and it is a sub-branch of several machine learning field with several complex series of algorithms. Deep learning models have their own architectural structures. Examples of these structures are Convolutional Neural Networks (CNN), Recurrent Neural Networks, Long Short-Term Memory Networks, Restricted Boltzmann Machines, Deep Belief Networks and Deep Autoencoders (Şeker et al., 2017). Among the neural networks, CNN has achieved remarkable success in image and audio processing applications, such that there are several studies in the literature that report CNN applications in the biomedical field.

6.3.1 CONVOLUTIONAL NEURAL NETWORK AND TRANSFER LEARNING ARCHITECTURES

CNNs are one of the most powerful types of deep neural networks. While CNN architectures were initially less preferable due to hardware deficiencies, the advent of graphical processing units with much more powerful computing capabilities than central processing units has led to a wide patronage and popularity in the literature (Grewal et al., 2018). The CNN architectures comprise neurons arranged in three dimensions (width, height and depth) and the presence of several layers. The neurons in each CNN layer are arranged in a layout suitable for 3D data analysis, and there is a conversion of a three-dimensional input into a three-dimensional output. Figure 6.1 shows a convolutional neural layer in which a three-dimensional input is converted into a 3D output (*CS231n Convolutional Neural Networks for Visual Recognition*, n.d.).

The main difference between CNN and the traditional architectures lies in the presentation of extracted features to traditional neural networks for analysis whereas raw data serve as input to CNN architectures. Structurally, CNN differs from other artificial neural networks in terms of its deep and different internal layers. The most important reason why CNN architectures are called deep is that it contains many interconnected hidden layers with different activation functions. The different basic interlayers present in CNN are the convolutional, the pooling and the fully connected layers. It is also necessary to include a classification layer in a typical CNN structure to obtain a classification decision. Layers such as ReLU and Dropout are commonly used to increase the performance of CNN architectures.

The convolutional layer comprises filters, with specific dimensions, to create activation maps for the extraction of features from the input data (*CS231n Convolutional Neural Networks for Visual Recognition*, n.d.). Figure contained in the convolutional demo section of the *CS231n Convolutional Neural Networks for Visual Recognition* (n.d.)'s lecture notes presents a visual presentation of the convolutional process in a 3-dimensional convolution layer. As shown in the figure, a 3×3 filter, with a determined size, traverses the image while performing the convolution operation. In this layer, the size of the filter and the number of pixels to skip in each process can be determined by the researcher (Özkan İnik, n.d.).

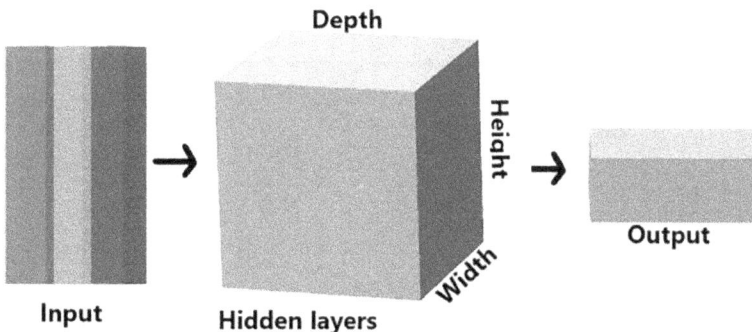

FIGURE 6.1 CNN configuration.

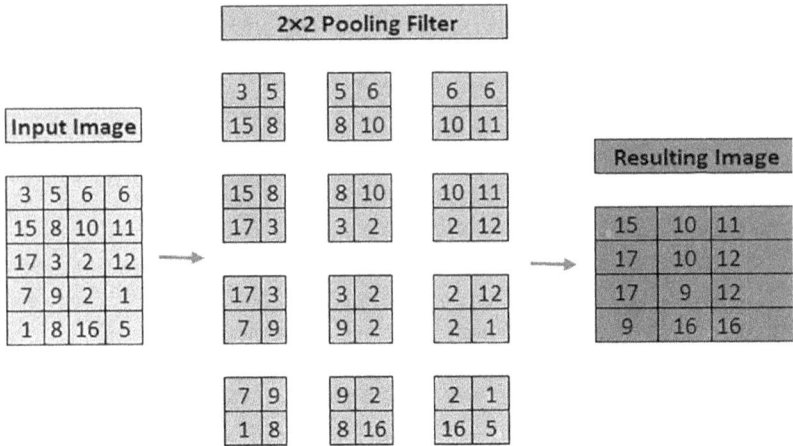

FIGURE 6.2   Maximum pooling for 5×5 image with 2×2 filter.

The purpose of adding pooling layer is to combine semantically similar properties. A typical pooling layer selects the maximum pixel from local units in the feature map created by convolution layer stage (Grewal et al., 2018). Briefly, the pooling layer decreases the number of parameters by sub-sampling. Figure 6.2 presents an example of a pooling layer process where the one-step maximum docking operations are applied to a 5×5 input image using a 2×2 filter.

Convolutional neural networks consist of two stages. The first stage, the feature extraction stage, comprise convolution and pooling layers, whereas the second stage consists of the classification section with softmax and fully connected layers (Şeker et al., 2017). The fully connected layer can be used more than once, but must be positioned before the last softmax layer. In the fully connected layer placed before the softmax layer, each neuron in the previous layer is connected to each neuron in the succeeding layer and there is an attempt to estimate the nearest class category (Şeker et al., 2017). An example of a fully connected layer is given in Figure 6.3.

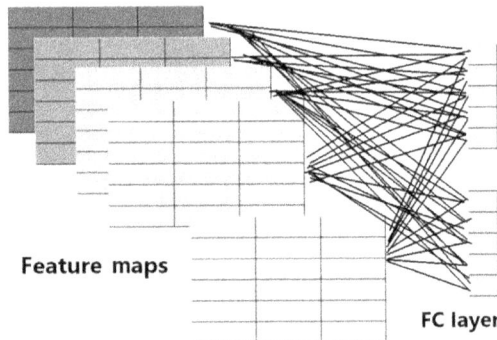

FIGURE 6.3   Fully connected layer.

6.3.2 TRANSFER LEARNING

Machine learning and data mining methods are a very large and highly successful field. However, there are some challenges associated with its successful application. Transfer learning methods have become the preferable method to resolve challenges associated with a very large data set (Pan & Yang, 2010; Weiss et al., 2016). Transfer learning can be thought of as a method of solving a problem by using previously acquired experiences. Using an example from human life, it is an inevitable fact that a veterinarian who is knowledgeable in animal anatomy will easily learn human anatomy in a shorter time than an individual who has never gained any knowledge of anatomy in his/her life (Pan & Yang, 2010). Similar to the example given, transfer learning is the training of deep neural networks with a large number of data to solve problems with fewer data. In recent years, various CNN-based deep neural network models, such as Alex Net (Krizhevsky et al., 2012), VGG (Simonyan & Zisserman, 2015), GoogleNet (Szegedy et al., 2015) or ResNet (He et al., 2016), used for transfer learning method, were trained with the large image database ImageNet, and have been employed for object classification and detection.

AlexNet, a CNN model developed by Krizhevsky et al. and initially released in 2010 with a revised version released in 2012, achieved the best top-5 error of 15.3% in the ImageNet ILSVRC-2012 competition (Krizhevsky et al., 2012). Their artificial neural network architecture consists of eight layers: three fully connected layers and five convolution layers each followed by the max-pooling layer and ends with a 1,000-class softmax layer. The architecture of their proposed artificial neural network requires an input image data with $227 \times 227 \times 3$ dimension.

Karen Simonyan and Andrew Zisserman, members of the Oxford University Visual Geometry Group, presented their VGG architecture which was adjudged second in the ImageNet ILSVRC competition in 2014, with an error rate of 7.3% (Simonyan & Zisserman, 2015). The architecture, which includes 16 layers (i.e., 13 convolutional layers and 3 fully connected), employs 5 pooling layers within some of the convolutional layers. The VGG network requires an input image data with $224 \times 224 \times 3$ dimension.

GoogleNet, presented by Szegedy et al., ranked 1st in the 2014 ILSVRC competition, with an error rate of 6.7% (Szegedy et al., 2015). The input data requirement of GoogleNet is $224 \times 224 \times 3$. Inception, a deep neural network architecture, was created by networking modules. Each module consists of different-sized convolutional and max-pooling processes. Although GoogleNet has a total of 22 layers, the use of size reduction modules reduced the 60 million parameters in AlexNet to 4 million. GoogleNet's size reduction module is shown in Figure 6.4.

Residual Networks (ResNet), launched by the Microsoft group, came up first in the 2015 ILSVRC competition, with an error rate of 3.6% (He et al., 2016). The network consists of 152 layers. Although it is presumed that the classification accuracy increases as the neural network deepens, a reverse negative relation is observed. To solve this problem, ResNet architecture has shortcut connections immediately after the residual values between the various layers. The scheme of these shortcut connections is given in Figure 6.5. Also, unlike the other architectures, an average pooling was used instead of max pooling.

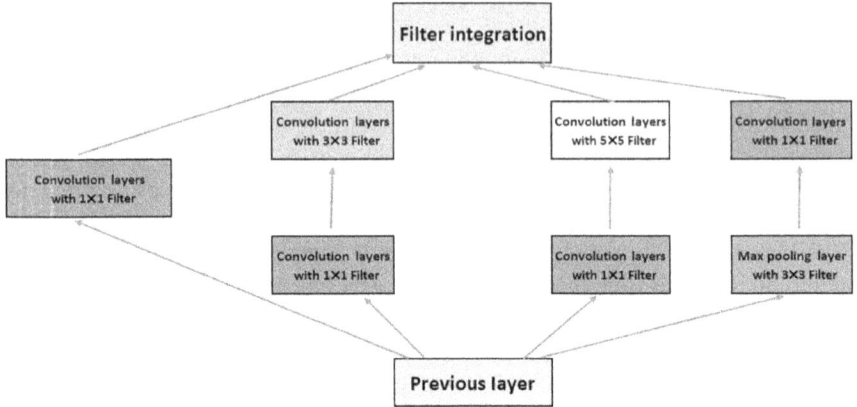

FIGURE 6.4 Inception size reduction module.

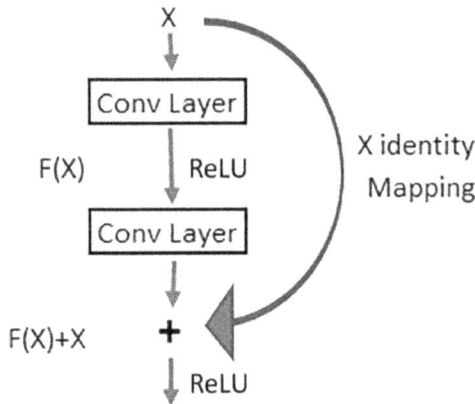

FIGURE 6.5 The building block of learning now.

6.4 LITERATURE REVIEW

The imaging techniques, which are the golden standard method to capture the retinal structure, and the most frequently employed field of the deep learning method are thoroughly discussed. In view of this information, the OCT imaging technique is an up-to-date and developing method with significant advantages in comparison to FFA imaging methods. Considering the increased rates of publications in 2019 with reference to 2018, publications involving Fundus imaging increased by 56% (*Scopus – Document Search Results | Signed In*, n.d.) whereas an increase of 115% was recorded for OCT publications (*Scopus – Document Search Results | Signed In*, n.d.). Additionally, considering the number of published studies involving CNN-based deep learning methods (as shown in Figure 6.6), this research area is rapidly evolving into a popular research area (*Scopus – Document Search Results | Signed In*, n.d.). Based on this information, this manuscript presents a thorough review of

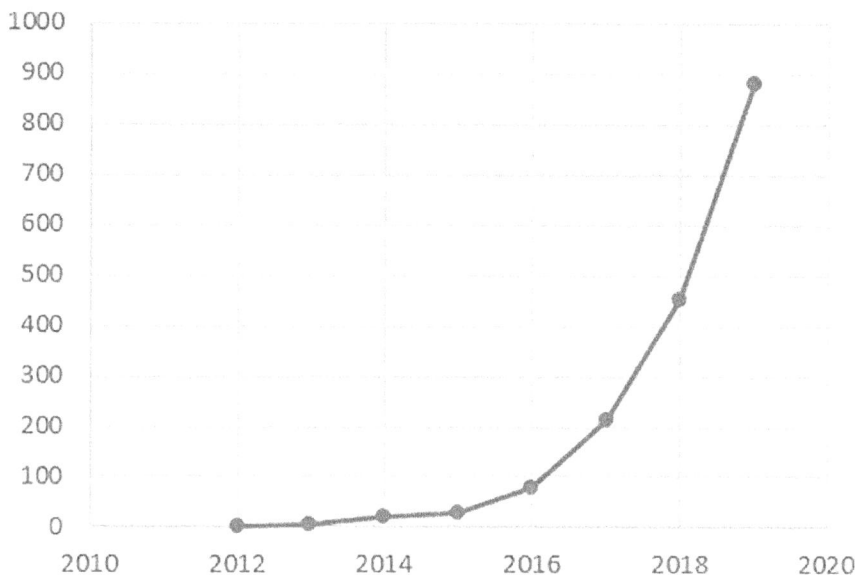

FIGURE 6.6   The number of publications in the biomedical field with deep learning in the last 8 years.

the above-mentioned retinal diseases using OCT images and CNN-based algorithms between 2019 and 2020.

In one of these studies Fengi Li et al. (2019) developed a CNN-based application to detect CNV, DME and dry-type AMD retinal diseases. The authors selected 5,319 OCT images of adult patients from the Shiley Eye Institute of the University of California San Diego, the California Retinal Research Foundation, Medical Center Ophthalmology Associates, the Beijing Tongren Eye Center and the Shanghai First People's Hospital between 2013 and 2017. A total of 109,312 images, selected for their experiments, were divided into four categories: CNV, DME, Drusen and normal. 37,546 images were taken from CNV patients, 11,599 images were obtained from DME patients, 11,599 images belonged to Drusen patients while there were 51,390 images of healthy individuals. After preprocessing of the images, a total of 1,000 images (where 250 images belonged to each category) chosen from 633 patients served as validation data set whereas the remaining data of 4,689 patients served as the training data set. A pre-trained VGG-16 CNN architecture, which had been pre-trained on the ImageNet database, was used in the study. By applying the transfer learning method, the weights of the VGG-16 network were re-trained using the retinal images taken from the patients and the desired settings were made. The authors reported a prediction accuracy of 98.6% for the diagnosis of retinal diseases using OCT images. A sensitivity of 97.8%, a specificity of 99.4% and an area of 100% under the ROC curve were also reported.

Sepna et al. (Mishra et al., 2019) employed OCT images and ResNet50 CNN architecture for the diagnosis of AMD and DME retinal diseases. The ResNet50 CNN was initially trained on the ImageNet database. Afterward, using the transfer learning method, the ResNet's trained weights were accordingly adjusted with training on the OCT images. The authors used the Duke (Rasti et al., 2018) and Neh (Wani et al., 2019) databases for their experiments. This study aimed to apply an approach called the multi-level dual-attention mechanism to CNN layers. Their proposed approach allowed their CNN model to learn both the noticeable rough features and the finer features of the input OCT images. The authors reported a 99.97% accuracy and 99.97% sensitivity for experiments with the Duke database, and a 99.62% accuracy and 99.62% sensitivity for the NEH database.

Ali Muhammed Alqudah (2020) worked on a new CNN architecture, called AOCT-NET, for the diagnosis of retinal diseases using OCT images. The proposed system was trained and tested on five main classes (AMD, CNV, DME, Drusen and Normal), where a total of 136,187 OCT images (belonging to the five categories) were obtained from the Zhang (Farsiu et al., 2014) and Farsiu (Srinivasan et al., 2014) databases. The authors selected 1,250 images for testing (with 250 images per each category). The remaining images, which were fed into their CNN, were divided into 70% for training and 30% for validation experiments. The proposed AOCT-NET has a total of 19 layers and was enriched using the adaptable moment ratio method. Their proposed method offered a higher accuracy at a lower computational cost. Their system attained 97.78% accuracy, 97.78% sensitivity and 97.778% specificity.

Vineeta Das et al. (2019) worked on a multi-scale deep feature fusion (MDFF)-based classification approach for the diagnosis of AMD, CNV and DME diseases. The method consists of three main steps: pre-processing, multi-scale spatial pyramid decomposition and classification using the MDFF based CNN. The OCT images of the retina, which have a natural curvature that varies between patients, can have adverse effects on classification performance. To prevent this situation, retina flattening was carried out by applying a graphic-based curvature method and the regions of interest within the image were cropped. Next, the images were resized, thereby completing the pre-processing step. In the second stage, the processed image was decomposed to obtain create multi-scale views of the image. These decomposed images served as input data to the MDFF-based classifier. Their proposed system performs classification according to four categories (CNV, DME, Drusen and Normal). They used the California San Diego (UCSD) database, which contains a total of 83,484 OCT images. These images were divided into two groups for the training and testing of their system. The authors choose 1,000 images from 633 patients (250 images per category) for their test experiments. Next, 80% of the remaining images served as the training set while 20% was used for validation. Their CNN structure was inspired by VGG16 architecture. The average sensitivity, specificity and accuracy obtained from testing their trained model on the test data set were 99.60%, 99.87% and 99.60%, respectively.

Vaghefi et al. (2020) proposed the training of a CNN architecture with different retinal images for the diagnosis of AMD disease. Initially, the individual groups of OCT, OCT-A and colored fundus images were sequentially fed to a CNN model. Next, the images were collectively fed into a CNN, and the experimental results from both experiments were analyzed. An accuracy of 94% was reported for the CNN training experiments with only OCT images while the experiments with only OCT-A produced a 91% diagnostic accuracy. The combination of OCT, OCT-A and colored fundus images produced an accuracy value of 96%. The authors modified the Inception-ResNet-V2 network to allow the simultaneous training on multiple image modalities. A total of 75 participants (with ethical approval from the Human Participants Ethics Committee of Auckland University) were included in the study. The participants were divided into three categories, namely, young healthy, elderly healthy and high-risk AMD. A comprehensive eye examination was performed for each participant. The macular status of patients in the AMD group was examined by an experienced specialist. The authors used the OCT device (Topcon DRI OCT Triton, Topcon Corporation, Tokyo, Japan) to acquire the images. The raw OCT, OCT-A and colored fundus images were exported using Topcon IMAGE net 6.0 software.

Naohiro et al. (Motozawa et al., 2019) studied the diagnosis of AMD disease using a two-computational deep learning model. In this study, two CNN models were created. The first model examined the OCT images for two categories: AMD and healthy. In the second transfer learning model, AMD-diagnosed images were classified as exudative and non-exudative. The authors also examined the effect of employing transfer learning on the speed of the model. The first CNN architecture recorded 100% sensitivity, 91.8% specificity and 99.0% accuracy for AMD diagnosis. The second CNN model successfully detected exudative cases with 98.4% sensitivity, 88.3% specificity and 93.8% accuracy. The authors reported that the inclusion of the transfer learning method in the second model increased the learning speed. The first CNN model was trained and validated with a total of 1,621 OCT images (1,382 AMD and 239 normal). The second transfer learning model was trained and validated using 721 AMD images with exudative changes and 661 AMD images without any exudative changes. The patient records of Kobe City Medical Center General Hospital were used in the study.

Sajib et al. (Saha et al., n.d.) investigated the automatic classification of biomarkers for AMD disease diagnosis. They discussed three main conditions (hyper-reflective foci, hyper-reflective foci in Drusen and sub-retinal Drusenoid deposits) that result in the AMD disease. Their image data set used for the training and testing of CNN models contained 19,584 OCT-B images obtained from 153 patients. These images were obtained from patients diagnosed with AMD at the Doheny Eye Center between 2010 and 2014. Three different CNN architectures (Inception-V3, ResNet50 and InceptionResNet50) were individually trained and tested for their experiments. They reported that accuracy values for the three pathologies ranged between 86% and 89%. The best results were obtained using the Inception ResNet50 architecture. This CNN network was able to detect sub-retinal Drusenoid deposits with 79%, 92% and 86% sensitivity, specificity and accuracy rates, respectively. The model recorded a 78% sensitivity and 100% specificity for hyper-reflective foci within Drusen, whereas hyper-reflective foci were successfully detected with 79% and 95% sensitivity and specificity, respectively.

Suhail et al. (Najeeb et al., n.d.) proposed the detection and classification of retinal diseases using OCT images. The study aimed to diagnose CNV, DME and Drusen diseases. In their proposed method, the open source OCT images of Kermany et al. (Farsiu et al., 2014) were used to train a CNN network. The training data set contained 83,484 images (37,205 CNV images, 11,348 DME images and 26,315 healthy eye images). In order to test the performance of their network model, 242 images from each category were reserved for testing. The authors used a basic CNN architecture. A review of their results shows that their proposed system can detect retinal diseases with a sensitivity of 95.66%.

Arka Bhowmil et al. (2019) employed OCT images for the detection of eye diseases and used transfer learning method in their CNN architecture. They investigated three groups of eye diseases: Drusen, DME and CNV. Their data set, downloaded from Kaggle, consisted of 84,495 grayscale OCT images. The data set was created using medical images from the University of California San Diego's Shiley Eye Institute, California Retinal Research Foundation, Medical Center Ophthalmology Associates, Shanghai Public Hospital and Beijing Tongren Eye Center. The pre-trained VGG16 and Inception-V3 neural networks were used as their CNN architecture. The authors used 4,000 images from the total data set of 1,000 images as their training data set for the categories: Druse, AMD, CNV and Normal, thus, shortening the time required for training their model. They used the remaining images in the data set to test the model. Their proposed approach produced an accuracy of 94% for test data and an accuracy of 99.94% for the training data set. According to their experimental results, the VGG16 architecture showed a better performance.

Kamble et al. (Chan et al., 2018) used the Inception-ResNet-V2 CNN architecture to detect DME disease from OCT images. They made some adjustments to the pre-trained architecture. The Inception-ResNet-V2 was trained using the public data sets from the Singapore Eye Research Institute. This trained model was tested with another data set published by the Chinese University Hong Kong. The proposed method provided a 100% diagnostic accuracy for DME disease. Additionally, the authors compared the results obtained from the Inception-ResNet-V2 network with the experimental results of the InceptionV3 and Resnet50 CNN architectures. From the comparative results, the authors commented on the superiority of Inception-ResNet-V2 architecture in comparison to the other two networks.

Weisen et al. (Wang et al., 2019) worked on a two-stream CNN model for the detection of wet AMD and dry AMD. In their approach, the CNN comprised a two-stream network to separately training using the OCT and fundus images. The pre-trained ResNet-18 network was used as the CNN architecture in the two models. A Loose Pair Training method was used for network training. With this method, the authors aimed to match an OCT image with another fundus image with the same effect. The authors reported that OCT-CNN outperformed Fundus-CNN with a 94.2% accuracy value in single-modal models. However, multi-modal CNN recognizes dry AMD and wet AMD at a higher accuracy.

Wang et al. (2020) trained two different CNN architectures to automatically detect the presence of CNV and perform segmentation of a detected CNV membrane. In accordance with the Helsinki Declaration, OCTA data sets with a wide range of signal strength index and containing data from retinal clinics at Oregon Eye and Science University, Portland, USA, and Shanxi Eye Hospital, Taiyuan, Shanxi, China, were used in the study. In their proposed method, two CNN architectures were combined. The first model was trained for CNV membrane identification and segmentation whereas the other model was employed for pixel-based vessel segmentation. The authors also used auto-encoder architecture in the CNN model which was employed for the membrane segmentation process. The authors employed a 3×3 sized atrous kernel instead of pooling layers to decrease the feature resolution. To send an input into the 2D CNN, the depth of the 3D structured retinal volumes was separately fed as a separate channel. After the structural and angiographic features were combined, they were fed to an auto-encoder. After the combination of the features, a single pooling layer was added, and a U-net-like architecture was applied to the decoder section. In the last layer of the CNV membrane segmentation architecture, a probability map of the CNV membranes was obtained using the softmax layer. In the vascular segmentation section, the probability map obtained from CNV membrane segmentation served as an input. Additionally, for the vascular segmentation architecture, the pooling layer of the CNV membrane segmentation architecture was replaced by the atrous kernel with reduced expansion rate to simplify the model. The authors reported a 100% precision, 95% specificity and an intersection ratio of 0.88 for their diagnostic model.

Xiaoming Xi et al. proposed a method that performs CNV segmentation using a multiscale CNN (MS-CNN-SP) with structure prior (Xi et al., 2019). The proposed method comprises two stages. In the first part, a structure prior learning was employed, whereas in the second part, a pre-trained multi-scale CNN structure was employed for CNV segmentation using the learned structure prior. The training and test images were decomposed into super-pixels. Next, features including density, texture and local information properties were extracted for each super-pixel. The global structure was trained on the super-pixels and shape regularity criteria (SRC). The spatial location of the CNV was determined from the previously trained global structure prior, and a local potential function was developed to compute the structure prior matrix. Subsequently, the original images were converted into images with enhanced clarity using the structure prior matrix. Different sizes of training patches were extracted from the enhanced images and used to train the multiscale pre-trained CNN model. All steps carried out during the training phase were repeated during the testing phase. The segmentation result was obtained through the combination of the segmentation results of the MS-CNN-SP models. 15 spectral-domain OCT images with CNV diagnoses were used in the study. A membrane similarity coefficient of 0.7806, a true positive volume ratio of 0.8024 and a false-positive volume ratio of 0.0036 were obtained using the MS-CNN-SP method. A comparison of the obtained results with a multi-scale CNN model without pre-learning revealed that the pre-learning method yielded approximately 28% more successful results (Table 6.1).

6.5 CONCLUSION

An alarmingly high number of recorded retinal disorders worldwide which results in blindness were observed. OCT and FFA imaging techniques are the two most preferred methods in the literature for the diagnosis of retinal diseases. Therefore, both OCT and FFA images and studies on the computer-aided automatic diagnosis and segmentation of these diseases play a very important role in the literature. With the recent technological advancement, deep learning models offer outstanding performances and outperform previous computer-aided diagnostic methods. In this study, comprehensive and detailed information is presented on the two most recent and very popular researches methods in the literature, by compiling automatic diagnosis and segmentation studies performed with CNN-based deep learning methods using OCT images, which is a more up-to-date and rapidly developing method compared to FFA. This review paves the way for other studies in this area and serves as a guide for the development of new methods.

TABLE 6.1
Review of the Retinal Diseases Detection Using OCT Images and CNN-Based Algorithms between 2019 and 2020

Article Name	Author Date	Method	Database	Journal	Results
Fully automated detection of retinal disorders by image-based deep learning	Li et al. (2019)	VGG-16	University of California San Diego, Shiley Eye Institute, California Retina Research Foundation, Medical Center Ophthalmology Associates, Beijing Tongren Eye Center and Shanghai First Public Hospital	*Graefe's Archive for Clinical and Experimental Ophthalmology*	98.6% accuracy 97.8% sensitivity, 99.4% specificity
Multi-level dual-attention-based CNN for macular OCT classification	Mishra et al. (2019)	ResNet50	Duke University, Neha University	*IEEE Signal Processing Letters*	99.97% accuracy, 99.97% sensitivity
MDFF for automated classification of macular pathologies from OCT images	Das et al. (2019)	MDFF-based CNN	University of California San Diego	*Biomedical Signal Processing and Control*	99.60% sensitivity, 99.87% specificity 99.60% accuracy
Multimodal retinal image analysis via deep learning for the diagnosis of intermediate dry AMD: a feasibility study	Vaghefi et al. (2020)	Inception-ResNet-V2	Auckland Optometry Clinic New Zealand, Auckland, Milford Eye Clinic	*Journal of Ophthalmology*	Accuracy value rising to 96%
OCT-based deep-learning models for classifying normal and AMD and exudative and non-exudative AMD changes	Motozawa et al. (2019)	CNN	Kobe City Medical Center General Hospital	*Ophthalmology and Therapy*	100% precision, 91.8% specificity, 99.0% accuracy

(Continued)

TABLE 6.1 (*Continued*)
Review of the Retinal Diseases Detection Using OCT Images and CNN-Based Algorithms between 2019 and 2020

Article Name	Author Date	Method	Database	Journal	Results
Automated detection and classification of early AMD biomarkers using deep learning	Saha et al. (2019)	Inception-V3 ResNet50 Inception-ResNet50	Doheny Eye Center	*Scientific Reports*	86%~89% Changing accuracy values
Classification of retinal diseases from OCT scans using convolutional neural networks	Suhail et al. (2019)	CNN	Kermany et al.	*International Conference on Electrical and Computer Engineering*	95.66% sensitivity
Eye disease prediction from OCT images with transfer learning	Bhowmik et al. (2019)	Inception V3	University of California San Diego, Shiley Eye Institute, California Retinal Research Foundation, Medical Center Ophthalmology Partners, Shanghai First Public Hospital Beijing Tongren Eye Center	In *International Conference on Engineering Applications of Neural Networks*	99.94% accuracy
Automated DME analysis using fine tuning with inception-resnet-v2 on OCT images	Kamble et al. (as pointed by Chan et al., 2018)	Inception-ResNet-V2	Singapore Eye Research Institute, China University of Hong Kong (CHUCK)	*2018 IEEE-EMBS Conference on Biomedical Engineering and Sciences (IECBES)*	100% accuracy

(*Continued*)

TABLE 6.1 (*Continued*)
Review of the Retinal Diseases Detection Using OCT Images and CNN-Based Algorithms between 2019 and 2020

Article Name	Author Date	Method	Database	Journal	Results
Two-stream CNN with loose pair training for multi-modal AMD categorization	Wang et al. (2019)	ResNet-18	Peking Union Medical College Hospital	*International Conference on Medical Image Computing and Computer-Assisted Intervention*	94.2% accuracy
Automated segmentation of CNV in OCT images using multi-scale CNNs with structure prior	Xi et al. (2019)	Multi-modal CNN		*Multimedia Systems*	dice similarity coefficient 0.7806, *true positive volume ratio 0.8024*
AOCT-NET: a convolutional network automated classification of multi-class retinal diseases using spectral-domain OCT images	Alqudah (2020)	AOCT-NET CNN	Zhang and Farsiu database	*Medical & Biological Engineering & Computing*	97.78% accuracy, 97.78% sensitivity 97.778% specificity
Automated diagnosis and segmentation of CNV in OCT angiography using deep learning	Wang et al. (2020)	Auto-Encoder CNN	Oregon Eye & Science University, Portland, Or, USA and Shanxi Eye Hospital, Taiyuan, Shanxi, Retina Clinics in PR China	*Biomedical Optics Express*	95% specificity, 100% sensitivity, 0.88 intersection

REFERENCES

Akram, M. U., & Nasim, A. (n.d.). Review of OCT and fundus images for detection of Macular Edema. *Ieeexplore.Ieee.Org*. Doi: 10.1109/IST.2015.7294517.

Alqudah, A. M. (2020). AOCT-NET: A convolutional network automated classification of multiclass retinal diseases using spectral-domain optical coherence tomography images. *Medical and Biological Engineering and Computing, 58*(1), 41–53. Doi: 10.1007/s11517-019-02066-y.

Arel, I., Rose, D., & Karnowski, T.P. (n.d., 2010, undefined). Research frontier: Deep machine learning--a new frontier in artificial intelligence research. *IEEE Computational Intelligence Magazine Dl.Acm.Org*. Retrieved March 26, 2020, from https://dl.acm.org/doi/abs/10.1109/MCI.2010.938364.

Bhowmik, A., Kumar, S., & Bhat, N. (2019). Eye disease prediction from optical coherence tomography images with transfer learning. *Communications in Computer and Information Science, 1000*, 104–114. Doi: 10.1007/978-3-030-20257-6_9.

Boulemtafes, A., Derhab, A., & Challal, Y. (n.d., 2020, undefined). A review of privacy-preserving techniques for deep learning. *Neurocomputing, Elsevier*. Retrieved March 26, 2020, from https://www.sciencedirect.com/science/article/pii/S0925231219316431.

Chan, G. C. Y., Julian, O., Charry, P., Kamble, R. M., Perdomo, O., González, F. A., Kokare, M., Müller, H., & Mériaudeau, F. (2018). Automated diabetic macular edema (DME) analysis using fine tuning with Inception-Resnet-v2 on OCT images. In *ieeexplore.ieee.org*. https://www.researchgate.net/publication/327833908.

Chhablanı, J., & Sudhalkar, A. (n.d.). It is important to know the strengths and weaknesses of imaging modalities and their unique uses for diagnosing different retinal diseases. In *retinatoday.com*. Retrieved March 26, 2020, from http://retinatoday.com/pdfs/0114RT_Imaging_Chhablani.pdf.

CS231n Convolutional Neural Networks for Visual Recognition. (n.d.). Retrieved March 10, 2020, from http://cs231n.github.io/convolutional-networks/.

Das, V., Dandapat, S., & Bora, P. K. (2019). Multi-scale deep feature fusion for automated classification of macular pathologies from OCT images. *Biomedical Signal Processing and Control, 54*, 101605. Doi: 10.1016/j.bspc.2019.101605.

Deng, L., & Yu, D. (2013). Deep learning: Methods and applications foundations and trends R in signal processing. *Signal Processing, 7*(2013), 197–387. Doi: 10.1561/2000000039.

Farsiu, S., Chiu, S. J., O'Connell, R. V., Folgar, F. A., Yuan, E., Izatt, J. A., & Toth, C. A. (2014). Quantitative classification of eyes with and without intermediate age-related macular degeneration using optical coherence tomography. *Ophthalmology, 121*(1), 162–172. Doi: 10.1016/j.ophtha.2013.07.013.

Grewal, P. S., Oloumi, F., Rubin, U., & Tennant, M. T. S. (2018). Deep learning in ophthalmology: A review. *Canadian Journal of Ophthalmology 53*(4), 309–313. Elsevier B.V. Doi: 10.1016/j.jcjo.2018.04.019.

He, K., Zhang, X., Ren, S., & Sun, J. (2016). *Deep residual learning for image recognition*. http://image-net.org/challenges/LSVRC/2015/.

Ishtiaq, U., Abdul Kareem, S., Abdullah, E. R. M. F., Mujtaba, G., Jahangir, R., & Ghafoor, H. Y. (2019). Diabetic retinopathy detection through artificial intelligent techniques: A review and open issues. *Multimedia Tools and Applications*, 1–44. Doi: 10.1007/s11042-018-7044-8.

Kermany, D. S., Goldbaum, M., Cai, W., Valentim, C. C. S., Liang, H., Baxter, S. L., ... Zhang, K. (2018). Identifying medical diagnoses and treatable diseases by image-based deep learning. *Cell, 172*(5), 1122–1131.e9. Doi: 10.1016/j.cell.2018.02.010.

Khochtali, S., Khairallah-Ksiaa, I., & Ben Yahia, S. (2016). Normal fundus fluorescein angiography. In *The Uveitis Atlas* (pp. 1–7). Springer India. Doi: 10.1007/978-81-322-2506-5_5-1.

Krizhevsky, A., Sutskever, I., & Hinton, G. E. (2012). *ImageNet classification with deep convolutional neural networks.* http://code.google.com/p/cuda-convnet/.

Li, F., Chen, H., Liu, Z., Zhang, X., & Wu, Z. (2019). Fully automated detection of retinal disorders by image-based deep learning. *Graefe's Archive for Clinical and Experimental Ophthalmology, 257*(3), 495–505. Doi: 10.1007/s00417-018-04224-8.

Li, F. F., Karpathy, A., & networks, J. J.-N. (n.d., 2016, undefined). *Stanford University CS231n: Convolutional Neural Networks for Visual Recognition.*

Mishra, S. S., Mandal, B., & Puhan, N. B. (2019). Multi-level dual-attention based CNN for macular optical coherence tomography classification. *IEEE Signal Processing Letters, 26*(12), 1793–1797. Doi: 10.1109/LSP.2019.2949388.

Moraes, G., Faes, L., & Pal, B. (n.d., 2018, undefined). Optical coherence tomography angiography: Principles and application in retinal diseases. *The Official Scientific Journal of Delhi Ophthalmological Society, Djo.Org.In.* Retrieved March 26, 2020, from https://www.djo.org.in/articles/29/1/Optical-Coherence-Tomography-Angiography.html.

Motozawa, N., An, G., Takagi, S., Kitahata, S., Mandai, M., Hirami, Y., Yokota, H., Akiba, M., Tsujikawa, A., Takahashi, M., & Kurimoto, Y. (2019). Optical coherence tomography-based deep-learning models for classifying normal and age-related macular degeneration and exudative and non-exudative age-related macular degeneration changes. *Ophthalmology and Therapy, 8*(4), 527–539. Doi: 10.1007/s40123-019-00207-y.

Najeeb, S., Sharmile, N., Khan, M., Sahin, I., Islam, M.T., & Bhuiyan, M.I.H. (n.d., 2018, undefined). Classification of retinal diseases from OCT scans using convolutional neural networks. *Ieeexplore.Ieee.Org.* Retrieved March 26, 2020, from https://ieeexplore.ieee.org/abstract/document/8636699/

Özkan, İ.N.İ.K. and Ülker, E. (n.d.). Derin Öğrenme ve Görüntü Analizinde Kullanılan Derin Öğrenme Modelleri. *Gaziosmanpasa Journal of Scientific Research.* Retrieved March 26, 2020, from http://dergipark.gov.tr/gbad.

Pan, S. J., & Yang, Q. (2010). A survey on transfer learning. *IEEE Transactions on Knowledge and Data Engineering, 22*(10), 1345–1359. Doi: 10.1109/TKDE.2009.191.

Rasti, R., Rabbani, H., Mehridehnavi, A., & Hajizadeh, F. (2018). Macular OCT classification using a multi-scale convolutional neural network ensemble. *IEEE Transactions on Medical Imaging, 37*(4), 1024–1034. Doi: 10.1109/TMI.2017.2780115.

Rawat, C. S., & Gaikwad, V. S. (n.d., 2014, undefined). Signal analysis and image simulation for optical coherence tomography (OCT) systems. In *2014 International Conference on Control, Instrumentation, Communication and Computational Technologies (ICCICCT)* Ieeexplore.Ieee.Org. Retrieved March 26, 2020, from https://ieeexplore.ieee.org/abstract/document/6993037/.

Saha, S., Nassisi, M., Wang, M., Lindenberg, S., Sadda, S., & Hu, Z.J. (n.d., 2019, undefined). Automated detection and classification of early AMD biomarkers using deep learning. *Scientific reports, Nature.Com.* Retrieved March 26, 2020, from https://www.nature.com/articles/s41598-019-47390-3.

Scopus - Document search results | Signed in. (n.d.). Retrieved March 10, 2020, from https://www.scopus.com/results/results.uri?numberOfFields=0&src=s&clickedLink=&edit=&editSaveSearch=&origin=searchbasic&authorTab=&affiliationTab=&advancedTab=&scint=1&menu=search&tablin=&searchterm1=biomedical+and+deep+learning&field1=TITLE_ABS_KEY&dateType=Publication_Date_Type&yearFrom=Before+1960&yearTo=Present&loadDate=7&documenttype=All&accessTypes=All&resetFormLink=&st1=biomedical+and+deep+learning&st2=&sot=b&sdt=b&sl=43&s=TITLE-ABS-KEY%28biomedical+and+deep+learning%29&sid=427dd9e938156a3a7c4553a11695de2b&searchId=427dd9e938156a3a7c4553a11695de2b&txGid=98a00cc9af040855857d115058797662&sort=plf-f&originationType=b&rr=.

Şeker A., Diri B., & Balik H. (2017). Derin Öğrenme Yöntemleri Ve Uygulamaları Hakkında Bir İnceleme. *Gazi Mühendislik Bilimleri Dergisi (GMBD), 3*(3), 47–64.

Simonyan, K., & Zisserman, A. (2015, September 4). Very deep convolutional networks for large-scale image recognition. *3rd International Conference on Learning
Representations, ICLR 2015- Conference Track Proceedings*, San Diego, CA.

Spaide, R., Klancnik, J., & Cooney, M.J. (n.d., 2015, undefined). Retinal vascular layers
imaged by fluorescein angiography and optical coherence tomography angiography.
JAMA ophthalmology, Jamanetwork.Com. Retrieved March 26, 2020, from https://
jamanetwork.com/journals/jamaophthalmology/article-abstract/1910581.

Srinivasan, P. P., Kim, L. A., Mettu, P. S., Cousins, S. W., Comer, G. M., Izatt, J. A., & Farsiu,
S. (2014). Fully automated detection of diabetic macular edema and dry age-related
macular degeneration from optical coherence tomography images. *Biomedical Optics
Express*, *5*(10), 3568. Doi: 10.1364/boe.5.003568.

Szegedy, C., Liu, W., Jia, Y., Sermanet, P., Reed, S., Anguelov, D., Erhan, D., Vanhoucke, V.,
& Rabinovich, A. (2015). *Going Deeper with Convolutions*, In *Proceedings of the IEEE
conference on computer vision and pattern recognition* (pp. 1–9), IEEE, USA.

Talisa, E., de Carlo M.D., Baumal, C.R. (n.d., 2016, undefined). Will OCT angiography
replace FA? *Retina Specialist, Retina-Specialist.Com*. Retrieved March 26, 2020, from
https://www.retina-specialist.com/article/will-oct-angiography-replace-fa.

Vaghefi, E., Hill, S., Kersten, H. M., & Squirrell, D. (2020). Multimodal retinal image analysis via deep learning for the diagnosis of intermediate dry age-related macular degeneration: A feasibility study. *Journal of Ophthalmology*. Doi: 10.1155/2020/7493419.

Varma, R., Bressler, N. M., Doan, Q. V., Gleeson, M., Danese, M., Bower, J. K., Selvin,
E., Dolan, C., Fine, J., Colman, S., & Turpcu, A. (2014). Prevalence of and risk factors for diabetic macular edema in the United States. *JAMA Ophthalmology*, *132*(11),
1334–1340. Doi: 10.1001/jamaophthalmol.2014.2854.

Wang, J., Hormel, T. T., Gao, L., Zang, P., Guo, Y., Wang, X., Bailey, S. T., & Jia, Y. (2020).
Automated diagnosis and segmentation of choroidal neovascularization in OCT angiography using deep learning. *Biomedical Optics Express*, *11*(2), 927. Doi: 10.1364/
boe.379977.

Wang, W., Xu, Z., Yu, W., Zhao, J., Yang, J., He, F., Yang, Z., Chen, D., Ding, D., Chen, Y.,
& Li, X. (2019). Two-stream CNN with loose pair training for multi-modal AMD cat-
egorization. *Lecture Notes in Computer Science (Including Subseries Lecture Notes
in Artificial Intelligence and Lecture Notes in Bioinformatics)*, *11764 LNCS*, 156–164.
Doi: 10.1007/978-3-030-32239-7_18.

Wani, M. A., Bhat, F. A., Afzal, S., & Khan, A. I. (2019). *Advances in Deep Learning. 57*. Doi:
10.1007/978-981-13-6794-6.

Weiss, K., Khoshgoftaar, T. M., & Wang, D. D. (2016). A survey of transfer learning. *Journal
of Big Data*, *3*(1), 9. Doi: 10.1186/s40537-016-0043-6.

Xi, X., Meng, X., Yang, L., Nie, X., Yang, G., Chen, H., Fan, X., Yin, Y., & Chen, X. (2019).
Automated segmentation of choroidal neovascularization in optical coherence tomog-
raphy images using multi-scale convolutional neural networks with structure prior.
Multimedia Systems, *25*(2), 95–102. Doi: 10.1007/s00530-017-0582-5.

Zhang, Y., Zhang, B., Fan, M., Gao, X., Wen, X., Li, Z., Zeng, P., Tan, W., & Lan, Y. (2020). The
vascular densities of the macula and optic disc in normal eyes from children by optical
coherence tomography angiography. *Graefe's Archive for Clinical and Experimental
Ophthalmology*, *258*(2), 437–444. Doi: 10.1007/s00417-019-04466-0.

7 Deep Learning vs. Super Pixel Classification for Breast Masses Segmentation

Mohammed El Amine Bechar and Nesma Settouti
University of Tlemcen

Inês Domingues
IPO Porto Research Centre (CI-IPOP)

CONTENTS

7.1 INTRODUCTION

The expansion and democratisation of medical imaging acquisition devices is now producing an incredible amount of patient-related data. Having access to this wealth of information opens the opportunity for various applications of computer-assisted diagnosis (CAD).

The underlying assumption of this chapter is that deep learning (DL) will provide additional information for the physician that would have been difficult to obtain with algorithms based on traditional solutions. Therefore, the main objective of this research is to study the feasibility of DL for the medical community to encourage the discovery of clinically relevant structures present in the data. More specifically, this work will focus on one sub-objective that addresses mass detection in mammography images.

The CAD of breast cancer is becoming more and more a necessity with the exponential growth in the number of mammograms performed each year (Kaushal et al. 2019, Zou et al. 2019, Tsochatzidis et al. 2019). There is currently significant interest in the diagnosis of breast masses and their classification. Indeed, the complexity and the difficulty encountered to discern them require the use of appropriate algorithms. In this work, segmentation methods adapted to breast pathology's are analysed.

The contributions of the present chapter include as follows:

- A comparative study of different segmentation techniques is carried out on INBreast database (Moreira et al. 2012).
- *Super-pixel-based segmentation*: The challenges of divergent inputs and high-dimensional characteristics relative to image data have made super-pixels key building blocks for many computer vision algorithms. The construction of super-pixels on the image makes it possible to extract information by manipulating local regions, while significantly reducing processing time (Bechar et al. 2019).
- *Segmentation by deep learning*: DL can learn patterns from visual inputs to identify classes of objects in an image. For image processing, the principle is often based on a Convolutional Neural Network (CNN) architecture.

The main objective of this work is to compare two segmentation techniques (CNN vs super-pixel-based segmentation). CNN is a modern technique dedicated to computer vision, whose success is due to the fact of automatic features extraction of images by neuronal training. In contrast, super-pixel-based segmentation is a traditional technique that consists of sub-dividing the image into super-pixels and calculating the features (such as Texture features) on each super-pixel thereafter to initiate training of a classifier and segmentation at the end.

The analysis of the different algorithms and of different methodologies is focused on answering a series of key questions such as: *Has deep learning superseded traditional computer vision? Is there still a need to study traditional computer vision techniques for the case of biomedical applications?* In the first place, we return to the classic segmentation by super-pixels classification, reflection will focus on the quality of super-pixel feature extraction, exploiting information from the grey level of the super-pixel. Secondly, we test the CNN performance such as U-Net (Ronneberger et al. 2015), Feature Pyramid Networks (FPN) (Lin et al. 2017) or LinkNet (Chaurasia and Culurciello 2017). Third, based on the evolution of research and trends, we consider which future is drawn for segmentation methods for breast pathology's. Finally, a series of key recommendations for the best suited choice method will emerge from this analysis.

The remaining of this document is outlined as follows. Section 7.2 provides an historical overview of the segmentation evolution, together with taxonomy, while

Section 7.3 dwells into the segmentation works made specifically on mass detection and segmentation in mammogram images from INBreast database.

In Section 7.4, the specific pipelines and methods are presented, while Section 7.5 illustrates the results. Finally, Section 7.7 draws the final conclusions and points to future work directions.

7.2 BACKGROUND

The segmentation is a central point in the processes of image interpretation and analysis. Although segmentation has already been the subject of much works, it generally remains very dependent on the nature and context of image exploitation. The particularity of segmentation lies in the fact that there is no one method that is suitable for all applications. As such, it has been the subject of several publications, in which researchers have attempted to provide various and varied solutions that often consider the nature of the processed images. Indeed, several research projects have focused on the development of diagnostic support systems to automatically detect lesions (micro-calcification's or masses); this can guide experts in the screening and diagnostic process, thus enabling better analysis of complex cases.

A wide range of work has been carried out in order to carry out the segmentation of the different breast cancer cells. However, this segmentation is still a difficult task for the following reasons (Goubalan 2016):

- The mammography image is generally low contrast. Thus, decision-making regarding the classification of the observed pixels as belonging to a given breast structure is accompanied by a certain degree of uncertainty.
- The suspect area may have unclear contours, which leads to ambiguity in the discrimination of lesion boundaries.
- Two parameters make the interpretation of the mammography image a difficult task. These parameters represent the size of the suspect area, which can be very small, and the great variability in the shapes it can take.

In the literature, different techniques of mammography image segmentation are often classified in three distinct families (Agarwal et al. 2019): conventional segmentation methods (region-based segmentation, contour-based segmentation and region clustering), model-based segmentation (pixel-based methods, pattern matching) and the DL techniques.

7.2.1 CONVENTIONAL SEGMENTATION METHODS

Conventional methods are more particularly materialised by region-based segmentation methods. Their purpose is to divide an image into several homogeneous disjoint and connected regions; they are based on the principle of homogeneity, which means that there must be at least one descriptor which, to a certain extent, remains uniform for all pixels belonging to the same region of the image.

The main advantage of the region growth method is its ability to manage spatial pixel information in a natural way. Nevertheless, this method is sensitive to the initialisation of seed points. Thus, its performance is very dependent on the choice of initial sprouts (Cheng et al. 2006).

Among the various existing works (Senthilkumar et al. 2010; Berber et al. 2013; Rouhi et al. 2015; Punitha et al. 2018; Min et al. 2019a, Shrivastava and Bharti 2020), some of them propose methods for automatic selection of seed points. Senthilkumar et al. (2010) use the Harris detector to perform automatic germ positioning to decide whether or not to add a pixel to the seed region, Melouah (2013) compare the similarity measure to a threshold value automatically generated from the cancerous areas as a prediction model. In Rouhi et al. (2015), segmentation is performed by automated region growing, where the threshold used for growth is calculated using a trained artificial neural network (ANN).

Mohamed et al. (2016) introduced a segmentation approach based on the principle of growing regions which outperform existing region growing technique in terms of accuracy. Their proposal consists on adding the orientation constraint along with existing constraint of original region growing method.

Recently, an Efficient Seeded Region Growing is proposed in Shrivastava and Bharti (2020) to spot breast cancer. Breast image pre-processing is based on several operations which can be summarised as: region of interest (ROI) extraction, image contrast adjustment, image noise reduction and image binarisation. In region growing, the starting points are calculated automatically and their coordinates are determined by the pixel intensity value. Finally, it is necessary to calculate a threshold value to proceed with the region growing.

The watershed is another approach based on region growth segmentation; it is inspired by tools developed in mathematical morphology. Among the powerful image segmentation techniques, we can find the Watershed and marker-controlled watershed. Generally, a fully automatic, marker-controlled watershed is applied to segment the mass region, then this segmentation is refined by level set as in Liu et al. (2011), Hefnawy (2013) and Chattaraj et al. (2017).

The difficulty associated with the region growth method lies in the definition of a relevant cut-off criterion that allows optimal segmentation of the regions to be segmented. Indeed, if the initial seed point is selected in a non-homogeneous region, this method will tend to produce strong variations, which will lead to a rapid halt in the growth of the region.

Historically, many segmentation techniques have emerged and continue to multiply and diversify (Dabass et al. 2019; Platania et al. 2017). Among them are contour-based segmentation methods, which approach segmentation as a search for boundaries between objects (anomalies) and background. They involve identifying pixel intensity transitions between regions to define the edges of the anomalies being searched for.

Contour-based segmentation methods for breast masses segmentation range from simple edge detection (Kozegar et al. 2018, Guo and Razmjooy 2019) to polynomial modelling (Paramkusham et al. 2015, Bhateja et al. 2016). Other approaches are based on the gradient (Zheng et al. 2013, Tello-Mijares et al. 2019) or graph-based approaches.

This later gain increasing popularity in breast masses segmentation and especially on BUS (Breast Ultrasound) images due to their advantages. Indeed, it provides a simple way to organise task-related prior and image information in a unified framework; it is flexible and suitable for expressing soft constraints among random variables; also, the computation based on graphical manipulation is very efficient (Huang et al. 2017).

In the graph-based method, the image is represented as a weighted and undirected graph. Usually, the similarity/dissimilarity between pixels is defined by an edge weight; this weight is calculated from a node associated with a pixel or group of pixels. Then, a criterion designed to model the good clusters is used to partition the graph (image) (Huang et al. 2017). Some popular algorithms of this category are graph cuts (Liu et al. 2015), robust graph-based (Huang et al. 2012, 2015, Luo et al. 2016), discriminative graph cuts (Zhang et al. 2010, Zhou et al. 2014), dynamic graph cuts (Angayarkanni et al. 2015), tree-based segmentation (Suhail et al. 2018, Divyashree et al. 2018) and segmentation-based object categorisation (Chang et al. 2015).

Among the contour-based segmentation, active contour-based segmentation methods have presenting considerable advantages in terms of the obtained structure (closed curve) and the quality of the contour. Nevertheless, these are semiautomatic methods where an initialisation is necessary to continue the evolution of the contour, which requires human intervention. To overcome this problem, the researchers use other methods to obtain an initial contour which is then refined using active contours. As an example, Anitha and Peter (2015) applied the Fuzzy C-Means (FCM) algorithm for initialisation. In Chakraborty et al. (2016), Sobel edge detection method is used as a prior step of active contour model for mammograms image segmentation. Recently, Ciecholewski (2017) make a comparison study between three active contours models: edge-based active contour model using an inflation/deflation force with a damping coefficient, a geometric active contour model and an active contour without edges; the qualitative and quantitative results show that the damping coefficient outperform methods presented in the literature. Active contours have also been applied in other work on ultrasound images (Jumaat et al. 2011, Lotfollahi et al. 2018) and in digital tomosynthesis of the breast.

In order to address the shortcomings of the region growth method and contour-based segmentation methods, hybrid approaches have been developed to allow the advantages of each to be leveraged to address the weaknesses of the other. Indeed, traditional methods of region growth have the disadvantage of having a difficulty in positioning borders. Therefore, the association with a contour-based segmentation method aims to address this limitation.

7.2.2 MODEL-BASED SEGMENTATION METHODS

Model-based segmentation is a method that has a training phase during which the objects to be detected are training automatically by the computer-aided detection system. This system is capable of classify or detect new images considering into account the content of the image like those observed during the training phase. During this training phase, the system learns from images with masses, their probable location as well as the variation in the shape and size of the masses. On images of the training base with no contain lesions, the system can learn descriptors that represent healthy tissue.

In model-based segmentation, the sample can be represented by a pixel, a group of pixels, an object in the image or the full image. Depending on the application, each pixel in the image is classified into different regions. As an example, it is possible to classify the different regions of a mammography image as lesion or not. We distinguish two categories of classification methods: unsupervised or clustering and supervised classifications.

Clustering methods: The unsupervised classification, known as automatic, or clustering, consists in identifying the different classes naturally without any prior knowledge. The objective, in this case, is to identify a structure in the images based on their contents. The images are assigned to the different classes estimated according to two essential criteria which are the great homogeneity of each class and the good separation between the classes.

Among the clustering methods, the most commonly used method is the K-means algorithm, which is at the same time easy to implement and has low complexity. In mammography, it has been used to generate initial segmentation and then these initial results were enhanced by incorporating contour information (Yang et al. 2012, Elmoufidi et al. 2015), while Yuan et al. (2019) applied it to a set of descriptors extracted through wavelets. We also report Markov field segmentation markov random field (MRF), the strength of MRFs resides in their ability to model joint probabilities as local spatial interactions, thereby introducing information about local dependencies between pixels into the algorithm. Various applications in different format of breast cancer images were registered, as magnetic resonance (MR) and tomosynthesis images (Shafer et al. 2011), mammogram images (El Idrissi El Kaitouni et al. 2018) and thermography images (Mahmoudzadeh et al. 2015).

Another unsupervised classification method is the Self-Organising Map (SOM). An SOM is a network of neurons that through a competitive unsupervised process is capable of projecting large data sets into two-dimensional space (Chen et al. 2000, Rickard et al. 2004, Marcomini and Schiabel 2015, Marcomini et al. 2016). The advantage of this method is the robustness to the initial conditions of the K-means algorithm. However, the computation time allowing the construction of SOM is important.

The main disadvantage of the cited clustering segmentation techniques is that they ignore the spatial arrangement of pixels. They identify the classes of pixels present in the image and assign each pixel a label indicating the class to which it belongs. Thus, pixels belonging to a class may form several non-adjacent regions in the image, but sharing the same properties.

Hierarchical methods (Shi et al. 2018, Ramadijanti et al. 2018, Hazarika and Mahanta 2019) have the interesting property of preserving spatial and neighbouring information among segmented regions. It provides a region-oriented scale-space, i.e., the segmentation at coarser levels is nested with respect to those at finer levels. Likewise, the FCM algorithm is a fuzzy extension of the k-means algorithm and allows each object in the image to be associated with a class using a fuzzy membership function (Feng et al. 2017, Chowdhary and Acharjya 2018, Vald´es-Santiago et al. 2018).

Supervised methods: Image segmentation by supervised training methods or classification is derived from the multi-dimensional data classification domain. It defines a partition of the image into a set of classes such that each class gathers pixels having vectors of characteristics (colours or often reduced to grey level) as similar as possible and that the classes are as distinct as possible from each other. Generally, these segmentation methods do not take into account the spatial arrangement of the pixels and consider only the feature vector used. It identifies the classes of pixels present in the image and assigns each pixel a label indicating the class to which it belongs. Thus pixels belonging to a class may form several non-adjacent regions in the image but sharing the same statistical properties. A segmentation into regions is only obtained after analysing the connectivity of the pixels in the labelled image.

Unlike unsupervised methods, supervised approaches require a database of labelled images which will be used to train the classifier. Methods based on supervised training have aroused strong interest in the field of breast tumour segmentation (Bozek et al. 2009, Ganesan et al. 2013b, Huang et al. 2017, Wang 2017). There are many supervised and semi-supervised methods that have been proposed in recent years to help practitioners make decisions.

Supervised classification methods include Linear Discriminant Analysis (Liu et al. 2010, Li et al. 2016), ANNs (Ganesan et al. 2013a, Rouhi et al. 2015, Punitha et al. 2018), Decision Tree (Mohanty et al. 2012), Naive Bayes (Domingues and Cardoso 2014, Karabatak 2015, Udayakumar et al. 2017), Bayesian Network (Mahersia et al. 2016), K-Nearest Neighbour (Karahaliou et al. 2014), Support Vector Machines (SVM) (de Lima et al. 2016), (Raghavendra et al. 2016) and Random Forest (Dong et al. 2015, Dhungel et al. 2015a, Martel et al. 2016, Vogl et al. 2019).

Unlike the previously cited approaches which work at the pixel scale, the recent approaches use a low-level segmentation of the image, where the pixels are grouped in small homogeneous regions called super-pixels. These super-pixels make it possible to considerably reduce the number of visual primitives to manipulate, by creating sets of adjacent pixels whose colours are similar.

Super-pixels have gradually attracted researchers, attention and have been used for a long time as a first step towards segmentation because it makes it possible to accelerate the computational time and allows to produce excellent contour quality. In Daoud et al. (2016), a fully automatic algorithm is proposed to decompose ultrasound images into a set of homogeneous super-pixels; this algorithm is based on the method of Normalised Cuts (NCuts) combined with texture analysis, and the segmentation of BUS image is accurate using boundary-based and region-based information. Later, the same authors (Daoud et al. 2019) proposed an extended study to the application of the Simple Linear Iterative Clustering (SLIC) algorithm to improve super-pixels. This study investigated the effect of super-pixel number on recall ratio. Xi et al. (2017) developed a prior knowledge learning model based on super-pixel and SVM to generate the prior knowledge image according to the learned abnormal information. *Always for BUS images segmentation:* Huang and Huang (2018) proposed a novel method based on SLIC super-pixel classification, where from each super-pixel, features are extracted including grey histogram, grey level co-occurrence matrix and co-occurrence matching of local binary pattern (LBP); next, the multi-layer perceptron is applied to classify each super-pixel, and the segmentation result is the fusion of the classified super-pixels. Huang et al. (2020) expanded their study to semantic classification of super-pixels, where SLIC is firstly used to generate the super-pixels. Second, feature extraction is applied to calculate features on each super-pixel as textures and LBP. The initial segmentation is obtained by classifying each super-pixel using the back propagation neural network classifier. Then, a K Nearest Neighbour (KNN)-based approach is designed to refine the segmentation result.

Cong et al. (2014) focuses on systematic analyses for the performance of SLIC algorithm, compared with normalised cuts and turbopixels algorithm from the indicators of computational speed, boundary recall and boundary accuracy, and super-pixel uniformity for BUS image segmentation. Comparison results demonstrate that SLIC algorithm should be one of the deserved research domain in the future.

In Yu et al. (2015), an automatic breast dynamic contrast enhanced MR (DCE-MR) tumour segmentation framework was developed and validated, which leveraged intensity, geometric and textural information of super-pixels, and the topology of pixel-wise graph for tumour segmentation. Recently, Hong et al. (2019) proposes an algorithm for segmenting breast MR images by an improved density clustering algorithm. First, the superpixel clustering algorithm (SLIC) is used to divide the image into a certain number of ultrapixel regions. Next, the density peaks clustering (DPC) algorithm optimised by uncertain number neighbours and allocation strategy in K Nearest Neighbour DPC (KNN-DPC) is used to effectively segment the MR image. Sun et al. (2018) proposed a semi-supervised Breast Tumour Segmentation based on super-pixel strategies. At first, an approximate area of tumours in a magnetic resonance imaging (MRI) (namely approximate area) is delineate, by segmenting an MRI based on Otsu threshold method to remove low intensity pixels, and used SLIC super-pixel method to over-segment MRIs. After that, group super-pixels based on the DBSCAN technique in terms of mean intensities and positions of super-pixels. Finally, classify tumour patches to locate tumours in the original image by using an Adaboost-M1 classification algorithm based on 20 texture features and mean intensity levels of patches.

Despite the contribution and the significant improvement brought by super-pixels to model-based segmentation approaches, the fact remains that they are unable to take into account the great variation in mammography mass shapes, as (Carneiro et al. 2015) and (Dhungel et al. 2015b) have recognised. In addition, their performance and robustness is highly dependent on the size and content of the data set, which must be as large and varied as possible; something that is difficult to achieve in medical imaging. The consequence is that the quality of the contour segmentation that these approaches provide is very rough and does not allow an objective assessment of the nature of the mass.

To date, the use of automatic deep-learning image processing techniques represents the most promising direction for breast cancer segmentation.

7.2.3 Deep Learning Techniques

As with the approaches mentioned above, traditional segmentation methods have major limitations that do not promote their deployment in the clinic to perform critical tasks. If an approach is successful, it requires a significant amount of execution time or human interaction. If the approach is automatic and does not require a learning mechanism, it is very sensitive to image noise.

For methods requiring a learning mechanism, a detection phase is almost mandatory because segmentation performance is closely linked to it. Moreover, the choice of features to be extracted is problematic because even this restricts the scope of the method to a specific type of images, where the classifier learns a feature of the structure to be segmented and not its global representation. It also limits the application of this type of method in the case of anatomical structures that are deformed.

The success of DL methods in performing image classification has expanded their use to solve more complex tasks including segmentation by interpreting it as either a regression or discrimination problem. In fact, DL methods, especially CNNs (also known as ConvNets), have gained lots of attentions to medical image segmentation as they help overcome computer-aided diagnosis systems limitations (Litjens et al. 2017, Shen et al. 2017, Hesamian et al. 2019, Domingues et al. 2019, Minaee et al. 2020). We review a number of recent works on Breast Tumours Segmentation Algorithms and cite the most relevant ones.

In Benjelloun et al. (2018), breast tumour segmentation was resolved by the application of deep neural network based on the **U-net** architecture. This architecture improved the principle of the Fully Convolutional Neural Network; the advantage of **U-net** is the operation of concatenation of the feature maps after up-sampling, allowing a better learning of the image representation. For BUS imaging, Almajalid et al. (2018) proposed a modified and improved framework based on DL architecture U-Net. A multi-U-net algorithm is applied in Kumar et al. (2018) to segment suspicious breast masses on ultrasound imaging. To improve the U-Net segmentation performance, Li et al. (2018) developed a Conditional Residual U-Net; also Zhuang et al. (2019) proposed RDAU-NET (Residual Dilated Attention Gate) architecture to segment the lesions in BUS images. The model is based on the classical U-Net network, where simple neural units are replaced by residual units in order to improve the information at the periphery as well as the performance of the network.

Always with U-Net model, Vakanski et al. (2019) employ attention on blocks to introduce visual salience to force learning feature representations that prioritise spatial regions with high levels of salience on BUS images. Schreier et al. (2019) proposed a combination of the U-Net and the ResNet named BibNet for Breast CT image segmentation. The network inherits its basic shape from the U-Net architecture, but connections on all resolution levels are added. These connections process the image and are interconnected with layers of higher and lower resolution levels.

Instead of DL-based models developed for mammography mass segmentation that focus on extracted patches, Sun et al. (2020) proposed a new architecture, AUNet for segmentation of breast masses, it is based on an asymmetrical encoder-decoder structure that uses an effective up-sampling block and attention-guided dense-up-sampling block (AU block) to compensate the loss information caused by bi-linear up-sampling.

In Ragab et al. (2019), a well-known deep convolutional neural network (DCNN) architecture named **AlexNet** is used as the feature extraction tool whereas the last fully connected (FC) layer is connected to the SVM classifier to obtain better accuracy. Jung et al. (2018) proposed a mass detection model based on RetinaNet demonstrating that the implemented model achieves comparable or better performance than more complex state-of-the-art models including the two-stage object detector. In Chiao et al. (2019), mask regions with convolutional neural network (Mask R-CNN) were developed for breast lesions segmentation with ultrasound images.

In Wang et al. (2017), super-pixel-based local binary pattern is proposed to obtain breast tumour candidates as pre-processing to the CNN to avoid complicated feature extraction as well as elevate the accuracy and efficiency.

Semantic segmentation is the task of classifying each and every pixel in an image into a class; in Yap et al. (2019), an end-to-end DL Approach using Fully Convolutional Networks (FCNs), namely, FCN-AlexNet, FCN-32s, FCN-16s and FCN-8s, is proposed for semantic segmentation of BUS lesions. Besides, Shen et al. (2019) proposed also an end-to-end DL approach based on two popular CNN structures, the VGG network and the residual network (Resnet) which are typically constructed by stacking convolutional layers on top of the input, followed by one or more FC layers to join with the classification output for mammography image segmentation.

On another side, Dhungel et al. (2015a, 2017b) have shown an interest on the generative graphical model for Automated Lesion Detection and Segmentation of Breast masses in mammography images. The multi-scale deep belief network (**m-DBN**) classifier is used for a pixel-wise classification over an image grid using input regions of a fixed size at various scales, by next a cascade of deep CNNs and random forest classifiers are applied for false positive reduction stage. As well, a conditional Generative Adversarial Network (**cGAN**) was proposed by Singh et al. (2018, 2020) to segment a breast tumour within a ROI in a mammogram. In Singh et al. (2019), an atrous convolution layer with channel attention and channel weighting is combined to a **cGAN** model in order to enhance the discriminant ability of feature representations at multi-scale in BUS images.

Recent breast cancer detection and classification models have been analysed in the form of a comparative study. The comparative analysis of Hamed et al. (2020) shows that the recent highest accuracy models based on simple breast cancer detection and the classification architectures are You Only Look Once (YOLO) and RetinaNet. Agarwal et al. (2019) compare performances of patch-based CNN methods: VGG16, ResNet50 and InceptionV3 for automated mass detection in full-field digital mammograms. Results show that the InceptionV3 obtains the best performance for classifying the mass and non-mass breast region. Finally, various surveys (Rao et al. 2018, Abdelhafiz et al. 2019) were conducted to review the breast image segmentation solutions proposed in the past decade. All agreed that breast segmentation is still an open and challenging problem and require further investigations for mammography.

7.3 RELATED WORK

A literature search was performed using Google Scholar, on April 29th 2020, by extracting all of the works that cite the INBreast database paper (Moreira et al. 2012). The retrieved papers were trimmed to include only works that use INBreast in the experimental setting and that concern simultaneously mass detection and segmentation. Moreover, all works not written in English were excluded.

The first work attempting mass detection using INBreast was Koozegar et al. (2013) and Kozegar et al. (2013), where an algorithm inspired by binary search was proposed, reaching a sensitivity of 87% (the algorithm missed 15 masses) with a false positive rate per image (FPI) of 3.67. In Domingues (2014), an iris filter was used achieving a sensitivity of 38% with 5 FPI. A dual-view analysis is made in Amit et al. (2015), providing an area under the Receiver Operating Characteristic (ROC) curve of 0.94, and sensitivity of 87% at 90% specificity of detection. Min et al. (2017) use multi-scale morphological filtering combined with self-adaptive cascade of random forests, achieving 0.94 of average sensitivity at 1.99 FPI. In his Master's dissertation, Oliveira (2018) tests three methods, Graph-Based Visual Saliency, Watershed and Iris Filter, concluding that saliency achieves better performances with 5 FPI, 0.686 true positive rate (TPR), an area overlap of 0.396, a combined measure of 0.560, and a Dice score of 0.520. In Min et al. (2019a), region candidate selection by multi-scale morphological sifting combined with cascaded learning techniques is used, achieving 0.90 average sensitivity at 0.9 FPI. Belhaj Soulami et al. (2020) assess the performance of several evolutionary algorithms, with invasive weed optimisation achieving best results in fatty (0.45 Cohens Kappa, 0.46 correlation, 0.01 FPI, 0.12 false negative rate – FNR) and fatty-glandular (0.45 Cohen's Kappa, 0.48 correlation, 0.01 FPI, 0.12 FNR) breast tissue categories, artificial bee colony being best for dense breasts (0.38 Cohens Kappa, 0.40 correlation, 0.02 FPI, 0.25 FNr), and genetic algorithm for extremely dense breast tissue (0.30 Cohen's Kappa, 0.23 correlation, 0.01 FPI, 0.28 FNR). Fuzzy level sets are used in Sasikala et al. (2020) with accuracy of 79.1%, at sensitivity of 75.5% and specificity of 84.8%.

Several conclusions can be drawn from the above analysis. For one, it is clear that there is not a "winner" technique in what refers to non-DL methods. All the works use different techniques. Another observation is that super-pixel classification, as to be used in the present work, has not been attempted yet. Concerning evaluation metrics, there is also not a clear consensus, with Recall (or sensitivity) and FPI being more frequently used. Overall, non-DL methods seem to have Recalls between 38% and 94% with a number of FPI between 0.9 and 5, and Dice of 0.520.

Using DL, and to the best of our knowledge, the first work was the one in Domingues and Cardoso (2013) where an auto-encoder was used, but no quantitative results are presented. In Dhungel et al. (2015a), a cascade of DL and random forest classifiers is used achieving a TPR of 0.96 at 1.2 FPI. Dhungel et al. (2017a) break the problem into three parts, detection, segmentation and classification, detecting 90% of masses at 1 FPI, having a Dice score of around 0.85 for segmentation of the correctly detected masses, and sensitivity of 0.98 at specificity of 0.7 for binary classification. In Al-antari et al. (2018), the problem was also subdivided in the same stages, although different deep learning techniques were used for each stage, reaching 98.96% of detection accuracy; 92.97% of segmentation accuracy, 92.69% Dice (F1-score) and 86.37% Jaccard similarity; and 95.64% classification accuracy with 94.78% AUC and 96.84% F1-score. The model used in Cerqueira (2018) extends the RetinaNet architecture by adding additional outputs obtaining an Average Precision of 0.62 at an Intersection over Union (IoU) threshold of 0.5. In Diaz et al. (2018), the resnet-50 CNN architecture pre-trained with the ImageNet database is used achieving 0.92 accuracy with an AUC of 0.98, 17 false negatives and 843 false positives. Ribli et al. (2018) use Faster R-CNN, achieving a sensitivity of 0.9 at 0.3 FPI. The popular U-Net is used in Wang (2018), with 0.2503 Dice score, 0.3239 precision, 0.4026 recall, 0.2703 IoU, 0.3848 average precision and 0.4618 average recall. A unified framework for whole-mammogram classification and segmentation is presented in Zhang et al. (2018) with Dice score of 0.85. Hamidinekoo et al. (2019) use Conditional GANs with a U-Net-based structure as a generator and a convolutional PatchGAN classifier as the discriminator, with accuracy of 34%, precision of 34%, recall of 32%, an F-score of 0.33, Dice score of 0.33 and Hausdorff distance of 8.33. In Min et al. (2019b), a mass detection-segmentation based on Mask R-CNN is used after pseudo-colour image generation, achieving 0.90 average TPR at 0.9 FPI and 0.88 average Dice similarity for mass segmentation. In his PhD thesis, (Gao (2019) and Gao et al. (2020) jointly address detection, segmentation and classification, achieving 0.91 TPR at 3.67 FPI and 0.76 Dice score. In Shen et al. (2020b), a two-stage framework is derived with suspicious region localisation and multi-context multi-task learning, with 0.919 TPR at 0.12 FPI. In Yan et al. (2019), mass segmentation is performed directly, without any pre-detection, using multi-scale cascade of deep convolutional encoder-decoders, with Dice, sensitivity and specificity of 70.04%, 72.19% and 99.61%, respectively. Sun et al. (2020) use an attention-guided dense up-sampling network (AUNet), achieving a Dice score of 79.1%, sensitivity of 80.8%, relative area difference of 37.6% and Hausdorff distance of 4.04. The chapter (Al-antari et al. 2020) presents a CAD system based on YOLO for detection, FrCN for segmentation, and InceptionResNet-V2 for classification, reaching 97.27% accuracy at 0.25 FPI, 93.93% Matthewss correlation coefficient (MCC), and 98.02 F1 for detection and 92.36% Dice, 85.81% Jaccard, 92.94% sensitivity, 92.47% specificity, 92.69% accuracy, 92.70% AUC, 85.36% MCC for segmentation. Tardy and Mateus (2020) design a training process based on a modified U-Net using both benign and malignant data for training, with Dice score of 0.59. Shen et al. (2020a) propose an unsupervised domain adaptation framework with adversarial learning and have reached 0.8522 area under the free-response ROC curve and 0.8788 TPR at 0.5 FPIs. In Yan et al. (2020), mass detection is performed by YOLO extended by integrating multi-scale predictions, while segmentation is achieved with a convolutional encoder-decoder network with nested and dense skip connections attaining Dice of 80.44%.

When looking at the state-of-the-art on the use of DL for mass detection and segmentation, similar conclusions to the ones made for the non-DL methods can be drawn. There is not a method that is consistently used with virtually all papers using different techniques. While some authors have tested U-Net based architectures, as is done in the present work, we note that FPN and LinkNet have not been experimented with before. Concerning numerical results, Dice scores vary between 0.2503 and 0.9269, IoU between 0.2703 and 0.5, Recall (or sensitivity) between 32% and 98%, and Precision between 0.3239 and 0.62.

7.4   METHODS

Accurate diagnoses of diseases depend on image acquisition and interpretation. Although machine learning is widely used for computer vision applications, traditional machine learning algorithms for image interpretation rely heavily on experts for several tasks such as extraction of ROI. Machine learning has evolved over the last few years by its ability to shift through complex and big data.

Advances in DL have turned the world of healthcare upside down. Proof of this is the multiple applications of DL in medical imaging applications brought in annual challenges around the word.

Faced with these findings, a question arises: *is it the end of classical machine learning methods for the segmentation of medical images?* In this chapter, we propose a comparative study between these two components in the context of the segmentation of masses in breast images.

For traditional machine learning approach, we study a super-pixel-based classification process, obverse to three different architectures of CNNs which are presented below.

7.4.1 SUPER-PIXEL-BASED SEGMENTATION

Currently, two concepts are at the origin of notable advances:

- Super-pixels, which are a way of summarising the information contained in an image;
- Supervised machine learning, which includes a series of methods capable of learning to predict behaviour or classify data, based on a few examples.

Segmentation by super-pixel classification is a technique commonly used in various fields, particularly in the medical field. Several works (Ilesanmi et al. 2020, da Silva et al. 2020, Cheng et al. 2013, Wang et al. 2020) have exploited super-pixel-based algorithms to segment and classify regions of interest.

The challenges of divergent inputs and high-dimensional characteristics in relation to samples have made super-pixels key building blocks for many computer vision algorithms. A super-pixel is an image patch, which allows for better alignment of intensity edges than a rectangular patch. It captures redundancy in the image and reduces the complexity of subsequent processing. Indeed, the super-pixel can cause substantial acceleration in processing time, since the number of super-pixels in an image ranges from 25 to 2500, as opposed to the hundreds of thousands of pixels in an image. Beyond the construction of super-pixels on the image, it allows to work locally on the extracted information while reducing processing time considerably.

In this work, we propose a super-pixel-based segmentation framework for breast masses as a classical method to be compared to DL approaches. The proposed process is divided into four steps as illustrated in Figure 7.1.

- Step 1: Image pre-processing;
- Step 2: Generate the super-pixel breast images by the Simple Linear Iterative Clustering algorithm;
- Step 3: Super-pixel Feature extraction, based on first-order statistics (FOS);
- Step 4: Super-pixel classification with Random Forests.

Pre-processing: In this work, we apply contrast-limited adaptive histogram equalisation (CLAHE) (Yadav et al. 2014) on breast cancer images as a pre-processing step.

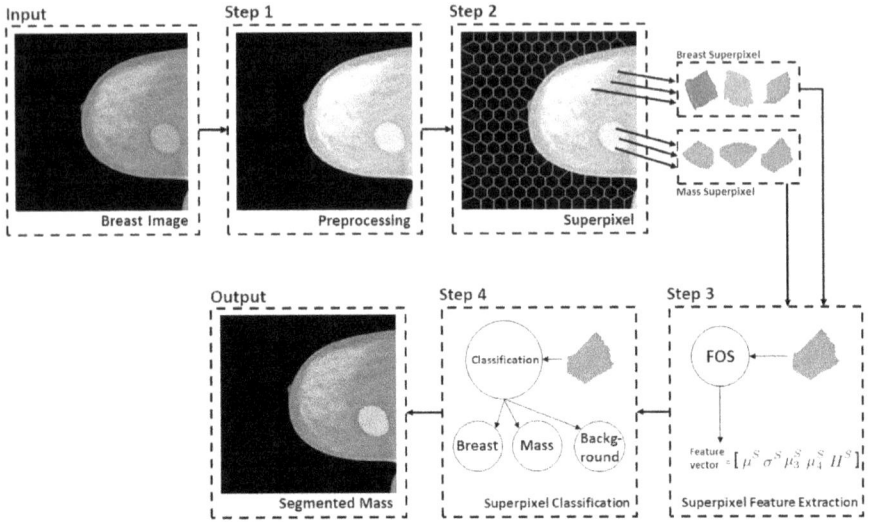

FIGURE 7.1 Super-pixel-based segmentation framework for breast masses.

This method was originally proposed for the enhancement of low-contrast medical images (Pisano et al. 1998, Jintasuttisak and Intajag 2014).

The CLAHE method is based on the histogram equalisation to enhance each contextual region. The steps of this technique are detailed in Ma et al. (2018).

In short, the CLAHE method consists of homogenising the distribution of pixels and amplifying the intensity by clipping the histogram at an user-defined value called clip-limit. The clipping level reflects the amount of noise in the histogram and the degree of contrast enhancement. The input image is divided into non-overlapping contextual regions called tiles, whose size is set by the user, generally at 8.

Super-pixels by SLIC: The SLIC algorithm (Achanta et al. 2012) is probably one of the most famous methods for cutting an image into super-pixels. Its general algorithm is as follows:

1. Pixels are initially grouped into rectangular and regular super-pixels.
2. Each super-pixel is described by its average colour and the location of its barycentre.
3. Each pixel is reassigned to the super-pixel it is closest to in terms of colour and location
4. Steps 2 and 3 are repeated until the super-pixels are stable.

The speed of SLIC and the quality of the results it produces have ensured its immense popularity in computer vision methods. Several implementations of this algorithm are available. We will use the one from the Scikit-image library.

In addition to the image, two parameters are supplied to the SLIC function: the number of desired super-pixels (n segments) and a compactness parameter, which measures the influence of the location of the pixel in relation to its colour.

In this work, several sizes of super-pixels are tested. High compactness favours regular super-pixels, close to the initial rectangles. Generally, it is recommended to give a value between 10 and 20. Beyond that, the super-pixels produced tend not to follow the edges of objects.

Super-Pixel Feature Extraction: Feature extraction is a component of image processing that often goes hand in hand with classification. Indeed, to establish a classification rule (supervised or unsupervised), it is generally based on a set of numerical criteria describing the object or the observed phenomenon. The same is applicable at the super-pixel level.

In this step, we will describe each super-pixel by five numerical values representing the FOS which correspond to mean level, variance, third and four statistical moments, and entropy.

Mean: Mean is formulated in Equation (7.1), where image intensity is usually represented by a mean value.

$$\mu_s = \sum_{i \in sp}^{n} p_i H(p_i) \tag{7.1}$$

with n being the number of distinctive grey levels, p_i is the grey value of the ith pixel in superpixel S and $H(p_i)$ is the normalised histogram.

Variance: Variance corresponds to the intensity variation around the mean (Equation 7.2).

$$\sigma^s = \sqrt{\sum_{i \in SP}^{n} \left(P_i - \mu^s\right)^2 H(P_i)} \tag{7.2}$$

The third and four statistical moments: The third and four statistical moments are very powerful attributes. A moment μ_{ij} is a weighted sum of all pixels according to their positions in the image. In 1962, the seven moments of Hu were proposed (Hu 1962); in our work, we use μ_3^S and μ_4^S moments applied to super-pixels S as shown in Equations (7.3) and (7.4), respectively.

$$\mu_3^S = \sigma^{s-3} = \sqrt{\sum_{i \in SP}^{n} \left(P_i - \mu^s\right)^{-3} H(P_i)} \tag{7.3}$$

$$\mu_4^S = \sigma^{s-4} = \sqrt{\sum_{i \in SP}^{n} \left(P_i - \mu^s\right)^{-4} H(P_i)} - 3 \tag{7.4}$$

Entropy: Entropy is a measure of histogram consistency, where the histogram uniformity is measured (Equations 7.5).

$$H^S = -\sum_{i \in SP}^{n} P_i \log_2[\mathrm{H}(P_i)] \tag{7.5}$$

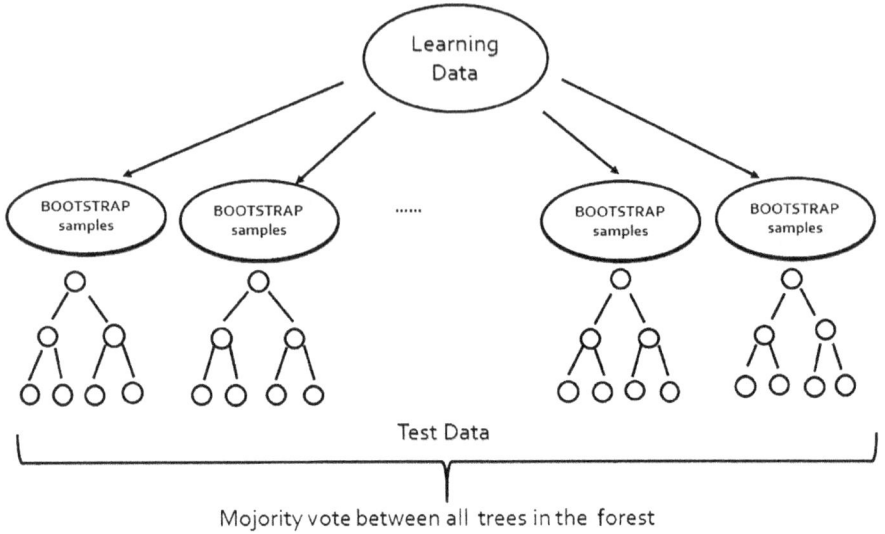

FIGURE 7.2   Schematic illustration of the random forest algorithm.

Super-Pixel Classification: In recent years, ensemble methods have become one of the most popular lines of research as they allow adding the global behaviour to the individual behaviour, which significantly improves the obtained performance in classification compared to classical methods, i.e. the use of a single classifier. Among the most fundamental ensemble methods, the random forest as a non-parametric statistical method is the most used in the current literature. Applied to many classification and regression problems, this method has demonstrated its high performance capacity, high robustness as well as its ability to preserve data variability with low time cost. Introduced by L. Breiman (2001), the main idea of the algorithm as described in Figure 7.2 is based on the aggregation of a collection of independent and identically distributed decision trees on bootstrap samples of the same size formed from the original input data.

7.4.2 DEEP LEARNING APPROACH

Segmentation and automatic recognition have become an important contribution in computer aided diagnosis. The traditional method is based on techniques for extracting and selecting information such as edges, colours, and textures from the image. CNNs are modern and efficient segmentation methods, which have been widely applied in medical image segmentation.

CNNs were initiated by Fukushima (1980) in the Neocognitron, based on the hierarchical receptive field model of the visual cortex. Waibel et al. (1989) developed a CNN model with shared weights and back-propagation training for phoneme recognition, and Lecun et al. (1998) proposed a CNN architecture for document recognition.

The CNNs consist mainly of a number of layers, each with a role to play.

Three of the main types of layers include as follows:

1. Convolutional layers, a filter is convoluted with the image to extract features of the image.
2. ReLu layers, which applies an activation function to feature maps.
3. Pooling layers, to apply a reduction of spatial information on the feature maps.

The layers are connected together to form a pyramid, the higher level layers extract global features and the deep layers extract detail features. Several works have proposed CNN architectures to address the issue of segmentation. In this work, we made a selection of architectures to study them.

U-Net: Ronneberger et al. (2015) has become a reference in many biomedical image segmentation tasks. Figure 7.3 illustrates the architecture of the network. U-Net architecture consists of five encoding layers and five decoding layers. The difference between the encoding and the decoding unit is the concatenation of the feature maps and the up-convolution layer. The role of the decoding unit is to return to the starting image which represents the result of the segmentation.

FPN: Lin et al. (2017) proposed an architecture called FPN; this CNN network is based on a pyramid construction. The construction of the pyramid involves a bottom-up pathway, a top-down pathway and lateral connections, as introduced in Figure 7.4.

Bottom-up pathway: The bottom-up pathway is the feed-forward computation of convolution of the input image; this pathway has to calculate a feature hierarchy consisting of feature maps at several scales. The creation of the pyramid is done by the last convolution layer of each stage, which represents the reference set of feature maps. The strongest features will be extracted on the deepest layer of each stage.

Top-down pathway and lateral connections: The role of the top-down pathway is to bring together the different feature maps of the pyramid by up-sampling spatially coarser, but semantically stronger, feature maps from higher pyramid levels. The up-sampling features are enhanced with features from the bottom-up pathway via

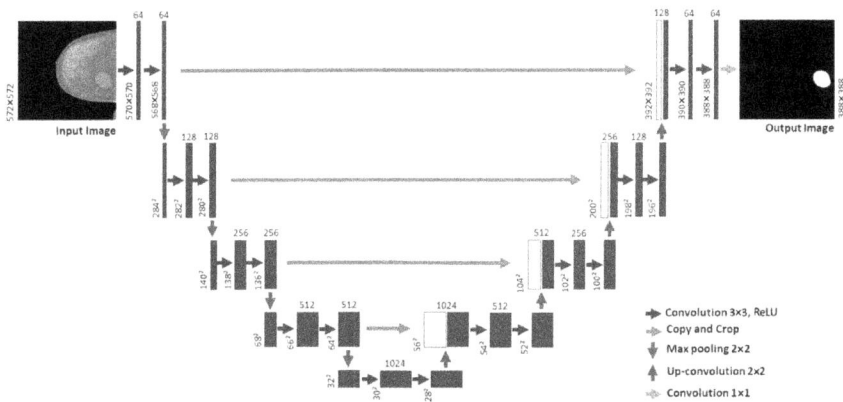

FIGURE 7.3 Schematic representation of the U-Net network.

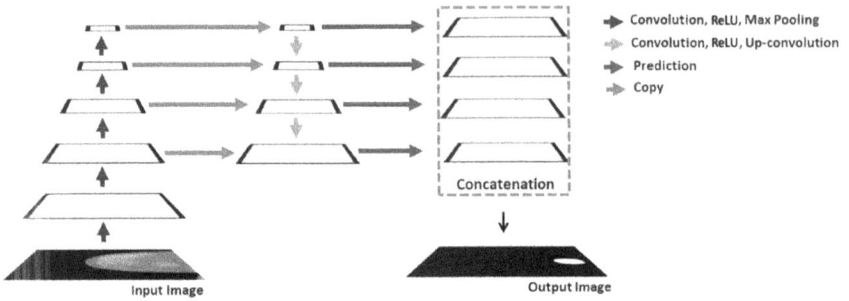

FIGURE 7.4 Schematic representation of the FPN network.

lateral connections. The lateral connection is proposed to merge feature cards from the bottom-up pathway and the top-down pathway.

LinkNet: Chaurasia and Culurciello (2017) proposed a LinkNet architecture to exploit encoder representations for efficient semantic segmentation. It is a simple architecture that looks a lot like the UNET architecture, which deviates in two parts (encoder and decoder part).

Figure 7.5 illustrates the architecture of LinkNet, the encoding part is made up of four encoding blocks and the same for the decoding part. The architecture begins with a convolution block on the input image with a kernel of size 7 7, a stride of two and spatial max-pooling.

Convolutional layer details encoder and decoder blocks that are provided in Figure 7.6. The novelty of LinkNet lies in the way in which the connection between

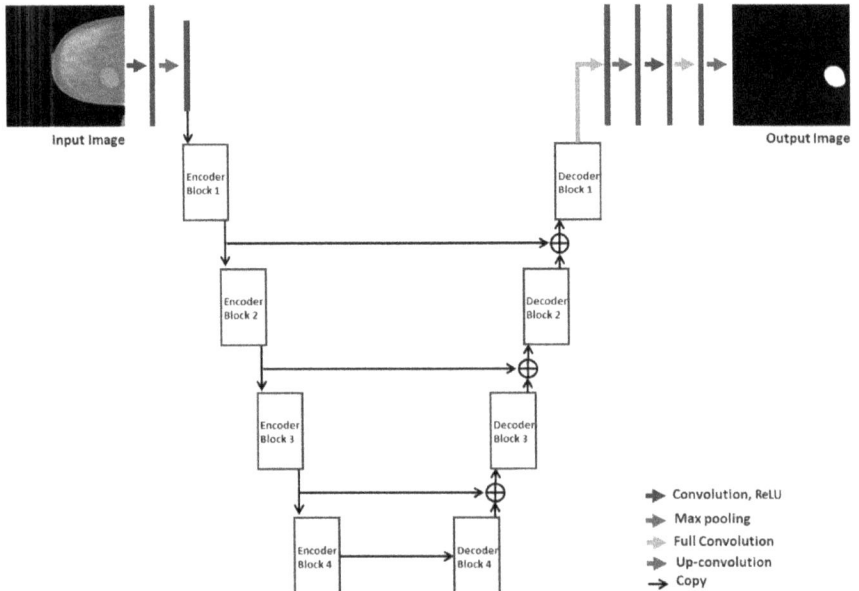

FIGURE 7.5 Schematic representation of the LinkNet network.

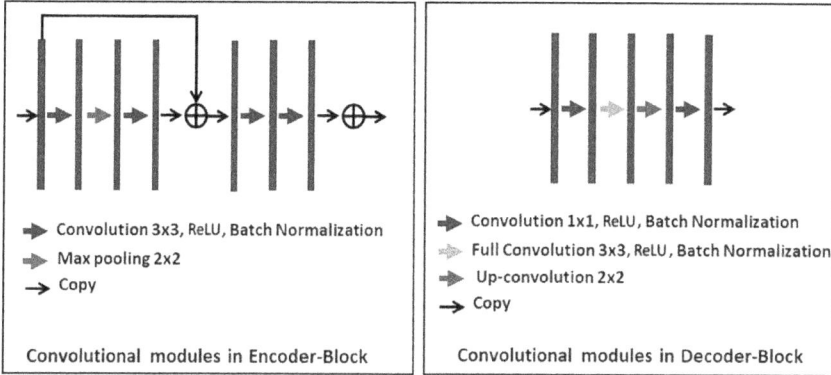

FIGURE 7.6 Convolutional modules in encoder and decoder block.

encoder and decoder blocks. This connection has to retrieve spatial information that was lost during down-sampling operations in the encoder block.

7.4.3 EXPERIMENTAL SETTING

This section focuses on the experimental setting. We start by describing the database, then we detail the implementation details, and finally, we list the used evaluation metrics.

Database experiments were performed using the INBreast database (Moreira et al. 2012).

INBreast gathers data from 205 breasts with mediolateral oblique (MLO) and craniocaudal (CC) views (making a total of 410 images). Images area ranges from 8 to 14 10^6 pixels^2 (average area of 11 10^6 pixels^2) with an average height of 2.9 10^3 and an average width of 3.6 10^3 (Domingues et al. 2012). The database includes examples of normal mammograms, mammograms with masses, mammograms with calcifications, architectural distortions, asymmetries and images with multiple findings (Domingues 2014). INBreast also comes with annotations, detailed contours of the findings, made by a specialist radiologist in the field and validated by a second specialist (Domingues 2014).

In this work, we are interested in the segmentation of breast masses. For this, we have selected only the images bearing a breast mass for our experiments. The data set was split into 61 images for training, 7 for validation and 12 for testing. Each image in our experiments has been resized to 512×512 pixels.

Implementation details: For segmentation by super-pixel classification, we need to adjust the pre-processing and SLIC algorithm. The SLIC algorithm requires a configuration of the number of super-pixels and the compactness; we carried out several tests to choose the optimal configuration which is 500 for super-pixel and 0.05 for compactness.

Following super-pixel feature extraction, we realised that the extracted features are highly unbalanced between mass and breast features. Indeed, we exploit artificial intelligence techniques to solve this problem. We have used in our experiments the synthetic minority over-sampling technique (Chawla et al. 2002) to balance the data.

For the segmentation by CNN, we applied data augmentation to enrich the training set. The training calculation was carried out by exploiting the resources of COLAB[1] provided by GOOGLE.

A Github repository provides all implementation details which the code and the additional materials publicly available in.[2]

Evaluation Metrics: For the evaluation and comparison of the different proposed methods, four widely used metrics in the medical segmentation imaging field are applied to assess the utility of automatic segmentation of images to delineate isolated tumour masses in mammography images.

Dice Coefficient (D_C): The Dice coefficient (D_C) is a measure of similarity. This coefficient is used in statistics to determine the similarity between two samples. For the segmentation evaluation, the coefficient gives the similarity between the segmentation result Y and ground truth $\hat{Y}$. The Dice coefficient is calculated as

$$D_c = \frac{2\left|Y \cap \hat{Y}\right|}{|Y| + |\hat{Y}|}$$

The D_c coefficient is always between 0 (criteria must be met) and 1 (acceptable match).

Intersection-Over-Union or Jaccard Index (IoU): The Intersection-Over-Union (IoU) is the ratio between the cardinality (size) of the intersection of the considered sets and the cardinality of the union of the sets. It allows to evaluate the similarity between sets and to measure the accuracy of an object detector on a data set.

$$IoU(Y\hat{Y}) = \frac{Y \cap \hat{Y}}{Y \cup \hat{Y}}$$

It should be noted that in segmentation tasks, the IoU is preferred over accuracy as it is not affected by the class imbalance that is inherent in foreground/background segmentation tasks.

Recall (or sensitivity): Recall is the proportion of relevant items proposed among all relevant items:

$$\text{Recall} = \frac{\text{TP}}{\text{TP} + \text{FN}}$$

Precision (or positive predictive value): Precision is the proportion of relevant items among the set of items proposed:

    with

$$\text{Precision} = \frac{\text{TP}}{\text{TP} + \text{FP}}$$

---

[1] https://www.colab.research.google.com
[2] https://github.com/MEABECHAR/Deep-learning-vs
  -Superpixel-classification-for-breast-masses-segmentation

- *TP* (True Positives): number of positive pixels classified as positive.
- *FP* (False Positives): number of negative pixels classified as positive.
- *FN* (False Negatives): number of negative pixels classified as positive.

7.5   RESULTS

In this section, we first provide a detailed experimental study on super-pixel-based segmentation which concerns the compromise between the number of super-pixel and compactness. Then, we provide the quantitative and qualitative performance of the Unet, FPN and LinkNet DL -based segmentation models and super-pixel-based segmentation.

7.5.1   SUPER-PIXELS-BASED SEGMENTATION

The process of super-pixels-based segmentation is divided into several steps. The super-pixel calculation is a fundamental step in this process; the number and the compactness of super-pixel are the most important parameters to study because they can influence the segmentation results.

In the first part, we perform a qualitative analysis of the compactness on several mass images. The number of super-pixels has been fixed at 500 and we have varied the compactness between 0.01, 0.05, 0.5 and 5. Figure 7.7 shows an example of a super-pixel calculation.

The qualitative analysis of several mass images has shown that the best value for compactness that generates better super-pixel quality while preserving the contours of the breast mass is 0.05. We estimate that it is the optimal value of the compactness which delimits well the breast mass as is shown in Figure 7.7; this value will be used to carry out our experiments.

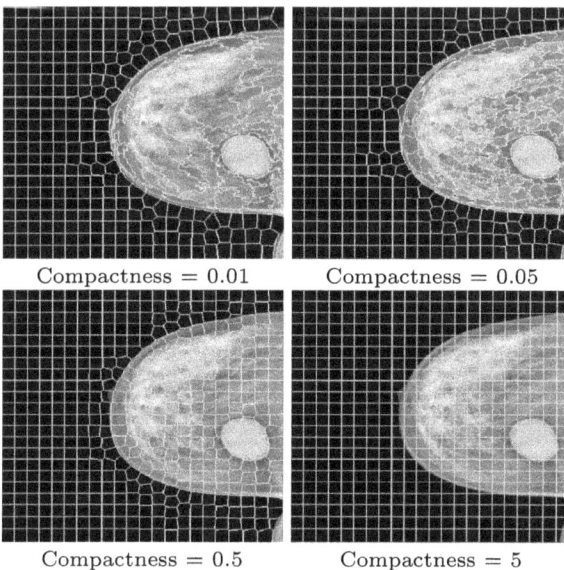

FIGURE 7.7   An example of a super-pixel calculation with different compactness values.

TABLE 7.1
Super-Pixels-Based Segmentation Results

Super-Pixels Number	D_c	IoC	Recall	Precision
100	0.069	0.059	0,059	0.082
200	0.351	0.267	0.504	0.378
300	0.390	0.277	0.539	0.384
400	0.427	0.310	0.583	0.403
500	0.491	0.353	0.702	0.441
600	0.363	0.258	0.485	0.300
700	0.349	0.238	0.534	0.316
800	0.340	0.232	0.518	0.314
900	0.339	0.230	0.454	0.327
1,000	0.300	0.197	0.499	0.262

In the second part, we studied what number of super-pixels should be used to achieve the best segmentation results. In this experiment, we studied the segmentation of different super-pixel values on our experimentation data. The compactness was fixed at 0.05 and we varied the number of super-pixels, and the segmentation results are shown in Table 7.1. The comparison of these results shows that the segmentation results are less efficient if we reduce or increase the number of super-pixels. However, the best segmentation result was obtained by a generation of 500 super-pixels as shown in Figure 7.8.

7.5.2 DEEP LEARNING MODELS

We set out to study the performance of breast mass segmentation by machine learning; we made a comparison between a traditional segmentation technique (super-pixel-based segmentation) and a modern segmentation technique (segmentation by CNN). The results of this comparison are summarised in Table 7.2 (see page 144); the quantitative results clearly show that modern methods performance outperforms the traditional method performance. Some examples of segmentation outputs can be seen in Figure 7.8. If the mass is easy to segment, the traditional technique can effectively solve the segmentation (Example: Image 1 in Figure 7.8), but the segmentation fails if the mass is difficult to segment (Example: Images 2 and 3 in Figure 7.8).

Indeed, the quantitative and qualitative results obtained by modern techniques show the effectiveness and robustness of CNN in the segmentation of breast masses, the U-Net network has given better results in comparison with FPN and LinkNet network, because the U-Net network is originally proposed to solve medical problems.

7.6 GENERAL SYNTHESIS

One of the main advantages of DL is that it does not require structured data. The system works from several layers of neural networks, so it is able to work from unstructured data. This approach is particularly suitable for complex tasks, where not all

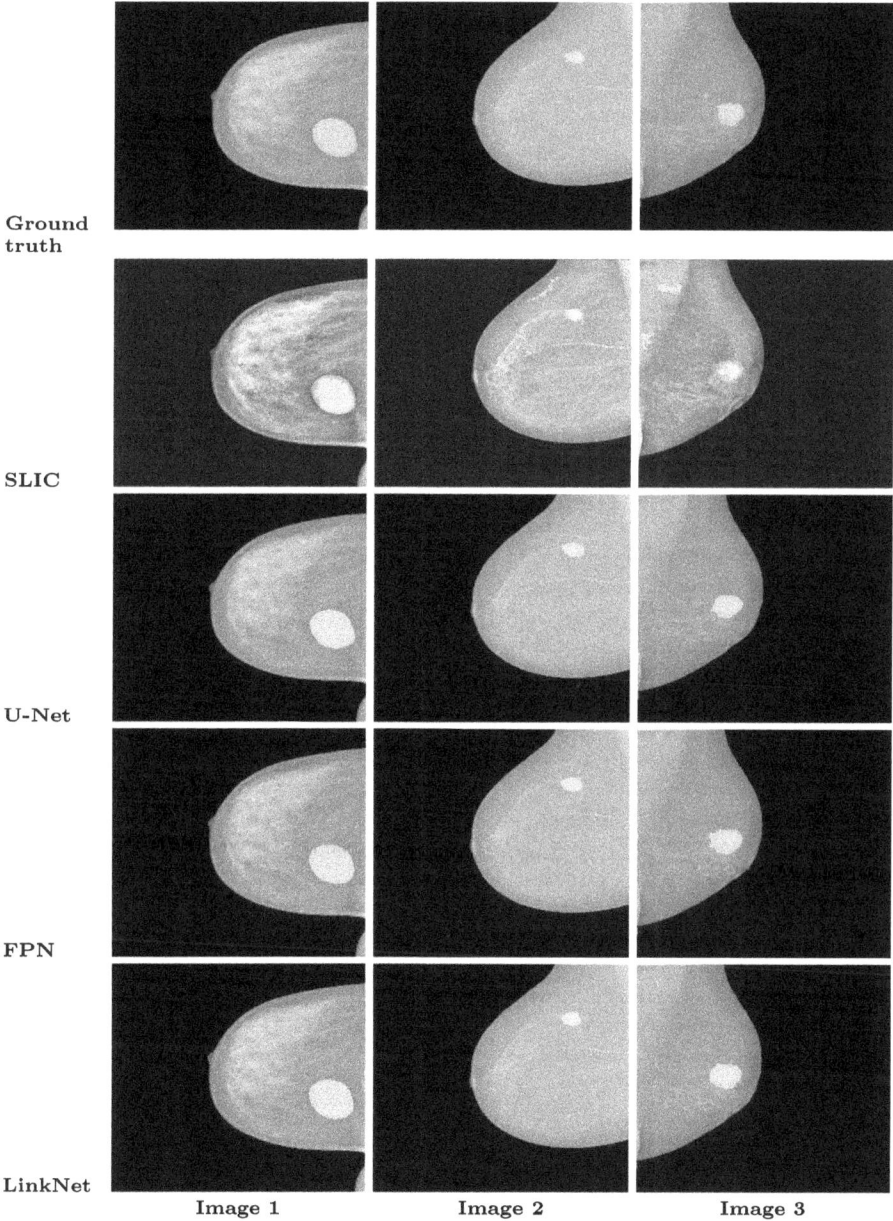

FIGURE 7.8 Results of automatic segmentation.

aspects of the objects to be processed can be categorised beforehand. Indeed, traditional machine learning algorithms almost always require structured data, whereas DL networks rely on layers of the ANNs. In addition, the technology required for DL is more sophisticated. It requires more IT resources and is significantly more expensive than traditional machine learning techniques (Marcus 2019).

TABLE 7.2

Comparison of Results Algorithm Dice Coefficient IoU Recall Precision

Algorithm	Dice Coefficient	IoU	Recall	Precision
SLIC	0.491	0.353	0.702	0.441
U-Net	0.833	0.722	0.947	0.757
FPN	0.712	0.603	0.852	0.619
LinkNet	0.796	0.677	0.945	0.695

Table 7.3 summarises the main differences between traditional machine learning techniques and DL techniques. However, Marcus (2019) presents several concerns for DL and temper some irrational exuberance to consider what we might need to move forward for a more generalised systems.

For segmentation task, we study here two approaches: *superpixel-based methods* and *DL approaches*. The first one is an approach seen as the result of a classification of super-pixels. A super-pixel is a local and coherent mid-level structure. It has a spatial support that is noticeably more consistent but less regular in shape than that of a patch (regularly shaped area). Several works have proved that these approaches allow building relevant segmentation, and this thanks to the contribution of super-pixels that build clear groupings from the point of view of appearance, geometry and semantics.

The second one is the DL models through its CNNs and the success it shows in image segmentation due to its performance and its ability to generalise on various data. This capability is conditional on the availability of a large amount of annotated data, which is very difficult to obtain in the medical context where the restriction of access to medical images is a serious obstacle.

Form his study, G. Marcus (2019) suggest that DL model must be supplemented by other techniques if we reach an artificial general intelligence.

TABLE 7.3

Traditional Machine Learning Techniques and Deep Learning Techniques Comparison

	Traditional machine Learning Techniques	DL
Data organisation	Structured data	Unstructured data
Database	Controllable	Large-scale data
Training	Human training required	Need to fix architecture for autonomous learning
Algorithm	Various Machine Learning Algorithm, (Neural Network includes)	Only Neural Network Algorithms
Applications	Simple routine actions	Complex tasks

Recent studies proposed to combine the previous literature DL models efforts in accurate biomedical image segmentation with a super-pixel strategy since that combination removes the need for low-level feature engineering. Generally, most works (Blanco et al. 2020, Albayrak and Bilgin 2018, Qin et al. 2018) applied super-pixels as a pre-segmentation method, where it can significantly reduce algorithmic complexity while ensuring interactive time.

Blanco et al. (2020) combines DL models with super-pixel-driven segmentation methods for dermatological ulcers. The proposed approach adopts a divide-and-conquer strategy through only a few labelled images, from which hundreds of thousands of super-pixels can be automatically extracted and used for the training of CNNs. In Albayrak and Bilgin (2018), super-pixels are used as pre-segmentation algorithm to perform segmentation of renal cell carcinoma on WSI images. Each super-pixel obtained in the first stage was resized to be used as a regular input image to the proposed CNN algorithms. The results showed that super-pixel segmentation algorithm combined with CNN algorithm could perform accurate results in segmentation of histopathological images. A super-pixel-based and boundary sensitive convolutional neural network pipeline was developed in Qin et al. (2018) for automated liver segmentation. The CNN framework is based on super-pixels and the saliency maps from CT images. The entropy-based saliency map is used to guide the patch sampling and only keeping informative patches by eliminating the redundant ones; this will result in a decreasing training patch size, leading to significantly improved computational efficiency and robustness.

Based on the assumptions that super-pixel images are visually perceivable to humans, but the conventionally trained DL model (trained using only raw images) often performs poorly when working on super-pixel images. Zhang et al. (2019) proposed a new super-pixel-based data augmentation method that consistently improve the performance of state-of-the-art FCNs for 2D and 3D biomedical image segmentation.

Rather than working on the pixel grid directly, Zohourian et al. (2018) also make the choice of using super-pixels to reduce the computational complexity as pre-segmentation step and feed image descriptors extracted from these regions into a CNN for real-time segmentation of road systems. For classification task, in Gonzalo-Martin et al. (2016), super-pixels were applied as a strategy to reduce CNN time classification of remote sensing images. The idea behind the combination of super-pixels with CNN is that super-pixels are expected to maintain all the characteristics of a reduced environment inside of the area learned by a CNN which saves considerable time.

Jampani et al. (2018) initiate to incorporate super-pixels into deep network by proposing a new differentiable model for super-pixel sampling that leverages deep networks for learning super-pixel segmentation. This combination of a deep network with superpixels forms an end-to-end trainable super-pixel algorithm which is called super-pixel sampling network.

To answer our initial question: *are we facing the end of traditional machine learning segmentation methods?* We can say that the context and the challenges of the application are always essential for the choice of the appropriate approaches. However, from the study carried out, it is obvious that the contribution of super-pixels is not negligible; we believe that in the future, the segmentation of mammography images through convolutional networks using paired super-pixels aims at a better precise localisation of tumour structures.

7.7 CONCLUSIONS AND FUTURE WORK

We presented a comparative study between a traditional and a modern technique for breast masses segmentation. In the traditional technique, we have studied a super-pixels-based segmentation process which is divided into several steps, pre-processing, super-pixel generation, super-pixel feature extraction and super-pixel classification. In the modern technique, we have studied different CNN architecture for segmentation; it is a completely automatic technique to calculate features.

The segmentation of the breast mass was carried out on the INBreast database; the obtained results show that the CNN methods clearly surpass the classical method. The effectiveness of CNN methods relies on the ability of convolution in training and extracting relevant features which results in better segmentation. The failure of the traditional method in segmentation can be explained by the quality of the used features which are not effective in distinguishing between mass and breast super-pixels.

The deep-learning neural network was able to realise the accurate segmentation of the breast mass. The super-pixel method retained the mass boundary information to a large extent. In the future, we will further investigate this work by combining the advantages of super-pixel and the power of deep-learning; this combination can be carried out according to different strategies, like the superpixel in pre-processing or the superpixel is integrated into the convolutional layers of the network. We would like to design a new convolutional layer based on the super-pixel to make a more accurate segmentation model.

ACKNOWLEDGMENTS

The authors would like to thank the Directorate-General of Scientific Research and Technological Development (Direction Générale de la Recherche Scientifique et du Développement Technologique, DGRSDT, URL: www.dgrsdt.dz, Algeria) for the financial assistance towards this research.

REFERENCES

Abdelhafiz, D., Yang, C., Ammar, R., and Nabavi, S. (2019). Deep convolutional neural networks for mammography: advances, challenges and applications. *BMC Bioinformatics*, 20(S11): 281.

Achanta, R., Shaji, A., Smith, K., Lucchi, A., Fua, P., and Susstrunk, S. (2012). Slic superpixels compared to state-of-the-art superpixel methods. *IEEE Transactions on Pattern Analysis and Machine Intelligence*, 34(11): 2274– 2282.

Agarwal, R., Diaz, O., Llad'o, X., Yap, M. H., and Mart'i, R. (2019). Automatic mass detection in mammograms using deep convolutional neural networks. *Journal of Medical Imaging*, 6(03): 1.

Al-antari, M. A., Al-masni, M. A., Choi, M.-T. T., Han, S.-M. M., and Kim, T.-S. S. (2018). A fully integrated computer-aided diagnosis system for digital X-ray mammograms via deep learning detection, segmentation, and classification. *International Journal of Medical Informatics*, 117(June): 44–54.

Al-antari, M. A., Al-masni, M. A., and Kim, T.-S. (2020). Deep learning computer-aided diagnosis for breast lesion in digital mammogram. In Eds. Gobert LeeHiroshi Fujita, *Deep Learning in Medical Image Analysis*, pp. 59–72. Springer, Cham.

Albayrak, A. and Bilgin, G. (2018). A hybrid method of superpixel segmentation algorithm and deep learning method in histopathological image segmentation. In Innovations in Intelligent Systems and Applications (INISTA), pp. 1–5. IEEE, Thessaloniki.

Almajalid, R., Shan, J., Du, Y., and Zhang, M. (2018). Development of a deep-learning-based method for breast ultrasound image segmentation. In *17th IEEE International Conference on Machine Learning and Applications (ICMLA)*, pp. 1103–1108, Orlando, FL, USA.

Amit, G., Hashoul, S., Kisilev, P., Ophir, B., Walach, E., and Zlotnick, A. (2015). Automatic dual-view mass detection in full-field digital mammograms. In *International Conference on Medical Image Computing and Computer Assisted Intervention*, pp. 44–52. Springer, Cham.

Angayarkanni, S. P., Kamal, N. B., and Thangaiya, R. J. (2015). Dynamic graph cut based segmentation of mammogram. *SpringerPlus*, 4(1): 591.

Anitha, J. and Peter, J. D. (2015). Mass segmentation in mammograms using a kernel-based fuzzy level set method. *International Journal of Biomedical Engineering and Technology*, 19(2): 133.

Bechar, M. E. A., Settouti, N., Daho, M. E. H., Adel, M., and Chikh, M. A. (2019). Influence of normalization and color features on super-pixel classification: application to cytological image segmentation. *Australasian Physical & Engineering Sciences in Medicine*, 42(2): 427–441.

Belhaj Soulami, K., Kaabouch, N., Saidi, M. N., and Tamtaoui, A. (2020). An evaluation and ranking of evolutionary algorithms in segmenting abnormal masses in digital mammograms. *Multimedia Tools and Applications*, 79: 18941–18979.

Benjelloun, M., Adoui, M. E., Larhmam, M. A., and Mahmoudi, S. A. (2018). Automated breast tumor segmentation in DCE-MRI using deep learning. In *4th International Conference on Cloud Computing Technologies and Applications (Cloudtech)*, pp. 1–6. IEEE, Brussels.

Berber, T., Alpkocak, A., Balci, P., and Dicle, O. (2013). Breast mass contour segmentation algorithm in digital mammograms. *Computer Methods and Programs in Biomedicine*, 110(2): 150–159.

Bhateja, V., Misra, M., and Urooj, S. (2016). Non-linear polynomial filters for edge enhancement of mammogram lesions. *Computer Methods and Programs in Biomedicine*, 129: 125–134.

Blanco, G., Traina, A. J., Traina Jr., C., Azevedo-Marques, P. M., Jorge, A. E., de Oliveira, D., and Bedo, M. V. (2020). A superpixel-driven deep learning approach for the analysis of dermatological wounds. *Computer Methods and Programs in Biomedicine*, 183: 105079.

Bozek, J., Mustra, M., Delac, K., and Grgic, M. (2009). *A Survey of Image Processing Algorithms in Digital Mammography*, pp. 631–657. Springer Berlin Heidelberg, Berlin, Heidelberg.

Breiman, L. (2001). Random forests. *Machine Learning*, 45: 5–32

Carneiro, G., Nascimento, J., and Bradley, A. P. (2015). Unregistered multiview mammogram analysis with pre-trained deep learning models. In *Medical Image Computing and Computer-Assisted Intervention (MICCAI)*, pp. 652–660. Springer, Cham.

Cerqueira, R. D. (2018). *New Learning Strategies in Deep Models for Breast Cancer Screening*. Mestrado integrado em engenharia inform´atica e computa¸cao, Universidade do Porto, Porto.

Chakraborty, S., Bhowmik, M. K., Ghosh, A. K., and Pal, T. (2016). Automated edge detection of breast masses on mammograms. In *IEEE Region 10 Conference (TENCON)*, pp. 1241–1245, Singapore.

Chang, H., Chen, Z., Huang, Q., Shi, J., and Li, X. (2015). Graph-based learning for segmentation of 3D ultrasound images. *Neurocomputing*, 151: 632–644.

Chattaraj, A., Das, A., and Bhattacharya, M. (2017). Mammographic image segmentation by marker controlled watershed algorithm. In *IEEE International Conference on Bioinformatics and Biomedicine (BIBM)*, pp. 1000–1003, Kansas City, MO.

Chaurasia, A. and Culurciello, E. (2017). Linknet: Exploiting encoder representations for efficient semantic segmentation. In *IEEE Visual Communications and Image Processing (VCIP)*, pp. 1–4.

Chawla, N. V., Bowyer, K. W., Hall, L. O., and Kegelmeyer, W. P. (2002). Smote: synthetic minority over-sampling technique. *Journal of Artificial Intelligence Research*, 16: 321–357.

Chen, D.-R., Chang, R., and Huang, Y. L. (2000). Breast cancer diagnosis using self-organizing map for sonography. *Ultrasound in Medicine & Biology*, 26: 405–411.

Cheng, H., Shi, X., Min, R., Hu, L., Cai, X., and Du, H. (2006). Approaches for automated detection and classification of masses in mammograms. *Pattern Recognition*, 39(4): 646–668.

Cheng, J., Liu, J., Xu, Y., Yin, F., Wong, D. W. K., Tan, N., Tao, D., Cheng, C., Aung, T., and Wong, T. Y. (2013). Superpixel classification based optic disc and optic cup segmentation for glaucoma screening. *IEEE Transactions on Medical Imaging*, 32(6): 1019–1032.

Chiao, J.-Y., Chen, K.-Y., Liao, K. Y.-K., Hsieh, P.-H., Zhang, G., and Huang, T.-C. (2019). Detection and classification the breast tumors using mask R-CNN on sonograms. *Medicine*, 98(19):e15200.

Chowdhary, C. L. and Acharjya, D. P. (2018). Segmentation of mammograms using a novel intuitionistic possibilistic fuzzy C-mean clustering algorithm. In Panigrahi, B. K., Hoda, M. N., Sharma, V., and Goel, S., editors, *Nature Inspired Computing*, pp. 75–82, Springer Singapore, Singapore.

Ciecholewski, M. (2017). Malignant and benign mass segmentation in mammograms using active contour methods. *Symmetry*, 9(11): 277.

Cong, J., Wei, B., Yin, Y., Xi, X., and Zheng, Y. (2014). Performance evaluation of simple linear iterative clustering algorithm on medical image processing. *Bio-Medical Materials and Engineering*, 24(6): 3231–3238.

da Silva, G. L. F., Diniz, P. S., Ferreira, J. L., Franca, J. V. F., Silva, A. C., de Paiva, A. C., and de Cavalcanti, E. A. A. (2020). Superpixel-based deep convolutional neural networks and active contour model for automatic prostate segmentation on 3d MRI scans. *Medical & Biological Engineering & Computing*, 58(9): 1947–1964.

Dabass, J., Arora, S., Vig, R., and Hanmandlu, M. (2019). Segmentation techniques for breast cancer imaging modalities-a review. In *9th International Conference on Cloud Computing, Data Science & Engineering (Confluence)*, pp. 658–663. IEEE, India

Daoud, M. I., Atallah, A. A., Awwad, F., and Al-Najar, M. (2016). Accurate and fully automatic segmentation of breast ultrasound images by combining image boundary and region information. In *IEEE 13th International Symposium on Biomedical Imaging (ISBI)*, pp. 718–721, Prague.

Daoud, M. I., Atallah, A. A., Awwad, F., Al-Najjar, M., and Alazrai, R. (2019). Automatic superpixel-based segmentation method for breast ultrasound images. *Expert Systems with Applications*, 121: 78–96.

de Lima, S. M., da Silva-Filho, A. G., and dos Santos, W. P.(2016). Detection and classification of masses in mammographic images in a multikernel approach. *Computer Methods and Programs in Biomedicine*, 134(C): 11–29.

Dhungel, N., Carneiro, G., and Bradley, A. P. (2015a). Auto-mated mass detection in mammograms using cascaded deep learning and random forests. In *International Conference on Digital Image Computing: Techniques and Applications (DICTA)*, pp. 1–8. IEEE, Clayton VIC.

Dhungel, N., Carneiro, G., and Bradley, A. P. (2015b). Deep learning and structured prediction for the segmentation of mass in mammograms. In Navab, N., Hornegger, J., Wells, W. M., and Frangi, A., editors, *Medical Image Computing and Computer-Assisted Intervention (MICCAI)*, pp. 605–612. Springer International Publishing, Cham, India.

Dhungel, N., Carneiro, G., and Bradley, A. P. (2017a). A deep learning approach for the analysis of masses in mammograms with minimal user intervention. *Medical Image Analysis*, 37: 114–128.

Dhungel, N., Carneiro, G., and Bradley, A. P. (2017b). Fully automated classification of mammograms using deep residual neural networks. In *IEEE 14th International Symposium on Biomedical Imaging (ISBI)*, pp. 310–314.

Diaz, O., Marti, R., Llado, X., and Agarwal, R. (2018). Mass detection in mammograms using pre-trained deep learning models. In Krupinski, E. A., editor, *14th International Workshop on Breast Imaging (IWBI)*, p. 12. SPIE, Atlanta, GA.

Divyashree, B., R, A., M, N., and Kumar, G. H. (2018). Novel approach to locate region of interest in mammograms for Breast cancer. *CoRR, abs/1811.0*.

Domingues, I. (2014). *An Automatic Mammogram System: From Screening to Diagnosis*. Phd, Universidade do Porto, Porto.

Domingues, I. and Cardoso, J. S. (2013). Mass detection on mammogram images: a first assessment of deep learning techniques. In *19th Portuguese Conference on Pattern Recognition (RecPad)*, p. 2, Lisbon.

Domingues, I. and Cardoso, J. S. (2014). Using Bayesian surprise to detect calcifications in mammogram images. In *36th Annual International Conference of the IEEE Engineering in Medicine and Biology Society*, pp.1091–1094, Chicago, IL.

Domingues, I., Pereira, G., Martins, P., Duarte, H., Santos, J., and Abreu, P. H. (2019). Using deep learning techniques in medical imaging: a systematic review of applications on CT and PET. *Artificial Intelligence Review*, 53(6), 4093–4160.

Domingues, I. C., Cardoso, J., and Cardoso, P. (2012). Identification of benign breasts during mammogram screening. In *Proceedings of 18th Portuguese Conference on Pattern Recognition (RECPAD)*, Porto.

Dong, M., Lu, X., Ma, Y., Guo, Y., Ma, Y., and Wang, K. (2015). An efficient approach for automated mass segmentation and classification in mammograms. *Journal of Digital Imaging*, 28(5): 613–625.

El Idrissi El Kaitouni, S., Abbad, A., and Tairi, H. (2018). A breast tumors segmentation and elimination of pectoral muscle based on hidden markov and region growing. *Multimedia Tools and Applications*, 77(23): 31347–31362.

Elmoufidi, A., El Fahssi, K., Jai-Andaloussi, S., and Sekkaki, A. (2015). Automatically density based breast segmentation for mammograms by using dynamic K-means algorithm and Seed Based Region Growing. *IEEE International Instrumentation and Measurement Technology Conference (I2MTC)*, pp. 533–538, Pisa.

Feng, Y., Dong, F., Xia, X., Hu, C.-H., Fan, Q., Hu, Y., Gao, M., and Mutic, S. (2017). An adaptive Fuzzy C-means method utilizing neighboring information for breast tumor segmentation in ultrasound images. *Medical Physics*, 44(7): 3752–3760.

Fukushima, K. (1980). Neocognitron: A self-organizing neural network model for a mechanism of pattern recognition unaffected by shift in position. *Biological Cybernetics*, 36(4): 193–202.

Ganesan, K., Acharya, R. U., Chua, C. K., Min, L. C., Mathew, B., and Thomas, A. K. (2013a). Decision support system for breast cancer detection using mammograms. *Proceedings of the Institution of Mechanical Engineers, Part H: Journal of Engineering in Medicine*, 227(7): 721–732.

Ganesan, K., Acharya, U. R., Chua, C. K., Min, L. C., Abraham, K. T., and Ng, K.-H. (2013b). Computer-aided breast cancer detection using mammograms: A review. *IEEE Reviews in Biomedical Engineering*, 6: 77–98.

Gao, F. (2019). *Novel Deep Learning Models for Medical Imaging Analysis*. Doctor of philosophy, Arizona State University, Tempe.

Gao, F., Yoon, H., Wu, T., and Chu, X. (2020). A feature transfer enabled multi-task deep learning model on medical imaging. *Expert Systems with Applications*, 143: 112957.

Gonzalo-Martin, C., Garcia-Pedrero, A., Lillo-Saavedra, M., and Menasalvas, E. (2016). Deep learning for superpixel-based classification of remote sensing images. In GEOBIA: Solutions and Synergies. University of Twente Faculty of Geo-Information and Earth Observation (ITC), Enschede.

Goubalan, S. (2016). *Contributions a l'analyse d'images m'edicales pour la reconnaissance du cancer du sein*. PhD thesis, Traitement du signal et de l'image [eess.SP]. Universit'e Paris-Saclay, Gif-sur-Yvette.

Guo, G. and Razmjooy, N. (2019). A new interval differential equation for edge detection and determining breast cancer regions in mammography images. *Systems Science & Control Engineering*, 7(1): 346–356.

Hamed, G., Marey, M. A. E.-R., Amin, S. E.-S., and Tolba, M. F. (2020). Deep learning in breast cancer detection and classification. In Hassanien, A.-E., Azar, A. T., Gaber, T., Oliva, D., and Tolba, F. M., editors, *International Conference on Artificial Intelligence and Computer Vision (AICV)*, pp. 322–333. Springer International Publishing, Cham.

Hamidinekoo, A., Denton, E., and Zwiggelaar, R. (2019). Automated mammogram analysis with a deep learning pipeline. *arXiv*, pp. 1–5.

Hazarika, M. and Mahanta, L. B. (2019). A hierarchical spatial fuzzy C means algorithm for mammographic mass segmentation. *International Journal of Computer Sciences and Engineering*, 7(1): 84–88.

Hefnawy, A. (2013). An improved approach for breast cancer detection in mammogram based on watershed segmentation. *International Journal of Computer Applications*, 75(15): 26–30.

Hesamian, M. H., Jia, W., He, X., and Kennedy, P. (2019). Deep learning techniques for medical image segmentation: Achievements and challenges. *Journal of Digital Imaging*, 32(4): 582–596.

Hong, F., Jing, Y., Cun-cun, H., Ke-zhen, Z., and Ruo-xia, Y. (2019). A fast density peak clustering algorithm optimized by uncertain number neighbors for breast MR image. *Journal of Physics: Conference Series*, 1229: 012024. IOP Publishing.

Huang, Q., Huang, Y., Luo, Y., Yuan, F., and Li, X. (2020). Segmentation of breast ultrasound image with semantic classification of superpixels. *Medical Image Analysis*, 61: 101657.

Huang, Q., Luo, Y., and Zhang, Q. (2017). Breast ultrasound image segmentation: a survey. *International Journal of Computer Assisted Radiology and Surgery*, 12(3): 493–507.

Huang, Q., Yang, F., Liu, L., and Li, X. (2015). Automatic segmentation of breast lesions for interaction in ultrasonic computer-aided diagnosis. *Information Sciences*, 314: 293–310.

Huang, Q.-H., Lee, S.-Y., Liu, L.-Z., Lu, M.-H., Jin, L.-W., and Li, A.-H. (2012). A robust graph-based segmentation method for breast tumors in ultrasound images. *Ultrasonics*, 52(2): 266–275.

Huang, Y. and Huang, Q. (2018). A superpixel- classification-based method for breast ultrasound images. In *5th International Conference on Systems and Informatics (ICSAI)*, pp. 560–564. IEEE, Nanjing.

Ilesanmi, A. E., Idowu, O. P., and Makhanov, S. S. (2020). Multiscale superpixel method for segmentation of breast ultrasound. *Computers in Biology and Medicine*, 125: 103879.

Jampani, V., Sun, D., Liu, M.-Y., Yang, M.-H., and Kautz, J. (2018). Superpixel samping networks. In *European Conference on Computer Vision (ECCV)*, Springer, Heidelberg.

Jintasuttisak, T. and Intajag, S. (2014). Color retinal image enhancement by rayleigh contrast-limited adaptive histogram equalization. In *14th International Conference on Control, Automation and Systems (ICCAS)*, pp. 692–697. IEEE, Seoul.

Jumaat, A. K., Rahman, W. E. Z. W., Ibrahim, A., and Mahmud, R. (2011). Segmentation and characterization of masses in breast ultrasound images using active contour. In *IEEE International Conference on Signal and Image Processing Applications (ICSIPA)*, pp. 404–409, Kuala Lumpur.

Jung, H., Kim, B., Lee, I., Yoo, M., Lee, J., Ham, S., Woo, O., Kang, J., Id, H. J., Kim, B., Lee, I., Yoo, M., Lee, J., Id, S. H., Woo, O., and Kang, J.(2018). Detection of masses in mammograms using a one-stage object detector based on a deep convolutional neural network. *PLOS One*, 13(9):e0203355.

Karabatak, M. (2015). A new classifier for breast cancer detection based on Naïve Bayesian. *Measurement*, 72: 32–36.

Karahaliou, A., Skiadopoulos, S., Boniatis, I., Sakellaropoulos, P., Likaki, E., Panayiotakis, G., and Costaridou, L. (2014). Texture analysis of tissue surrounding microcalcifications on mammograms for breast cancer diagnosis. *The British Journal of Radiology*, 80(956): 648–656.

Kaushal, C., Bhat, S., Koundal, D., and Singla, A. (2019). Recent trends in computer assisted diagnosis (CAD) system for breast cancer diagnosis using histopathological images. *IRBM*, 40(4): 211–227.

Koozegar, E., Soryani, M., and Domingues, I. (2013). A new local adaptive mass detection algorithm in mammograms. In *International Conference on Bio-inspired Systems and Signal Processing*, pp. 133–137. SciTePress Science and and Technology Publications, Barcelona.

Kozegar, E., Soryani, M., Behnam, H., Salamati, M., and Tan, T. (2018). Mass Segmentation in Automated 3-D Breast Ultrasound Using Adaptive Region Growing and Supervised Edge-Based Deformable Model. *IEEE Transactions on Medical Imaging*, 37(4): 918–928.

Kozegar, E., Soryani, M., Minaei, B., and Domingues, I. (2013). Assessment of a novel mass detection algorithm in mammograms. *Journal of Cancer Research and Therapeutics*, 9(4): 592.

Kumar, V., Webb, J. M., Gregory, A., Denis, M., Meixner, D. D., Bayat, M., Whaley, D. H., Fatemi, M., and Alizad, A. (2018). Automated and real- time segmentation of suspicious breast masses using convolutional neural network. *PLOS One*, 13(5):e0195816.

Lecun, Y., Bottou, L., Bengio, Y., and Haffner, P. (1998). Gradient- based learning applied to document recognition. *Proceedings of the IEEE*, 86(11): 2278–2324.

Li, H., Chen, D., Nailon, W. H., Davies, M. E., and Laurenson, D. (2018). Improved breast mass segmentation in mammograms with conditional residual U-Net. In *Lecture Notes in Computer Science (including subseries Lecture Notes in Artificial Intelligence and Lecture Notes in Bioinformatics)*, Vol. 11040 LNCS, pp. 81–89. Springer.

Li, Y., Chen, H., Wei, X., Peng, Y., and Cheng, L. (2016). Mass classification in mammograms based on two-concentric masks and discriminating texton. *Pattern Recognition*, 60(C): 648–656.

Lin, T., Dollr, P., Girshick, R., He, K., Hariharan, B., and Belongie, S. (2017). Feature pyramid networks for object detection. In *IEEE Conference on Computer Vision and Pattern Recognition (CVPR)*, pp. 936–944, Honolulu, HI.

Litjens, G., Kooi, T., Bejnordi, B. E., Setio, A. A. A., Ciompi, F., Ghafoorian, M., van der Laak, J. A., van Ginneken, B., and S'anchez, C. I. (2017). A Survey on deep learning in medical image analysis. *arXiv*, 42(1995): 60–88.

Liu, J., Chen, J., Liu, X., Chun, L., Tang, J., and Deng, Y. (2011). Mass segmentation using a combined method for cancer detection. *BMC Systems Biology*, 5(Suppl 3):S6.

Liu, L., Qin, W., Yang, R., Yu, C., Li, L., Wen, T., and Gu, J. (2015). Segmentation of breast ultrasound image using graph cuts and level set. In *IET International Conference on Biomedical Image and Signal Processing (ICBISP)*, pp. 1–4, Beijing.

Liu, X., Liu, J., Zhou, D., and Tang, J. (2010). A benign and malignant mass classification algorithm based on an improved level set segmentation and texture feature analysis. In *4th International Conference on Bioinformatics and Biomedical Engineering*, pp. 1–4. IEEE, Granada.

Lotfollahi, M., Gity, M., Ye, J. Y., and Mahlooji Far, A. (2018). Segmentation of breast ultrasound images based on active contours using neutrosophic theory. *Journal of Medical Ultrasonics*, 45(2): 205–212.

Luo, Y., Han, S., and Huang, Q. (2016). A novel graph-based segmentation method for breast ultrasound images. In *International Conference on Digital Image Computing: Techniques and Applications (DICTA)*, pp. 1–6. IEEE, Gold Coast.

Ma, J., Fan, X., Yang, S. X., Zhang, X., and Zhu, X. (2018). Contrast limited adaptive histogram equalization-based fusion in yiq and hsi color spaces for underwater image enhancement. *International Journal of Pattern Recognition and Artificial Intelligence*, 32(07): 1854018.

Mahersia, H., Boulehmi, H., and Hamrouni, K. (2016). Development of intelligent systems based on Bayesian regularization network and neuro- fuzzy models for mass detection in mammograms: A comparative analysis. *Computer Methods and Programs in Biomedicine*, 126: 46–62.

Mahmoudzadeh, E., Montazeri, M., Zekri, M., and Sadri, S. (2015). Extended hidden Markov model for optimized segmentation of breast thermography images. *Infrared Physics & Technology*, 72: 19–28.

Marcomini, K. D., Carneiro, A. A. O., and Schiabel, H. (2016). Application of artificial neural network models in segmentation and classification of nodules in breast ultrasound digital images. *International Journal of Biomedical Imaging*, 2016: 1–13.

Marcomini, K. D. and Schiabel, H. (2015). Investigating automatic techniques in segmentation accuracy of masses in digital mammography images. In *World Congress on Medical Physics and Biomedical Engineering*, pp. 199–202. Springer, Cham, India.

Marcus, G. (2019). Deep learning: A critical appraisal. arxiv 2018. *arXiv preprint arXiv:1801.00631.*

Martel, A. L., Gallego-Ortiz, C., and Lu, Y. (2016). Breast segmentation in MRI using Poisson surface reconstruction initialized with random forest edge detection. In Styner, M. A. and Angelini, E. D., editors, *Medical Imaging: Image Processing*, vol. 9784, p. 97841B. International Society for Optics and Photonics, SPIE.

Melouah, A. (2013). *A Novel Region Growing Segmentation Algorithm for Mass Extraction in Mammograms*, Springer International Publishing, Cham, pp. 95–104, India.

Min, H., Chandra, S. S., Crozier, S., and Bradley, A. P. (2019a). Multi-scale sifting for mammographic mass detection and segmentation. *Biomedical Physics & Engineering Express*, 5(2): 025022.

Min, H., Chandra, S. S., Dhungel, N., Crozier, S., and Bradley, A. P. (2017). Multi-scale mass segmentation for mammograms via cascaded random forests. In *IEEE 14th International Symposium on Biomedical Imaging (ISBI)* p. 113–117, Melbourne.

Min, H., Wilson, D., Huang, Y., Liu, S., Crozier, S., Bradley, A. P., and Chandra, S. S. (2019b). Fully automatic computer-aided mass detection and segmentation via pseudo-color mammograms and Mask R-CNN. *arXiv*, pp. 1–14.

Minaee, S., Boykov, Y., Porikli, F., Plaza, A., Kehtarnavaz, N., and Terzopoulos, D. (2020). No Title.

Hu, M.-K. (1962). Visual pattern recognition by moment invariants. *IRE Transactions on Information Theory*, 8(2): 179–187.

Mohamed, I., Jeberson, W., and Bajaj, H. (2016). Improved region growing based breast cancer image segmentation. *International Journal of Computer Applications*, 135(8): 1–4.

Mohanty, A. K., Senapati, M. R., Beberta, S., and Lenka, S. K.(2012). Texture-based features for classification of mammograms using decision tree. *Neural Computing and Applications*, 23(3–4): 1011–1017.

Moreira, I. C., Amaral, I., Domingues, I., Cardoso, A., Cardoso, M. J., and Cardoso, J. S. (2012). INbreast: Toward a full-field digital mammographic database. *Academic Radiology*, 19(2): 236–248.

Oliveira, M. S. (2018). *Automatic Detection of Anatomical Structures and Breast Cancer Diagnosis on X-Ray Mammography.* Master's degree in computer science, Universidade do Porto, Porto.

Paramkusham, S., Shivakshit, P., Rao, K., and Rao, B. P. (2015). A new features extraction method based on polynomial regression for the assessment of breast lesion Contours. In *International Conference on Industrial Instrumentation and Control (ICIC)*, pp. 579–583. IEEE, Pune.

Pisano, E. D., Zong, S., Hemminger, B. M., DeLuca, M., Johnston, R. E., Muller, K., Braeuning, M. P., and Pizer, S. M. (1998). Contrast limited adaptive histogram equalization image processing to improve the detection of simulated spiculations in dense mammograms. *Journal of Digital imaging*, 11(4): 193.

Platania, R., Shams, S., Yang, S., Zhang, J., Lee, K., and Park, S.-j. (2017). Automated breast cancer diagnosis using deep learning and region of interest detection (BC-DROID). In *8th ACM International Conference on Bioinformatics, Computational Biology, and Health Informatics (ACM-BCB)*, pp. 536–543, New York, ACM Press.

Punitha, S., Amuthan, A., and Joseph, K. S. (2018). Benign and malignant breast cancer segmentation using optimized region growing technique. *Future Computing and Informatics Journal*, 3(2): 348–358.

Qin, W., Wu, J., Han, F., Yuan, Y., Zhao, W., Ibragimov, B., Gu, J., and Xing, L. (2018). Superpixel-based and boundary-sensitive convolutional neural network for automated liver segmentation. *Physics in Medicine & Biology*, 63(9): 095017.

Ragab, D. A., Sharkas, M., Marshall, S., and Ren, J. (2019). Breast cancer detection using deep convolutional neural networks and support vector machines. *PeerJ*, 7:e6201.

Raghavendra, U., Rajendra Acharya, U., Fujita, H., Gudigar, A., Tan, J. H., and Chokkadi, S. (2016). Application of gabor wavelet and locality sensitive discriminant analysis for automated identification of breast cancer using digitized mammogram images. *Applied Soft Computing*, 46: 151–161.

Ramadijanti, N., Barakbah, A., and Husna, F. A. (2018). Automatic breast tumor segmentation using hierarchical K-means on mammogram. In *International Electronics Symposium on Knowledge Creation and Intelligent Computing (IES-KCIC)*, pp. 170–175. IEEE.

Rao, C. H., Naganjaneyulu, P. V., Satyaprasad, K., Dist, G., Pradesh, A., C. Hemasundara Rao, P. V. N., Satyaprasad, K., Rao, C. H., Naganjaneyulu, P. V., Satyaprasad, K., Dist, G., and Pradesh, A. (2018). Automated detection, segmentation and classification using deep learning methods for mammograms-a review. *International Journal of Pure and Applied Mathematics*, 119(16): 5209–5249.

Ribli, D., Horv́ath, A., Unger, Z., Pollner, P., and Csabai, I. (2018). Detecting and classifying lesions in mammograms with Deep Learning. *Scientific Reports*, 8(1): 4165.

Rickard, H., Tourassi, G., Eltonsy, N., and Elmaghraby, A. (2004). Breast segmentation in screening mammograms using multiscale analysis and self- organizing maps. In *26th Annual International Conference of the IEEE Engineering in Medicine and Biology Society*, vol. 3, pp. 1786–1789.

Ronneberger, O., Fischer, P., and Brox, T. (2015). U-Net: Convolutional networks for biomedical image segmentation. In *Lecture Notes in Computer Science*, vol. 9351, pp. 234–241. Springer.

Rouhi, R., Jafari, M., Kasaei, S., and Keshavarzian, P. (2015). Benign and malignant breast tumors classification based on region growing and CNN segmentation. *Expert Systems with Applications*, 42(3): 990–1002.

Sasikala, S., Ezhilarasi, M., and Arun Kumar, S. (2020). Detection of breast cancer using fusion of MLO and CC view features through a hybrid technique based on binary firefly algorithm and optimum-path forest classifier. In *Applied Nature-Inspired Computing: Algorithms and Case Studies*, pp. 23–40. Springer, Singapore.

Schreier, J., Attanasi, F., and Laaksonen, H. (2019). A full-image deep segmenter for CT images in breast cancer radiotherapy treatment. *Frontiers in Oncology*, 9: 677.

Senthilkumar, B., Umamaheswari, G., and Karthik, J. (2010). A novel region growing segmentation algorithm for the detection of breast cancer. In *IEEE International Conference on Computational Intelligence and Computing Research*, pp. 1–4.

Shafer, C. M., Seewaldt, V. L., and Lo, J. Y. (2011). Validation of a 3D hidden-Markov model for breast tissue segmentation and density estimation from MR and tomosynthesis images. In *Biomedical Sciences and Engineering Conference: Image Informatics and Analytics in Biomedicine*, pp. 1–4. IEEE.

Shen, D., Wu, G., and Suk, H.-i. (2017). Deep learning in medical image analysis. *Annual Review of Biomedical Engineering*, 19(1): 221–248.

Shen, L., Margolies, L. R., Rothstein, J. H., Fluder, E., McBride, R. B., and Sieh, W. (2019). Deep learning to improve breast cancer detection on screening mammography. *Scientific Reports*, 9(1): 12495.

Shen, R., Yao, J., Yan, K., Tian, K., Jiang, C., and Zhou, K. (2020a). Unsupervised domain adaptation with adversarial learning for mass detection in mammogram. *Neurocomputing*, 393(Mmd): 27–37.

Shen, R., Zhou, K., Yan, K., Tian, K., and Zhang, J. (2020b). Multicontext multitask learning networks for mass detection in mammogram. *Medical Physics*, 47(4): 1566–1578.

Shi, P., Zhong, J., Rampun, A., and Wang, H. (2018). A hierarchical pipeline for breast boundary segmentation and calcification detection in mammograms. *Computers in Biology and Medicine*, 96: 178–188.

Shrivastava, N. and Bharti, J. (2020). Breast tumor detection in digital mammogram based on efficient seed region growing segmentation. *IETE Journal of Research*, 0(0): 1–13.

Singh, V. K., Rashwan, H. A., Abdel-Nasser, M., Sarker, M. M. K., Akram, F., Pandey, N., Romani, S., and Puig, D. (2019). An efficient solution for breast tumor segmentation and classification in ultrasound images using deep adversarial learning. *CoRR*, abs/1907.0.

Singh, V. K., Rashwan, H. A., Romani, S., Akram, F., Pandey, N., Sarker, M. M. K., Saleh, A., Arenas, M., Arquez, M., Puig, D., and Torrents-Barrena, J. (2020). Breast tumor segmentation and shape classification in mammograms using generative adversarial and convolutional neural network. *Expert Systems with Applications*, 139: 112855.

Singh, V. K., Romani, S., Rashwan, H. A., Akram, F., Pandey, N., Sarker, M. M. K., Abdulwahab, S., Torrents-Barrena, J., Saleh, A., Arquez, M., Arenas, M., and Puig, D. (2018). Conditional generative adversarial and convolutional networks for X-ray breast mass segmentation and shape classification. *Lecture Notes in Computer Science (including subseries Lecture Notes in Artificial Intelligence and Lecture Notes in Bioinformatics)*, 11071 LNCS: 833–840.

Suhail, Z., Denton, E. R. E., and Zwiggelaar, R. (2018). Treebased modelling for the classification of mammographic benign and malignant microcalcification clusters. *Multimedia Tools and Applications*, 77(5): 6135–6148.

Sun, H., Li, C., Liu, B., Liu, Z., Wang, M., Zheng, H., Dagan Feng, D., and Wang, S. (2020). AUNet: attention-guided dense-upsampling networks for breast mass segmentation in whole mammograms. *Physics in Medicine & Biology*, 65(5): 055005.

Sun, L., He, J., Yin, X., Zhang, Y., Chen, J.-H., Kron, T., and Su, M.-Y. (2018). An image segmentation framework for extracting tumors from breast magnetic resonance images. *Journal of Innovative Optical Health Sciences*, 11(04): 1850014.

Tardy, M. and Mateus, D. (2020). Improving mammography malignancy segmentation with well designed training process. In *Medical Imaging with Deep Learning*, pp. 1–4.

Tello-Mijares, S., Woo, F., and Flores, F. (2019). Breast cancer identification via thermography image segmentation with a gradient vector flow and a convolutional neural network. *Journal of Healthcare Engineering*, 2019: 1–13.

Tsochatzidis, L., Costaridou, L., and Pratikakis, I. (2019). Deep learning for breast cancer diagnosis from mammograms a comparative study. *Journal of Imaging*, 5(3): 37.

Udayakumar, E., Santhi, S., and Vetrivelan, P. (2017). An investigation of Bayes algorithm and neural networks for identifying the breast cancer. *Indian Journal of Medical and Paediatric Oncology*, 38(3): 340.

Vakanski, A., Xian, M., and Freer, P. (2019). Attention enriched deep learning model for breast tumor segmentation in ultrasound images. *arXiv preprint arXiv:1910.08978*.

Vald´es-Santiago, D., Quintana-Mart´ınez, R., Le´onMec´ıas, A´., and Baguer D´ıaz-Roman˜ach, M. L. (2018). Mammographic mass segmentation using fuzzy c-means and decision trees. In Perales, F. J. and Kittler, J., editors, *Articulated Motion and Deformable Objects*, pp. 1–10, Cham. Springer International Publishing.

Vogl, W.-D., Pinker, K., Helbich, T. H., Bickel, H., Grabner, G., Bogner, W., Gruber, S., Bago-Horvath, Z., Dubsky, P., and Langs, G. (2019). Automatic segmentation and classification of breast lesions through identification of informative multiparametric PET/MRI features. *European Radiology Experimental*, 3(1): 18.

Waibel, A., Hanazawa, T., Hinton, G., Shikano, K., and Lang, K. J. (1989). Phoneme recognition using time-delay neural networks. *IEEE Transactions on Acoustics, Speech, and Signal Processing*, 37(3): 328–339.

Wang, T. (2018). Adapting multiple datasets for better mammography tumor detection. *Master of Science Thesis*. KTH Royal Institute of Technology, School of Electrical Engineering and Computer Science (EECS), Sweden.

Wang, X. (2017). *Development of Segmentation Algorithms and Machine Learning Classification Methods for Characterization of Breast and Spine Tumors on MRI*. Master of science in biomedical engineering, University of California, Irvine.

Wang, X., Guo, Y., Wang, Y., and Yu, J. (2017). Automatic breast tumor detection in ABVS images based on convolutional neural network and superpixel patterns. *Neural Computing and Applications*, 31: 1069–1081.

Wang, Y., Qi, Q., and Shen, X. (2020). Image segmentation of brain MRI based on LTriDP and superpixels of improved SLIC. *Brain Science*, 10(2): 116.

Xi, X., Shi, H., Han, L., Wang, T., Ding, H. Y., Zhang, G., Tang, Y., and Yin, Y. (2017). Breast tumor segmentation with prior knowledge learning. *Neurocomputing*, 237(C): 145–157.

Yadav, G., Maheshwari, S., and Agarwal, A. (2014). Contrast limited adaptive histogram equalization based enhancement for real time video system. In *International Conference on Advances in Computing, Communications and Informatics (ICACCI)*, pp. 2392–2397. IEEE, Noida.

Yan, Y., Conze, P.-H., Decenciere, E., Lamard, M., Quellec, G., Cochener, B., and Coatrieux, G. (2019). Cascaded multi-scale convolutional encoder- decoders for breast mass segmentation in high-resolution mammograms. In *41st Annual International Conference of the IEEE Engineering in Medicine and Biology Society (EMBC)*, pp. 6738–6741, Berlin.

Yan, Y., Conze, P.-H., Quellec, G., Lamard, M., Cochener, B., and Coatrieux, G. (2020). Two-stage breast mass detection and segmentation system towards automated high-resolution full mammogram analysis. *arXiv*.

Yang, H., Christopher, L. A., Duric, N., West, E., and Bakic, P. (2012). Performance analysis of EM-MPM and K-means clustering in 3D ultrasound image segmentation. In *IEEE International Conference on Electro/Information Technology*, pp. 1–4, Chicago, IL.

Yap, M. H., Goyal, M., Osman, F. M., Mart´ı, R., Denton, E., Juette, A., and Zwiggelaar, R. (2019). Breast ultrasound lesions recognition: end-to-end deep learning approaches. *Journal of medical imaging (Bellingham, Wash.)*, 6(1): 11007.

Yu, N., Wu, J., Weinstein, S. P., Gaonkar, B., Keller, B. M., Ashraf, A. B., Jiang, Y., Davatzikos, C., Conant, E. F., and Kontos, D. (2015). A superpixel- based framework for automatic tumor segmentation on breast DCE-MRI. In Hadjiiski, L. M. and Tourassi, G. D., editors, *Medical Imaging: Computer-Aided Diagnosis*, vol. 9414, p. 941400. International Society for Optics and Photonics.

Yuan, G., Liu, Y., and Huang, W. (2019). Segmentation of MR breast cancer images based on DWT and K-means algorithm. *Journal of Physics: Conference Series*, 1229: 012025.

Zhang, J., Zhou, S. K., Brunke, S., Lowery, C., and Comaniciu, D. (2010). Database-guided breast tumor detection and segmentation in 2D ultrasound images. In Karssemeijer, N. and Summers, R. M., editors, *Medical Imaging: Computer-Aided Diagnosis*, vol. 7624, p. 762405. International Society for Optics and Photonics, SPIE.

Zhang, R., Zhang, H., and Chung, A. C. S. (2018). A unified mammogram analysis method via hybrid deep supervision. In *Image Analysis for Moving Organ, Breast, and Thoracic Images*, pp. 107–115. Springer.

Zhang, Y., Yang, L., Zheng, H., Liang, P., Mangold, C., Loreto, R. G., Hughes, D. P., and Chen, D. Z. (2019). SPDA: Superpixel-based data augmentation for biomedical image segmentation. In Cardoso, M. J., Feragen, A., Glocker, B., Konukoglu, E., Oguz, I., Unal, G., and Vercauteren, T., editors, *Machine Learning Research*, volume 102, pp. 572–587, PMLR, London.

Zheng, S.-W., Liu, J., and Liu, C.-C. (2013). A Random-Walk Based Breast Tumors Segmentation Algorithm for Mammograms. In *International Journal on Computer, Consumer and Control (IJ3C)*.

Zhou, Z., Wu, W., Wu, S., Tsui, P.-H., Lin, C.-C., Zhang, L., and Wang, T. (2014). Semi-automatic breast ultrasound image segmentation based on mean shift and graph cuts. *Ultrasonic Imaging*, 36(4): 256–276.

Zhuang, Z., Li, N., Joseph Raj, A. N., Mahesh, V. G. V., and Qiu, S. (2019). An RDAU-NET model for lesion segmentation in breast ultrasound images. *PLOS ONE*, 14(8):e0221535.

Zohourian, F., Antic, B., Siegemund, J., Meuter, M., and Pauli, J. (2018). Superpixel-based road segmentation for real-time systems using CNN. In *13th International Joint Conference on Computer Vision, Imaging and Computer Graphics Theory and Applications*, pp. 257–265. INSTICC, SCITEPRESS - Science and Technology Publications, Funchal-Madeira.

Zou, L., Yu, S., Meng, T., Zhang, Z., Liang, X., and Xie, Y. (2019). A technical review of convolutional neural network-based mammographic breast cancer diagnosis. *Computational and Mathematical Methods in Medicine*, 2019: 1–16.

8 Deep Learning for Disease Prediction in Public Health

Kurubaran Ganasegeran
Ministry of Health Malaysia

CONTENTS

8.1 INTRODUCTION

The primer of epidemiology is to determine the distribution and determinants of diseases across population worldwide (Frerot et al., 2018). Since primordial times, epidemiologists often rely on conventional data sets and surveillance data from sources like disease registries, census, large epidemiological surveys and clinical or administrative data to explore temporal relationships between variables of interests (Ganasegeran, Ch'ng, Aziz, & Looi, 2020). These resources were benchmarked as the most reliable, validated and useful instruments to yield evidence outcomes that could serve as a guide and dogma for public health physicians to plan community interventions, or craft appropriate policies to improve populations' well-being, increase survival rates, reduce co-morbidities, control disease outbreaks and prevent illness occurrence. However, these conventional data sources are retrospective in nature, resource intensive and have substantially long lag periods of time for data availability, thus restricting its capabilities to execute urgent analytical inferences for evidence synthesis (Ganasegeran, Ch'ng, Aziz, & Looi, 2020). With current public health emergency situations occurring worldwide, such as uncontrolled transmissions of infectious diseases like COVID-19 and the exponential rise of debilitating lifestyle diseases affecting populations across different strata of communities, it has become a necessity to retrieve real-time data to execute urgent analytical process for crafting appropriate public health interventions in the quest to control disease transmission and occurrence.

The process for yielding hypothetical results depends heavily on its "data culture." It employs traditional statistical approaches for two principal functions; the first is to describe the data or the sample, while the second is to reject the null hypothesis so that the alternative hypothesis could be accepted for meaningful real-life interpretations. Basic statistical test (descriptive statistics) often report frequency (whole numbers), relative frequency (percentages), mean (average), median (center number) or proportion of the variable of interests in the sample data. It gives an overall view of a particular disease or illness affecting a target population or the sample being studied. Such statistical approaches would provide an answer to the following questions:

1. How many people are being affected by the disease?
2. Who are the people being affected mostly? Is it men, women or children?
3. What is the proportion of men or women being affected by the disease?
4. In which age group is the disease more prevalent?
5. In which area or living circumstances has the disease spread the most?

In contrast, inferential statistics aim to explore associations, relationships or impact of a particular disease. This component is more crucial to biostatisticians and epidemiologists to plan needful interventions. It is an approach to principally reject the null hypothesis and accept the alternative hypothesis. This statistics of inference is particularly useful to:

1. Explore the effect size (how much is the disease affecting the community or the sample being studied?)

2. Determine associations (what factors are associated with the disease?)
3. Facilitate disease modeling (linear or logistic regression capabilities that could answer what attributes predict or are associated with the detection of the disease or outcomes?)

Effect sizes are yielded through parameters such as odds ratios, relative risks or risk ratios and hazards ratios based on the prevalence or incidence nature of the disease or outcomes data. It is often reported with the relevant effect estimates such as 95% confidence intervals, 95% credible intervals or 95% uncertainty intervals. Traditional epidemiological regression models could be classified based on the objective of the model; whether to predict a dependent variable or to determine the factors associated with the dependent variable from a list of independent variables (known as predictive modeling), or to determine the magnitude of an effect while exploring the related attributes on its' main outcome measure (known as explanatory models) (Wiemken & Kelley, 2020). These conventional statistical approaches pose great importance to public health physicians and epidemiologists, but they are compounded with certain limitations. First, they are limited to deliver key understandable messages to lay persons and they are succinctly not powered to provide robust estimates with the revolution of big public health data that incorporate informatics and data-intelligence to provide real-time estimates for emergency interventions from huge scale population coverage. Bellman's "curse of dimensionality" has become more crucial to ponder at this moment of time, given the rise of modern statistical methods and robust conceptual approaches with the revolution of computational data systems that are made available in the current healthcare practice (Bellman, 2015). With such newer modalities of resource data sets, research questions become more advanced and complex, making conventional mathematical algorithms and modeling assumptions more intricate and difficult to synthesize. This is due to raw data sets that are composed of a set of variables association that are anticipated to be highly nonlinear, thus catalyzing newer methods to be adopted during statistical analysis. The dawn of artificial intelligence (AI) has prompted the adoption of novel approaches using machine learning (ML) and deep learning (DL) concepts to analyze population health data, disease screening and diagnosis in the field of public health. These computational analytical techniques have emerged as the fundamentals to be applied in real-time big public health data, collectively called as data science.

8.2   BIG PUBLIC HEALTH DATA

Big data ubiquitously rose as a consequence of rapid digitalization. It is contemporarily conceptualized as "data sets that primarily exhibit extensive characteristics in terms of volume, variety, velocity and/or variability that require substantial scalable architecture for efficient storage, manipulation and analytical procedures (National Institute of Standards and Technology, 2015)." Since its inception, big data analytics was adopted across many subject matter specializations within the field of healthcare and medicine. One crucial specialization that requires fast and extensive reliable data to mould preventive health measures is public health medicine. But till date most epidemiological experts have yet to decipher the nomenclature of "big public health data." The five core public health domains which include non-communicable diseases (NCDs), communicable diseases, maternal and child health, environmental health and socio-behavioral medicine has been a point of great focus by researchers and practitioners worldwide to obtain fast and accurate data in view of current phenomenological rise of unprecedented disease outbreaks, debilitating health outcomes, risky health behaviors and newer health threats that require urgent interventions.

The taxonomy and applicability of big public health data are visualized in Figure 8.1. The bigness of big public health data could theoretically be divided according to the nature of the data sets (Mooney & Pejaver, 2018):

1. Wide data sets that have many columns
2. Tall data sets that have many rows
3. Mixture of both wide or tall data sets

8.3 ARTIFICIAL INTELLIGENCE IN PUBLIC HEALTH

AI is contextualized as "a branch of computer science that simulates intelligent behaviors as humans, but using machines (Kurzweil, 1990; Poole, Mackworth, & Goebel, 1998; Ganasegeran & Abdulraman, 2020)." Machines here refer to computers! The fundamental aim of AI is to replicate human intelligence functions synthetically, also called "computational intelligence (Lavigne, Mussa, Creatore, Hoffman, & Buckeridge, 2019)." While human brain functions are instantaneous to interpret an

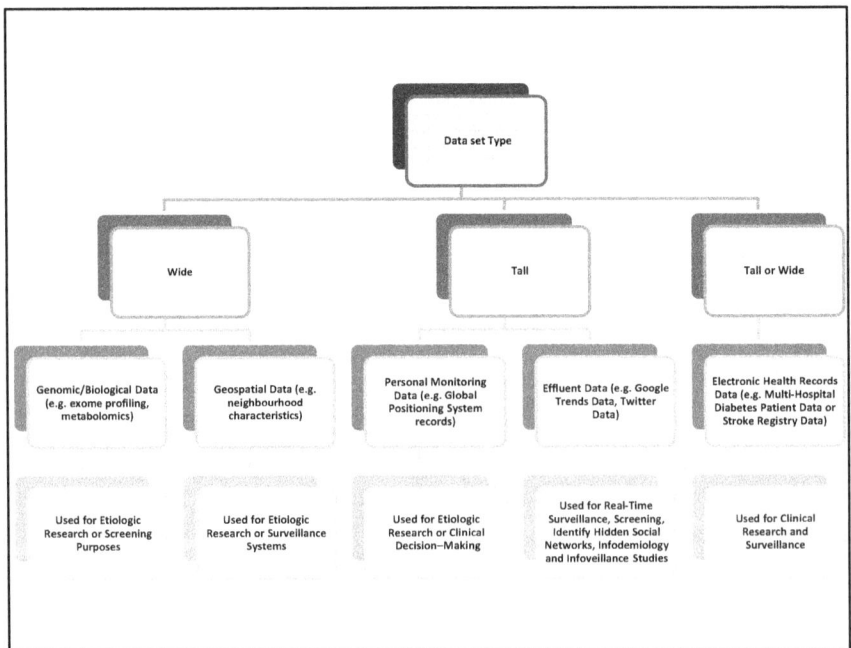

FIGURE 8.1   Functional taxonomy of big public health data.

environmental stimuli, object, image, noise or voice, AI executes similar tasks intelligently using mathematical algorithms from programmable computers to automate reactions (Ganasegeran & Abdulrahman, 2020). The primary difference between humans and AI here is that the former has emotions and feelings, while the latter do not! According to their architecture and functions, AI is sub-divided (Ayon & Islam, 2019; Ganasegeran & Abdulrahman, 2020) as follows:

1. *ML*: It is composed of machines that learn from prior experiences. ML is composed mainly of supervised learning (a system that use patterns of identified data) and unsupervised learning (a system that learns from patterns of data).
2. *DL*: It is a subset of ML constituting of artificial neural networks with more than one hidden layer. It has the capacity to carry out ample functions such as image recognition and natural language processing (NLP) with concurrent handling of massive information flow. The system has the capability to use large data sets for analytics. With multiple hidden layers between input and output, deep neural networks (DNN) employs a multitude of learning algorithms to yield the outcomes. Within the DNN, it has many elements or nodes which are interconnected similarly to human neurons. It is actually a replica of the synthetic version of the human brain architecture! Output accuracies solely depend on the structure's inter-unit connection strength. Within and in between of the numerous hidden layers, there are multiple neurons. A simple DNN architecture is exhibited in Figure 8.2. Across each layer of nodes, the output depends on the previous layer of output. The final output layer does not have an activated function because it represents the class labels.

The rise of data science analytics integrated within big public health data and AI applications has given rise to new statistical terminologies for interpretations (Table 8.1) as compared to traditional epidemiology and statistical terminologies.

With the adoption of data science that integrates the exploration of big public health data with AI methodologies and concepts, this chapter was written timely with the projected evolution of public health practice and research using intelligent

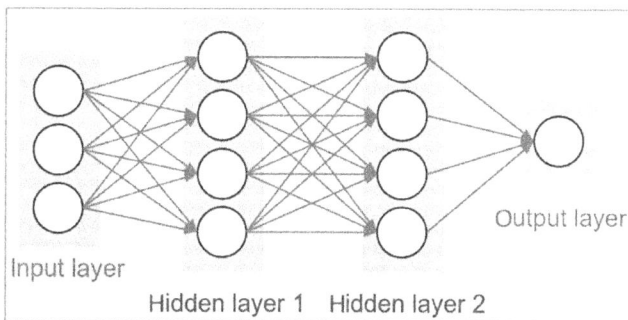

FIGURE 8.2   Architecture of deep neural network. (Ayon & Islam, 2019.)

TABLE 8.1

Important Conventional Terminologies Used in Epidemiology Equivalent to AI

Conventional Epidemiological and Statistical Terminologies	Equivalent to AI Terminologies
Dependent variable, outcome variable, or response variable	Label or class
Independent variable, predictor variable, or explanatory variable	Feature
2×2 table or contingency table	Confusion matrix
Sensitivity	Recall
Positive predictive value	Precision
Outcome group with highest frequency	Majority class
Outcome group with lowest frequency	Minority class
Proportion of cases in each category of the outcome variable (for categorical outcome)	Class balance
Exploratory analysis	Data mining
Qualitative or mixed – methods research with thematic content analysis	Natural language
Measurement error	Noisy labels

Source: Mooney and Pejaver (2018), Wiemken and Kelley (2020).

systems with modern, robust statistical applications for predicting, detecting and preventing diseases across populations worldwide. To be compliant with the chapter's intended aim and objective, this chapter will systematically appraise the utilization of AI, particularly DL for the prediction and detection of diseases from the public health approach. The chapter will illustrate examples of descriptors on the five core domains of public health, particularly NCDs, communicable diseases, maternal and child health, socio-behavioral medicine and environmental health for further exploration using data science, big public health data, AI and modern analytics concepts in the subsequent sections, and highlights potential strengths and limitations for practice.

8.4   DEEP LEARNING APPROACHES IN NON-COMMUNICABLE DISEASES PREDICTION

NCDs such as diabetes, hypertension, obesity/dyslipidemia and heart diseases have afflicted populations worldwide. In line with the industrial and technological revolution, population's lifestyle behaviors and dietary habits had changed concurrently. Most people adopted unhealthy eating habits due to lack of time as a consequence of busy work routines. Modern working conditions, which are highly tech savvy in nature, have changed routine work habits, forcing workers to adopt sedentary work patterns in office. These factors are attributed to lifestyle diseases such as diabetes, obesity/dyslipidemia and hypertension that subsequently cause more serious ailments such as ischemic heart diseases or stroke. Such diseases are currently the greatest public health threats to tackle as they cause significant co-morbidities, increased mortalities, reduced quality of life and escalated country's healthcare expenditures. What is more concerning to health systems and public health workers globally is that the majority of people across populations are undiagnosed with diabetes, hypertension and obesity/dyslipidemia. It is crucial to screen and detect populations being afflicted with these diseases early to plan proper management and control strategies in the quest to prevent debilitating ailments in the future. AI technologies through ML and DL algorithms have showed promising results to detect such diseases in a large scale within communities and populations worldwide, fast and accurately.

8.4.1 Diabetes

Diabetes is a chronic metabolic disease caused by progressive loss of β-cell insulin secretion as a consequence of insulin resistance (American Diabetes Association, 2020). The detection and diagnosis of diabetes are based on plasma glucose concentration and hemoglobin A1C. As diabetes is a disease that can cause a variety of complications such as retinopathy, nephropathy, neuropathy, heart diseases or stroke, the medical management for diabetes will concurrently screen these diseases to obtain relevant clinical parameters. They include findings from eye examinations, renal profiles, cardiac enzymes, lipid profiles, electrocardiogram readings and systolic and diastolic blood pressure readings. These data which are compiled as medical data sets have the capacity to be used for current detection and future prediction of diabetes using ML techniques.

Researchers from Bangladesh proposed the adoption of DNN with 5-fold and 10-fold cross-validation technique to detect diabetes using the Pima Indian Diabetes data set, available from an ML repository database (Ayon & Islam, 2019). Their findings showed that the proposed DL approach was feasible to predict diabetes. The yielded parameter of accuracy was 98.04%, sensitivity of 98.80% and specificity of 96.64% in the 5-fold cross-validation method. But the accuracy, sensitivity and specificity for the 10-fold technique were 97.11%, 96.25% and 98.8%, respectively. They concluded that the 5-fold cross-validation technique had better detection and prediction of diabetes, and much more feasible to be executed.

Investigators from Ontario, Canada, forecasted the incidence of diabetes from population health administrative data sets using ML techniques (Ravaut, Sadeghi, Leung, Volkovs, & Rosella, 2019). They used one of the largest health records compilations of patients available in their country which constituted the following variables: demographics (age, gender and ethnicities), lab investigations, drug effects, health system communications and hospital admission records. They subsequently performed the first large-scale complex ML algorithm with the aim to predict diabetes within communities for the next 1–10 years, without any additional screening of individuals. The following algorithms and techniques were employed:

1. *Logistic regression*: Used as the baseline.
2. *XGBoost*: Used for the main model, due to its capacity for high performance feature and handling of missing values.

3. *Highway network*: A relatively simple DNN architecture that has a temporal aspect with the capability to combine linear and non-linear output to provide greater modeling flexibility. This model yielded 14,944,001 parameters.

4. *CNN-LSTM* (Convolutional Neural Network - Long Short Term Memory): This model has a number of new features, consistent with the architecture proposed by Tonekaboni et al (2018). These include removing the maximum pooling as they have high potency to damage the performance. No dimensionality reduction was performed; instead batch normalization (Ioe & Szegedy, 2015) was added after each CNN layer, which increased the performance and convergence speed concurrently. Drop-out in the reference architecture was kept in the same place, i.e., after CNN layers. Two layers of LSTM were used. A three-layer perceptron followed by sigmoid was applied to perform binary prediction. This model yielded 22,744,136 parameters.

5. *LSTM-Seq2Seq*: An LSTM-based sequence to sequence architecture was borrowed from Sutskever, Vinyals, & Le (2014). It was used to reconstruct the concatenation of all features over time and applied a three layer perceptron on the encoder's last hidden layer to perform the prediction. Hence, this model is data-regularized due to the reconstruction cost that makes it different from the CNN-LSTM model. The investigators applied drop-out after each LSTM layer as advised by Zaremba, Sutskever, & Vinyals (2014). Teacher forcing (Williams & Zipser, 1989) was also applied to remove the reconstruction drift (bias) and increased the convergence speed. This model yielded 32,027,456 parameters.

After running the models, the investigators reached a test area under the curve (AUC) value of 80:3. Top fifteen features from the total 963 attributes yielded an AUC value of 79:1. The investigators successfully narrowed down important features from patient's laboratory investigations, insurance claims, having asthma, age and location for diabetes forecasting.

8.4.2 HYPERTENSION

Hypertension is a prevalent medical condition that is capable to lead serious complications such as ischemic heart disease, stroke or renal problems. Hypertension is diagnosed when systolic or diastolic blood pressure readings are elevated beyond the normal parameters of 120 or 80 mmHg, respectively (Whelton et al., 2018). Common risk factors of hypertension include advancing age, gender, obesity, stress, hyperlipidemia or family history of the disease. Uncertainties arise during diagnosis of hypertension, and such circumstances are due to incomplete clinical data or noisy data available within medical systems. ANN, an algorithm derived from DL method, has shown promising alternatives to conventional diagnostics; being powerful to detect hypertension in susceptible communities by eliminating or managing incomplete and noisy data sets.

LaFreniere, Zulkernine, Barber, and Mantin (2016) embarked on a work to identify risk factors attributed to hypertension from patients' medical records and demographic data. They used the Canadian Primary Care Sentinel Surveillance

Network dataset that consisted of approximately 185,371 patients and 193,656 controls. Required variables were extracted and analyzed using ANN to predict hypertension among individuals. Their model performance showed high accuracy for hypertension prediction, approximately 82%, concluding a promising alternative that ANN is useful to predict hypertension within the population, using big public health data sets.

8.4.3 Obesity

Evolutionary genomics has catalyzed biomedical research to transit small-scale research using conventional laboratory procedures into population-based studies by applying big data (Montanez et al., 2017). This prompted scientists to discover findings related to genetic variations associated with the risk of contracting diseases more accurately. Biomedical researchers will have the opportunity to deal with huge data sets, while encountering anticipated challenges related to data handling, processing and management through computational methods (Montanez et al., 2017). Genome-Wide Associated Studies (GWAS) reveals a variety of genomic loci related to complex traits across different populations worldwide. These studies will test huge number of genetic variants or a Single-Nucleotide Polymorphisms (SNPs) to explore associations within the trait of interests or common diseases encountered within the population, like obesity, diabetes or heart diseases (Burton et al., 2007; Hardy & Singleton, 2009; Visscher, Brown, McCarthy, & Yang, 2012; Fall & Ingelsson, 2014).

Emerging evidences postulated that genetic variations have important roles to determine individuals' susceptibility to diseases such as obesity. Obesity – a worldwide epidemic – catalyzes multiple morbidities such as diabetes, cardiovascular diseases (CVDs) and cancer. GWAS have identified multiple polymorphisms related to high Body Mass Index (BMI) and obesity. The most prevalent genetic variations encountered were Fat Mass Obesity-Associated and Melano-Cortin 4 Receptor (MC4R) (Scuteri et al., 2007; Wang et al., 2011). These findings were collected and compiled to create big databases such as the National Human Genome Research Institute Catalog (NHGRIC) or the GWAS database, motivating researchers to utilize data mining techniques to predict diseases (Montanez et al., 2017).

In their novel investigational approach, Montanez et al (2017) analyzed genetic variants from publicly available genetic profiles together with a manually crafted database – the NHGRIC. By applying data science techniques, genetic variants were identified from the collected participant profiles and subsequently indexed as a risk variant in the NHGRIC. These indexed genetic variants or SNPs were used as inputs through a series of ML algorithms to predict obesity. Participants BMI were classified into two; normal or with risks. Dimensionality reduction task was carried out to yield a string of 13 SNPs to be tested with various ML methods. The AUC values of the models were assessed. Techniques used include gradient boosting, generalized linear model, classification and regression trees, K-nearest neighbors, support vector machines (SVM), random forests (RFs) and multilayer perceptron neural network. They were evaluated based on their ability to identify the most important determinants like genetic variants, age or gender to classify an individual into the associated BMI class. SVM yielded the highest AUC value (90.5%).

In an innovative form, one study from the United States explored the following research question: How could CNN be useful to study the associations between built environment and obesity prevalence (Maharana & Nsoesie, 2018)? They proposed a technique to consistently measure the characteristics of the built environment (either natural or modified) and its association with the prevalence of obesity. Study design was cross-sectional in nature, and the CNN technique was employed to assess satellite images from Google Static Maps through Application Programming Interface. The features of the built environment across cities were extracted. Data on adult obesity prevalence were obtained from the Centers for Disease Control and Prevention's 500 Cities project.

Regression models were synthesized to explore the relationships between the features and obesity prevalence. The findings showed that neighborhood physical attributes such as parks, highways, green streets, crosswalks or housing types were associated with obesity prevalence. It was concluded that CNN has the ability to retrieve built environment characteristics from satellite images in the quest to explore health indicators.

8.4.4 Predicting Hypertension, Hyperglycemia and Dyslipidemia

As we apprehend, hypertension, hyperglycemia and dyslipidemia are diseases diagnosed based on blood pressure measurements, fasting blood glucose values and lipid profiles, respectively. These diseases are the primary risk factors for CVDs (Zhang et al., 2020). In recent decades, advancement in digital retinal photography and imaging techniques has facilitated scientists to recognize subtle changes in retinal blood vessels. Images from retinal fundus could enable us to detect early microcirculatory changes as a consequence of chronic diseases.

Retinal changes could be used to assess patient's risk for diabetes, hypertension or cardiovascular disease. Poplin et al. (2018) proved that changes in retina could point to significant CVD risks. As retinal fundus photography had shown promising results to detect early microcirculatory changes of chronic diseases, researchers from China-initiated efforts to develop neural network models for predicting hypertension, hyperglycemia, dyslipidemia and a range of risk factors using retinal fundus images, anthropometric parameters and biochemical result from 625 subjects (Zhang et al., 2020). The models in this study achieved an AUC of 0.880, 0.766 and 0.703 for predicting hyperglycemia, hypertension and dyslipidemia, respectively. These models also had an AUC > 0.7 for several blood erythrocyte parameters, including hematocrit, mean corpuscular hemoglobin concentration, and a cluster of CVD risk factors.

8.4.5 Cardiovascular Disease

CVDs such as coronary heart disease (CHD), cerebrovascular disease and rheumatic heart disease (RHD) are a major cause of morbidities and mortalities worldwide. Over 17.7 million people died in 2015 due to CVDs, accounting to almost 31% of all global deaths. Of these, approximately 7.4 million people died due to CHD alone (Alizadehsani et al., 2019). Although mortalities are high, chances of survival are better if diagnoses are made early. Scientists have devised appropriate models to predict patients at risks for contracting CHD using ML and data mining techniques from huge medical data sets

TABLE 8.2
Prediction and Detection of CVD using Different ML Algorithms

Works	Disease Studied	Techniques Used	Performance Accuracy
Tan, Teoh, Yu, and Goh (2009)	Heart disease	GA and SVM (hybrid approach)	84.07%
Parthiban and Srivatsa (2012)	Heart disease	SVM and NB	SVM – 94.6%; NB – 74%
Chaurasia and Pal (2013)	Heart disease	NB, J48 and Bagging	NB – 85.31%; J48–84.35%; Bagging – 85.03%
Vembandasamy, Sasipriya, and Deepa (2015)	Heart disease	NB	86.42%
Otoom, Abdallah, Kilani, Kefaye, and Ashour (2015)	Heart disease	BN, SVM and FT	BN – 85.5%; SVM – 85.1%; FT – 84.5%

Note: GA, Genetic Algorithm; SVM, Support Vector Machine; NB, Naive Bayes; FT, Functional Trees; BN, Bayes Net.

(Alizadehsani et al., 2019). Ayon, Islam, and Hossain, (2020) compared a number of AI techniques to predict CHD. They applied and tested a series of techniques, namely, Linear Regression (LR), SVM, DNN, Decision Tree, Naive Bayes (NB), and k-NN for comparative performance analytics in predicting CHD using heart disease data sets. They concluded that the technique with highest accuracy was DNN (98.15%), with sensitivity and precision accounted for 98.67% and 98.01% respectively in predicting CHD. Similarly, bulk of works have predicted CHD incidence from large data sets using a variety of ML algorithms and techniques as shown in Table 8.2.

8.5 DEEP LEARNING APPROACHES IN COMMUNICABLE DISEASES PREDICTION

The unprecedented threats of emerging and re-emerging infectious diseases like COVID-19 and the dengue epidemic to populations worldwide have called upon governments, healthcare and surveillance systems to enhance their pandemic preparedness capabilities. AI methodologies through ML and DL algorithms have offered new horizons to global public health systems to effectively forecast, predict, prevent and combat infectious diseases.

8.5.1 COVID-19 PANDEMIC

With the recent highly contagious COVID-19 pandemic, healthcare systems worldwide are struggling to contain the disease to further afflict populations at large; however, with the spectrum of unclear disease transmission dynamics, risk factors, treatment modalities and preventive measures, most healthcare systems are unable to cope with the exponential rise of positive cases and deaths occurred due to

COVID-19. Country resources were declining at an unexpected speed, bringing near collapse to governments and health care systems. With such rapid speed of infection rates, it was crucial for epidemiologists to yield mathematical prediction models to forecasts future anticipated cases to plan appropriate containment strategies towards flattening the epidemic curve. While conventional mathematical models are highly influenced by many extrinsic and intrinsic factors, AI systems using computational technologies were anticipated to be more accurate and reliable through the utilization of real-time big public health data and robust statistical procedures.

Researchers have developed an algorithmically driven system using DL approaches to predict COVID-19 transmission in India while determining the effectiveness of implemented preventive measures (Tomar & Gupta, 2020). The investigators used data-driven estimation methods, namely the LSTM and curve fitting for 30-day case predictions. They found significant accuracies in the prediction parameters (number of positive cases, recoveries and deaths) from the proposed method.

On another note, Alazab et al. (2020) analyzed the incidence of COVID-19 distribution using deep CNN from real-world data sets in Australia and Jordan. The proposed system examined chest radiographs to identify COVID-19 patients. Their results showed that chest radiographs were able to detect probable incidence of COVID-19, yet are conveniently and quickly available with low costs. The empirical findings obtained from 1,000 radiograph images of real patients confirmed that the proposed system was useful to detect COVID-19, with an F-measure range between 95% and 99%. Apart from the analysis, they forecasted COVID-19 incidence for the next seven days using three methods, namely, the prophet algorithm, autoregressive-integrated moving average model, and the LSTM to predict the numbers of COVID-19 detection, recoveries and mortalities. The prediction results exhibited promising performance and offered an average accuracy of 94.80% and 88.43% in Australia and Jordan, respectively. They concluded that the proposed system could significantly identify highly infected cities or coastal areas.

8.5.2 DENGUE OUTBREAK

The disproportionate spread of dengue outbreaks across endemic areas in most tropical and sub-tropical countries has been a major concern amongst epidemiologists and infectious disease specialists worldwide. Mathematical models projected that around fifty million infections occur throughout the year. Early diagnosis and forecasting future outbreaks coupled with identifying dengue hotspots through spatial epidemiology is crucial to control the outbreak. The applications of AI concepts and modern mathematical algorithms using ML and DL approaches have shown better accuracies in detecting and predicting dengue outbreaks. A group of investigators from Paraguay employed two ML techniques for comparisons, particularly the ANN and the SVM tools to detect the accuracies of dengue detection using data sets of dengue patients (Mello-Roman, Mello-Roman, Gomez-Guerrero, & Garcia-Torres, 2019). Classification models were yielded. Performance classification showed that the ANN multilayer perceptron had better results with 96% accuracy and sensitivity, and a specificity of 97%. In contrast, SVM had above 90% for accuracy, sensitivity and specificity.

8.6 DEEP LEARNING APPROACHES IN SOCIO-BEHAVIORAL MEDICINE

People's reactions, behavior and psychological repercussions during disease outbreaks and chronic health states are complex to decipher. DL methods and data science have enabled researchers to explore population's behavior, reactions and mental states during the course of an epidemic or chronic disease states to craft appropriate interventions and coping mechanisms. Apart from limited availability of neuro-biological data and series of time lags in conventional analytics, DL models have proven to be powerful in analyzing real-time mental health states of people through huge data sets available from centralized electronic health records (EHRs), wearable devices such as smartphone metadata and social media platforms such as "Twitter" or "Reddit."

8.6.1 PREDICTING MENTAL HEALTH STATES THROUGH MOBILE PHONES METADATA

Smartphones are embedded with sensor technologies which have extraordinary capacities to collect large volumes of data. While smartphones are a necessity within the human living environment, they are readily prepared to sense and collect various mental health variables that are available to a large degree. These sensor features available from GPS, calls or text messages could track movement patterns and social interactions to predict current or future mental health states (Canzian & Musolesi, 2015; Mehrotra, Hendley, & Musolesi, 2016; Abdullah et al., 2016).

For example, DL architecture analytics applied to smartphone metadata had the capability to determine psychological factors associated with sleep quality and stress (Sathyanarayana et al., 2016; Mikelsons, Smith, Mehrotra, & Musolesi, 2017), and to detect depression symptoms based on typing dynamics (Cao et al., 2017). Such approach is feasible as researchers could collect metadata on the duration of typing, speed and acceleration, allowing them to have more than 90% accuracy in detecting depressed individuals (Cao et al., 2017). With such approaches, it was possible to forecast future mental health states and disease dynamics. There were also efforts to track and predict future mental health states. A group of investigators forecasted severe depression on the basis of individual's mood, behavior diary and sleep pattern using the LSTM architecture (Suhara, Xu, & Pentland, 2017). They highlighted that these networks were capable to predict future psychological states.

8.6.2 PREDICTING MENTAL HEALTH STATES THROUGH SOCIAL MEDIA DATA

NLP, a DL technique is being used in healthcare systems to analyze EHRs for studying mental health conditions and people's risky behaviors on large scales. But these narratives in clinical records do not capture real-time experiences of patients; it is only a cross-section of the scenario and professional speculations during practice. Social media are currently being regarded as a real-time source to capture people's emotions, behaviors, feelings and psychology in the quest to analyze mental health repercussions in large communities or populations. Gkotsis et al. (2017) analyzed posts from Reddit (a social media platform) to recognize and classify posts related to mental disorders according to relevant themes. They employed neural networks to automatically recognize mental illness-related themes such as borderline personality disorder, bipolar disorder, schizophrenia, anxiety, depression, self-harm, suicide, addiction, alcoholism, opiates and autism spectrum disorder. They achieved an accuracy of 91.08%, with correct theme selection weighted an average accuracy of 71.37%. Their results have provided a novel method that has the ability to identify early psychological states for targeted interventions.

8.6.3 PUBLIC REACTIONS AND RESPONSES DURING OUTBREAKS

On-time apprehension of general public perceptions and reactions allow public health systems to intervene during outbreaks. Social media such as Twitter has provided novel alternatives for rapid evaluations of public responses during health crisis in large-scales. Twitter has facilitated users to post or read each other's tweets (Ganasegeran & Abdulrahman, 2020). Crucial information and geo-locate functions embedded within Twitter streams have allowed researchers to postulate and track Twitter users' reactions to forecast behaviors during health exigencies. Du et al. (2018) developed a hypothetical scheme to evaluate comprehensive public perceptions during measles outbreak in the USA based on Twitter data. They aimed to determine models' superiority in determining people's reactions during the outbreak by using either CNN or conventional ML techniques. Three dimensions were evaluated, particularly – theme discussions, analyzing expression of emotions and attitudes toward vaccination. A total of 1,154,156 tweets were analyzed. The performance yielded by the CNN framework was compared with other conventional ML and neural network models. Cohen kappa values from the CNN model were 0.78, 0.72 and 0.80 on the three respective dimensions, thus collectively outperformed all other classification frameworks.

8.7 DEEP LEARNING APPROACHES IN MATERNAL AND CHILD HEALTH DISEASE PREDICTION

8.7.1 MATERNAL HEALTH

Maternal health is conceptualized as the women's health during the period of gestation, child birth and post-partum period (Sahle, 2016). Countries worldwide aim to have the best maternal care services to prevent complications that could arise during pregnancy, labor or at puerperium to prevent maternal mortalities. Early detection of potential risk factors, morbidities or complications is crucial to facilitate appropriate treatment strategies to ensure that the wellbeing of the mother and the newborn is not compromised. The global Sustainable Development Goals aim to reduce the Maternal Mortality Ratio (MMR), ensuring that no countries in the world to have an MMR index double than that of global average (World Health Organization, 2019). Albeit many strategies and guidelines have been implemented, maternal mortality remains high, especially in low- and middle-income countries (LMICs). Approximately 810 women die daily as a consequence of complications that arise during pregnancy and childbirth (World Health Organization, 2019). Most of these deaths were preventable if complications such as eclampsia or pre-eclampsia, obstructed labor, ruptured uterus, infectious diseases like malaria and complications from abortion were detected early or handled by skilled professionals during the care of the mother and newborns (Tesfaye, Atique, Azim, & Kebede, 2019). Women in LMICs often seek delivery attendant services within their localities or proceed to deliver at home, which could be alarming if complications arise and no immediate management are executed (Tesfaye, Atique, Azim, & Kebede, 2019). It is important for pregnant mothers to seek consultations from skilled delivery service consultants for successful and uneventful deliveries.

It is crucial to understand what predicts the likelihood of pregnant mothers to use skilled delivery services. Such information is important to develop models that could assist public health practitioners to craft appropriate target interventions. Conventional available data, although being the "gold-standard" to understand the predictors of using skilled delivery services, are unable to forecast the future. Thus, the application of ML techniques using big public health data from maternal registries, records or surveillance data could be of great use to understand the current scenario, and to predict future phenomenon to mould targeted interventions to reduce maternal mortality.

A group of researchers from Ethiopia predicted skilled delivery service utilization by pregnant mothers using ML algorithms (Tesfaye, Atique, Azim, & Kebede, 2019). They used data from the 2016 Ethiopian Demographic and Health Survey (EDHS). They performed conventional LR analyses and the more robust model building of the Waikato Environment for Knowledge Analysis. Classification algorithms that include both ML and DL approaches such as J48, NB, SVM and ANN were utilized to yield prediction models. The yielded models were assessed for accuracies, sensitivities, specificities and the AUC. They found that 27.7% of pregnant women who received skilled delivery services were influenced based on the initial antenatal visit, birth order, television ownership, contraceptive use, healthcare cost, age of first birth and age of first sex. The J48 model had higher accuracy, sensitivity, specificity and AUC values as compared to other models (Tesfaye, Atique, Azim, & Kebede, 2019).

Postnatal care is another crucial aspect to prevent maternal mortality. By using data from the EDHS, Sahle (2016) applied Knowledge Discovery Data (KDD) to identify barriers of postnatal care in Ethiopia. J48 algorithm and JRip algorithms were employed to the dataset. It was found that accuracies for identifying delivery place, having professional personnel for delivery and women's age were attributed to postnatal care service utilization. The predictive model accounted for high accuracies, 93.97% for J48 algorithm and 93.93% for JRip algorithm. The study concluded that the rules generated by both algorithms were easily apprehended to predict outcomes easily (Sahle, 2016). The results obtained are highly valuable to craft, evaluate and update maternal health promotional policies.

8.7.2 CHILD HEALTH

Despite advancements in child health services, such as immunization programs to reduce child mortalities, there are still approximately 15,000 children under the age of five who die on a daily basis across LMICs (Roser, Ritchie, & Dadonaite, 2013). These mortalities are largely preventable and are caused by the most common etiologies such as diarrhea, malaria or malnutrition (Adegbosin, Stantic, & Sun, 2019). Basic medi-cal care services have the capacity to overcome these avoidable diseases among children. Under such circumstances, it is crucial to explore the health status of every child across different geographical and socio-economic levels. Conventional surveillance data may not effectively monitor the health coverage of every child and its impact across communities. Investigators from Australia predicted under-five mortality and its associated factors across twenty-one LMICs using DL methods by using data from the Demographic and Health Survey (DHS) (Adegbosin, Stantic, & Sun, 2019). They com-pared the efficacy of DL algorithms such as DNN, CNN, hybrid CNN-DNN and LR in predicting under-five mortality. Amongst the under-five mortality predictors identi-fied were breast feeding duration, household wealth index and maternal education. DL techniques (sensitivity and specificity values for: (a) DNN were 0.69 and 0.83, respec-tively; (b) CNN were 0.68 and 0.83, respectively; and (c) CNN-DNN were 0.71 and 0.83, respectively) were superior to LR with sensitivity and specificity values of 0.47 and 0.53, respectively, in classifying child survival (Adegbosin, Stantic, & Sun, 2019).

Another significant cause of childhood mortality is malnutrition. Researchers from India conducted a study to predict a model for malnutrition based on ML approaches by using available variables from the Indian Demographic and Health Survey data set and compared with the existing literature (Khare, Kavyashree, Gupta, & Jyotishi, 2017). The yielded results found that applying ML concepts have identified some attributes that were not identified within previous literature. An LR algorithm was conducted to explore further odds and probabilities affecting malnutrition in Indian children. They found significant correlates that could be useful to identify malnour-ished children in India based on LR algorithms yielded through AI concepts (Khare, Kavyashree, Gupta, & Jyotishi, 2017).

Many children across LMICs have not completed immunizations schedule, vac-cinated late or dropped out from on-going immunization schedule, thus alarming greater risk for vaccine preventable diseases and deaths. There is a crucial need to model and visualize risks of missed vaccinations from available big health data sets for vaccinators and public health advocates to identify children being missed from immunization coverage. ML technologies and data mining have shown promising outputs to identify children with missed immunizations. Chandir et al. (2018) con-ducted a feasibility study to determine children who are likely to be missed from immunization schedule. They developed an algorithm using longitudinal immuni-zation records, classified according to training and validation cohorts. ML models were yielded through RF, recursive partitioning, SVM and C-forests to predict the likelihood of each child that is expected to miss a subsequent immunization visit. Model performances were assessed. The RF model correctly predicted 8,994 cases of the total 11,889 cases available, yielding a 94.9% sensitivity and 54.9% specificity rates. The C-forest model, SVMs and recursive partitioning models improved pre-diction by achieving 352, 376 and 389 correctly predicted cases respectively, above the predictions made by the RF model. All models had a C-statistic of 0.75 or above, whereas the highest statistic (AUC 0.791, 95% CI 0.784-0.798) was observed in the recursive partitioning algorithm. The researchers concluded that predictive analytics can accurately identify children who are at a higher risk for defaulting on follow-up immunization visits (Chandir et al., 2018).

8.8   DEEP LEARNING APPROACHES IN ENVIRONMENTAL HEALTH DISEASE PREDICTION

Respiratory ailments such as acute respiratory tract infections or bronchitis are strongly correlated with environmental risk factors. Approximately seven million deaths that occur annually were attributed to atmospheric air pollution (Chen & Wu, 2019). Ozone (O_3), regarded as a secondary air pollutant formed by complex photochemical processes till date, has caused over 1.1 million deaths worldwide, with almost 20% of them being attributed to respiratory diseases or co-morbidities (Malley et al., 2017). Predicting and forecasting air quality or pollution exposures that are stratified across different geographical areas and populations are crucial to plan appropriate preventive measures from diseases that are highly attributable to pollutants or environmental particulate matter (PM). DL has emerged as a powerful computational tool to predict environmental hazards that could cause serious life-threatening diseases in exposed individuals. Environmental epidemiologists till date have executed classification, regression, clustering and association mining algorithms from big public health data sets through the application of DL algorithms to yield frameworks on the impact of pollution to people's health.

Investigators from Canada forecasted the quality of air using DL algorithms employed to time series data (Freeman, Taylor, Gharabaghi, & The, 2018). Air quality readings are continuously captured and retrieved from air monitoring stations. These data are collectively known as time series data sets. The captured information from the data sets is crucial to identify populations being exposed to hazardous PM, and to ensure if air pollutant index were compliant to local ambient air standards. To ensure reliable outcomes through statistical interpretation, the investigators forecasted an eight hour averaged O_3 concentrations through DL algorithms that employed the novel recurrent neural network (RNN) with LSTM approach.

Comparison architecture between simple feed-forward neural network and RNN is shown in Figure 8.3. The arrows between layers represent synaptic weights interconnecting each node (each layer can have different number of nodes except for the hidden layer, in which the nodes are static). RNN (Elman structure) has been used

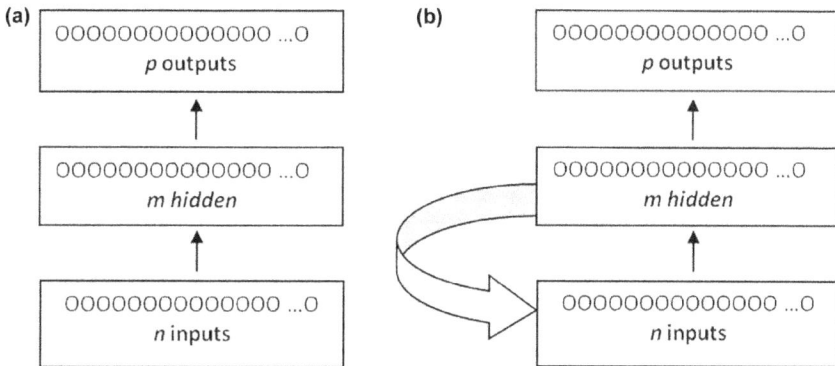

FIGURE 8.3 Comparison between simple feed-forward neural network (a) and recurrent "Elman" neural network (b).

with air station inputs to predict O_3 concentrations (Biancofiore et al., 2015) and $PM_{2.5}$ levels (Biancofiore et al., 2017). The implementation of such procedures are done through an LSTM approach; facilitating the trained network to operate without an "explode" or "vanish" parameters due to multiple learning efforts (Pascanu, Mikolov, & Bengio, 2013). The investigators used hourly air quality and meteorological data to train and forecast parameters up to seventy-two hours in length with minimal errors. LSTM was able to forecast the duration of continuous O_3 emissions. After adjusting for missing data and outliers, decision trees were used to identify input variables with highest degree of importance. The investigators concluded that the methodologies adopted in the current study would allow air managers to predict long range of air pollution concentration with key parametric observations without transforming or correcting the entire data set, thus facilitating real-time inputs and continuous forecasting.

Much recently, researchers from China explored the associations between environmental risk factors and acute respiratory diseases using DL method (Chen & Wu, 2019). By utilizing respiratory disease, air pollution and meteorological data sets from Beijing, they employed a cross-domain risk factors exploration, stratified according to age and gender to predict environmental hazards PM or pollutants that cause respiratory ailments. The conceptual analytical process is exhibited in Figure 8.4. DNN models in air pollution epidemiology with quantitative analyses were executed. The following results were yielded:

1. People aged ≥ 50 years were more likely to be sensitive to $PM_{2.5}$ pollution as compared to younger aged ones. Women aged ≥ 50 years were more sensitive to $PM_{2.5}$.
2. Men of all ages were more susceptible to PM_{10}.
3. Women aged < 50 years old were more sensitive to pollutants like SO_2 and NO_2.
4. Meteorological attributes like wind could advance the diffusion of PM and pollutants to reduce respiratory ailments.

The investigators concluded that such findings from the utilization of DL algorithms would assist to promote prevention strategies among populations towards environmental hazards (Chen & Wu, 2018).

8.9 STRENGTHS, LIMITATIONS AND FUTURE DIRECTION

In line with the revolution of big data and data science, it will be wise for public health researchers and practitioners to adopt newer analytical techniques by utilizing novel data sources. Such resources which are robust, valid and reliable have the ability to synthesize real-time evidences for policy making and to create newer knowledge to fill existing gaps in the literature. While these computational data resources have the capacity to develop latest infrastructures and methodologies to the public health workforce, they should be assured to be used ethically.

DL utilizes huge data sets and computational methods to synthesize results through automated classification (non-human operator dependent). Common techniques used

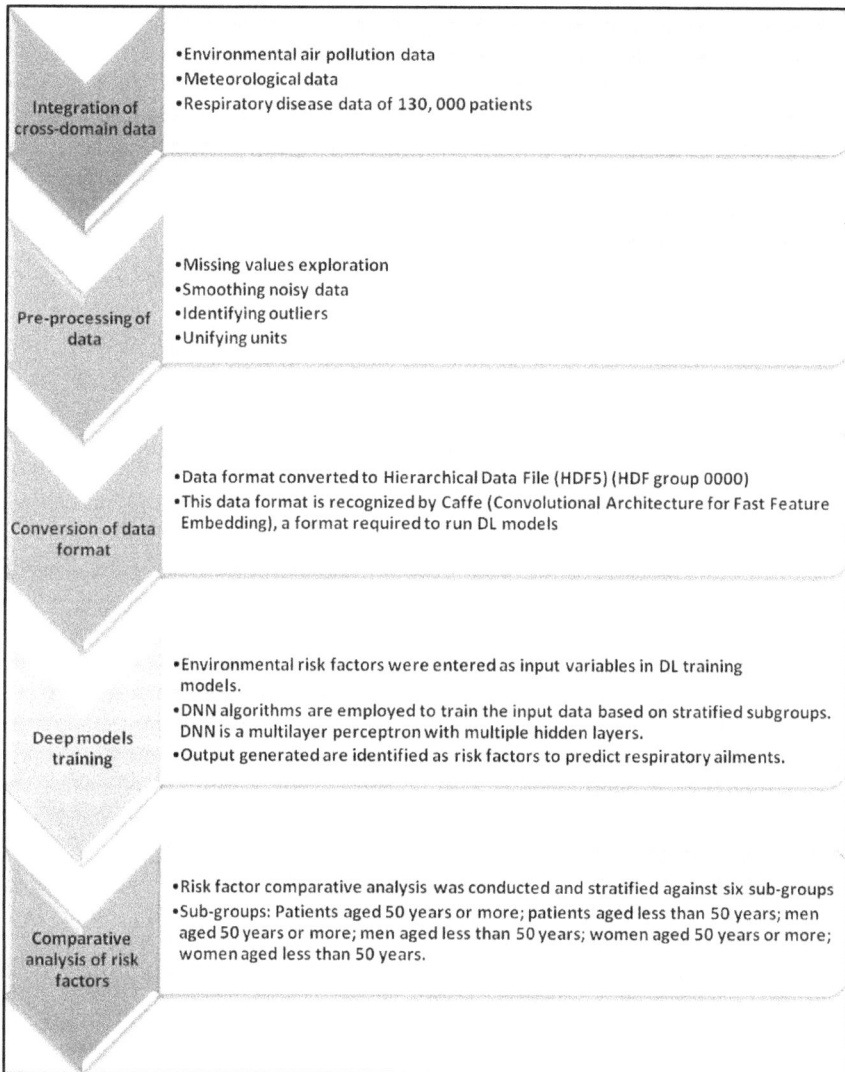

Integration of cross-domain data
- Environmental air pollution data
- Meteorological data
- Respiratory disease data of 130, 000 patients

Pre-processing of data
- Missing values exploration
- Smoothing noisy data
- Identifying outliers
- Unifying units

Conversion of data format
- Data format converted to Hierarchical Data File (HDF5) (HDF group 0000)
- This data format is recognized by Caffe (Convolutional Architecture for Fast Feature Embedding), a format required to run DL models

Deep models training
- Environmental risk factors were entered as input variables in DL training models.
- DNN algorithms are employed to train the input data based on stratified subgroups. DNN is a multilayer perceptron with multiple hidden layers.
- Output generated are identified as risk factors to predict respiratory ailments.

Comparative analysis of risk factors
- Risk factor comparative analysis was conducted and stratified against six sub-groups
- Sub-groups: Patients aged 50 years or more; patients aged less than 50 years; men aged 50 years or more; men aged less than 50 years; women aged 50 years or more; women aged less than 50 years.

FIGURE 8.4   Schema of stages in DNN structure.

are image classification and NLP (LeCun, Bengio, & Hinton, 2015). Such techniques are expected to gain increased momentum and applications in the near future as they are cost-effective (Lasko, Denny, & Levy, 2013). DL commonly uses ANN models which are intricate, but flexible to include unrestricted attributes for classifications or regressions. They are used for modeling non-linearity. As ANN models are computationally too invasive, extensive training are required to operate their algorithms, reducing wider adoption in local settings.

As we observe that DL approaches are gaining unprecedented popularity across all major public health domains, it has been regarded as an acceptance to fix global health issues that currently plague populations and communities – ranging from pandemic preparedness, lifestyle disease prevention, response toward health crises and environmental health hazards in comparison to conventional population-based approaches. However, with the rise of these smart-machines, resource-rich settings are challenged with the lack of expertise to build and update the knowledge base of expert systems. Concerns related to ownership of data and privacy settings using computational algorithms through AI were prevalent among practitioners and researchers. Resource-limited settings face substantial challenges due to poor internet infrastructure and connectivity.

Health crises and pandemics that are currently afflicting populations worldwide such as the COVID-19 outbreak, climate change, lifestyle changes and re-emergence of certain neglected tropical diseases has challenged public health workers worldwide to contain the spread of disease or health related states as a consequence of newer disease transmission dynamics or risk factors that were never encountered before. We want evidence now! We want a solution now! We need data now! The revolution of population health data science has offered new alternatives to conventional public health systems by integrating real-time data sets into sophisticated computational analyses to yield on time evidence for policy crafting. Despite this evolution, we lack the relevant expertise! The integration of computational technologies and big public health data is unavoidable within the current pace of practice, and we need two principal commitments to craft urgent public health interventions through robust analytic procedures; the first – we need to think like a computer (Tilson & Gebbie)! The second – we need to avoid systematic bias as we are required to handle secondary data (Kochenderfer, 2015)! We are going to deal with real-time continuous secondary data that would be huge to handle, and that require huge thinking capacity within a fast-working pace using statistical algorithms. To be in line with this evolution, we need new training and skills in addition to the conventional public health training and practice (Tilson & Gebbie, 2004)!

Big public health data and its analytical processes have fostered privacy concerns (Mai, 2016), with the fundamental issue on the possible revelation of personal information through online platforms (Bader, Mooney, & Rundle, 2016). The adoption of modern analytical approaches should be guaranteed by experts and stakeholders that privacy settings, security and anonymity of users are never compromised, and are facilitated with secured features.

8.10 CONCLUSION

It is undeniable that DL approaches in public health has enormous benefits to revolutionize populations health. Facilitating early disease detection, prediction, prevention and health promotion activities, DL algorithms through computational intelligence could be deployed to improve surveillance systems and public health outcomes. DL algorithms have ensured cost-effective methodologies through its modeling and predictive accuracy capabilities, varying from detection of outbreaks, health crises, lifestyle risk factors and health seeking behaviors using robust frameworks through expert systems and applications. While the revolution seems stunningly incredible, there are significant ethical and training concerns that are needed to be tackled before large scale implementations are made possible.

ACKNOWLEDGMENT

We thank the Ministry of Health Malaysia for the support to publish this chapter.

REFERENCES

Abdullah, S., Matthews, M., Frank, E., Doherty, G., Gay, G., & Choudhury, T. (2016). Automatic detection of social rhythms in bipolar disorder. *Journal of the American Medical Informatics Association, 23,* 538–543.

Adegbosin, A.E., Stantic, B., & Sun, J. (2019). Predicting under-five mortality across 21 low and middle-income countries using deep learning methods. *medRxiv,* Doi: 10.1101/19007583.

Alazab, M., Awajan, A., Mesleh, A., Abraham, A., Jatana, V., & Alhyari, S. (2020). COVID-19 prediction and detection using deep learning. *International Journal of Computer Information Systems and Industrial Management Applications, 12,* 168–181.

Alizadehsani, R., Roshanzamir, M., Abdar, M., Beykikhoshk, A., Khosravi, A., Panahiazar, M., et al. (2019). A database for using machine learning and data mining techniques for coronary artery disease diagnosis. *Scientific Data, 6,* 227.

American Diabetes Association. (2020). Classification and diagnosis of diabetes: standards of medical care in diabetes – 2020. *Diabetes Care, 43,* S14–S31.

Ayon, S.I., & Islam, M.M. (2019). Diabetes prediction: a deep learning approach. *International Journal of Information Engineering and Electronic Business, 2,* 21–27.

Ayon, S.I., Islam, M.M., & Hossain, M.R. (2020). Coronary artery heart disease prediction: a comparative study of computational intelligence techniques. *IETE Journal of Research,* Doi: 10.1080/03772063.2020.1713916.

Bader, M.D., Mooney, S.J., & Rundle, A.G. (2016). Protecting personally identifiable information when using online geographic tools for public health research. *American Journal of Public Health, 106,* 206–208.

Bellman, R. (2015). *Adaptive Control Processes: A Guided Tour.* Princeton, NJ: Princeton University Press.

Biancofiore, F., Verdecchia, M., Di Carlo, P., Tomassetti, B., Aruffo, E., Busilacchio, M., et al. (2015). Analysis of surface ozone using a recurrent neural network. *Science of the Total Environment, 514,* 379–387.

Biancofiore, F., Busilacchio, M., Verdecchia, M., Tomassetti, B., Aruffo, E., Bianco, S. et al. (2017). Recursive neural network model for analysis and forecast of PM10 and PM2:5. *Atmospheric Pollution Research, 8*(4), 652–659.

Burton, P.R., Clayton, D.G., Cardon, L.R., Craddock, N., Deloukas, P., & Duncanson, A. (2007). Genome-wide association study of 14,000 cases of seven common diseases and 3,000 shared controls. *Nature, 447*(7145), 661–678.

Canzian, L., & Musolesi, M. (2015). Trajectories of depression: unobtrusive monitoring of depressive states by means of smartphone mobility traces analysis. *Proceedings of the ACM International Joint Conference on Pervasive and Ubiquitous Computing.* ACM, 1293–1304, New York, NY.

Cao, B., Zheng, L., Zhang, C., Yu, P.S., Piscitello, A., & Zulueta, J., et al. (2017). DeepMood: modeling mobile phone typing dynamics for mood detection. *Proceedings of the 23rd ACM SIGKDD International Conference on Knowledge Discovery and Data Mining.* ACM, 747–755, New York, NY.

Chandir, S., Siddiqi, D.A., Hussain, O.A., Niazi, T., Shah, M.T., Dharma, V.K., et al. (2018). Using predictive analytics to identify children at high risk of defaulting from a routine immunization program: feasibility study. *JMIR Public Health and Surveillance, 4*(3), e63.

Chaurasia, V., & Pal, S. (2013). Data mining approach to detect heart disease. *International Journal of Advanced Computer Science and Information Technology, 2,* 56–66.

Chen, S., & Wu, S. (2019). Deep learning for identifying environmental risk factors of acute respiratory diseases in Beijing, China: implications for population with different age and gender. *International Journal of Environmental Health Research*, Doi: 10.1080/09603123.2019.1597836.

Du, J., Tang, L., Xiang, Y., Zhi, D., Xu, J., Song, H.Y., & Tao, C. (2018). Public perception analysis of Tweets during the 2015 measles outbreak: comparative study using convolutional neural network models. *Journal of Medical Internet Research, 20*(7), e236.

Fall, T., & Ingelsson, E. 2014. Genome-wide association studies of obesity and metabolic syndrome. *Molecular and Cellular Endocrinology, 382*(1), 740–757.

Freeman, B.S., Taylor, G., Gharabaghi, B., & The, J. (2018). Forecasting air quality time series using deep learning. *Journal of the Air & Waste Management Association, 68*(8), 866–886.

Frerot, M., Lefebvre, A., Aho, S., Callier, P., Astruc, K., & Aho Glele, L.S. (2018). What is epidemiology? Changing definitions of epidemiology 1978–2017. *Plos One, 13*(12), e0208442.

Ganaseggeran, K., & Abdulrahman, S.A. (2020). Artificial intelligence applications in tracking health behaviors during disease epidemics. In: D. J. Hemanth (Eds.), *Human Behaviour Analysis Using Intelligent Systems, Learning and Analytics in Intelligent Systems* (6th ed., pp. 141–155). Springer Nature Switzerland AG.

Ganaseggeran, K., Ch'ng, A.S.H., Aziz, Z.A., & Looi, I. (2020). Population's health information- seeking behaviors and geographic variations of stroke in Malaysia: an ecological correlation and time series study. *Scientific Reports, 10*, 11353.

Gkotsis, G., Oellrich, A., Velupillai, S., Liakata, M., Hubbard, T.J.P., Dobson, R.J.B., & Dutta, R. (2017). Characterisation of mental health conditions in social media using informed deep learning. *Scientific Reports, 7*, 45141.

Hardy, J., & Singleton, A. (2009). Genomewide association studies and human disease. *The New England Journal of Medicine, 360*(17), 1759–1768.

Ioe, S., & Szegedy, C. (2015). Batch normalization: accelerating deep network training by reducing internal covariate shift. *arXiv preprint, arXiv,* 1502.03167.

Khare, S., Kavyashree, S., Gupta, D.S., & Jyotishi, A. (2017). Investigation of nutritional status of children based on machine learning techniques using Indian demographic and health survey data. 7th international conference on advances in computing & communications. *Procedia Computer Science, 115*, 338–349.

Kochenderfer, M.J. (2015). *Decision Making Under Uncertainty: Theory and Application.* Cambridge, MA: MIT Press.

Kurzweil, R. (1990). *The Age of Intelligent Machines.* Cambridge, MA: MIT Press.

LaFreniere, D., Zulkernine, F., Barber, D., & Martin, K. (2016). Using machine learning to predict hypertension from a clinical dataset. *IEEE Symposium Series on Computational Intelligence (SSCI)*, pp. 1–7, Athens.

Lasko, T.A., Denny, J.C., & Levy, M.A. (2013). Computational phenotype discovery using unsupervised feature learning over noisy, sparse, and irregular clinical data. *PLoS One, 8*, e66341.

Lavigne, M., Mussa, F., Creatore, M.I., Hoffman, S.J., & Buckeridge, D.L. (2019). A population health perspective on artificial intelligence. *Healthcare Management Forum, 32*(4), 173–177.

LeCun, Y., Bengio, Y., & Hinton, G. (2015). Deep learning. *Nature, 521*, 436–444.

Maharana, A., & Nsoesie, E.O. (2018). Use of deep learning to examine the association of the built environment with prevalence of neighborhood adult obesity. *JAMA Network Open, 1*(4), e181535.

Mai, J-E. (2016). Big data privacy: the datafication of personal information. *The Information Society, 32,*192–199.

Malley, C.S., Henze, D.K., Kuylenstierna, J.C., Vallack, H.W., Davila, Y., Anenberg, S.C., et al. (2017). Updated global estimates of respiratory mortality in adults &$\geq$; 30 years of age attributable to long-term ozone exposure. *Environmental Health Perspectives, 125*(8), 087021.

Mehrotra, A., Hendley, R., & Musolesi, M. (2016). Towards multi-modal anticipatory monitoring of depressive states through the analysis of human-smartphone interaction. *Proceedings of the ACM International Joint Conference on Pervasive and Ubiquitous Computing.* ACM, 1132–1138, New York, NY.

Mello-Roman, J.D., Mello-Roman, J.C., Gomez-Guerrero, S., & Garcia-Torres, M. (2019). Predictive models for the medical diagnosis of dengue: a case-study in Paraguay. *Computational and Mathematical Methods in Medicine, 7307803,* 7.

Mikelsons, G., Smith, M., Mehrotra, A., & Musolesi, M. (2017). Towards deep learning models for psychological state prediction using smartphone data: challenges and opportunities. *arXiv preprint, arXiv,* 171106350.

Montanez, C.A.C., Fergus, P., Hussain, A., Al-Jumeily, D., Abdulaimma, B., Hind, J., et al. (2017). Machine learning approaches for the prediction of obesity using publicly available genetic profiles. *International Joint Conference on Neural Networks (IJCNN),* IEEE, Anchorage, AK, USA.

Mooney, S.J., & Pejaver, V. (2018). Big data in public health: terminology, machine learning, and privacy. *Annual Review of Public Health, 39,* 95–112.

National Institute of Standards and Technology. (2015). *NIST big data interoperability framework definitions (vol. 1). (NIST special publication 1500–1).* Retrieved from: http://nvlpubs.nist.gov/nistpubs/SpecialPublications/NIST.SP.1500-1.pdf.

Otoom, A.F., Abdallah, E.E., Kilani, Y., Kefaye, A., & Ashour, M. (2015). Effective diagnosis and monitoring of heart disease. *International Journal of Software Engineering and Its Applications, 9,* 143–156.

Parthiban, G., & Srivatsa, S.K. (2012). Applying machine learning methods in diagnosing heart disease for diabetic patients. *International Journal of Applied Information Systems, 3,* 25–30.

Pascanu, R., Mikolov, T., & Bengio, Y. (2013). On the difficulty of training recurrent neural networks. In *30th International Conference on Machine Learning,* Volume 28. W&CP. Retrieved from: http://proceedings.mlr.press/v28/pascanu13.pdf.

Poole, D.L., Mackworth, A.K., & Goebel, R. (1998). *Computational Intelligence: A Logical Approach* (vol. 1). New York, NY: Oxford University Press.

Poplin, R., Varadarajan, A.V., Blumer, K., Liu, Y., McConnell, M.V., Corrado, G.S., et al. (2018). Prediction of cardiovascular risk factors from retinal fundus photographs via deep learning. *Nature Biomedical Engineering, 2*(3), 158–164.

Ravaut, M., Sadeghi, H., Leung, K.K., Volkovs, M., & Rosella, L.C. (2019). Diabetes mellitus forecasting using population health data in Ontario, Canada. *Proceedings of Machine Learning Research, 85,* 1–18.

Roser, M., Ritchie, H., & Dadonaite, B. (2013). Child and infant mortality. Published online at OurWorldInData.org. Retrieved from: https://ourworldindata.org/child-mortality [Online Resource].

Sahle, G. (2016). Ethiopic maternal care data mining: discovering the factors that affect postnatal care visit in Ethiopia. *Health Information Science and Systems, 4,* 4.

Sathyanarayana, A., Joty, S., Fernandez-Luque, L., Ofli, F., Srivastava, J., & Elmagarmid, A., et al. (2016). Sleep quality prediction from wearable data using deep learning. *JMIR mHealth and uHealth, 4,* e125.

Scuteri, A., Sanna, S., Chen, W-M., Uda, M., Albai, G., & Strait, J. (2007). Genome-wide association scan shows genetic variants in the FTO gene are associated with obesity-related traits. *PloS Genetics, 3*(7), e115.

Suhara, Y., Xu, Y., & Pentland, A.S. (2017). Deepmood: forecasting depressed mood based on self-reported histories via recurrent neural networks. *Proceedings of the 26th International Conference on World Wide Web*, 715–724, Perth.

Sutskever, I., Vinyals, O., & Le, Q.V. (2014). Sequence to sequence learning with neural networks. *Advances in Neural Information Processing Systems*, 3104–3112.

Tan, K.C., Teoh, E.J., Yu, Q., & Goh, K.C. (2009). A hybrid evolutionary algorithm for attribute selection in data mining. *Journal of Expert System with Applications*, 36, 8616-8630.

Tesfaye, B., Atique, S., Azim, T., & Kebede, M.M. (2019). Predicting skilled delivery service use in Ethiopia: dual application of logistic regression and machine learning algorithms. *BMC Medical Informatics and Decision Making, 19*, 209.

Tilson, H., & Gebbie, K.M. (2004). The public health workforce. *Annual Review of Public Health, 25*, 341–356.

Tomar, A., & Gupta, N. (2020). Prediction for the spread of COVID-19 in India and effectiveness of preventive measures. *Science of the Total Environment, 728*, 138762.

Tonekaboni, S., Mazwi, M., Laussen, P., Eytan, D., Greer, R., Goodfellow, S.D., Goodwin, A., Brudno, M., & Goldenberg, A. (2018). Prediction of cardiac arrest from physiological signals in the pediatric ICU. *Machine Learning for Healthcare Conference*, 534–550.

Vembandasamy, K., Sasipriya, R., & Deepa, E. (2015). Heart diseases detection using naive Bayes algorithm. *International Journal of Innovative Science, Engineering & Technology, 2*, 441–444.

Visscher, P.M., Brown, M.A., McCarthy, M.I., & Yang, J. (2012). Five years of GWAS discovery. *The American Journal of Human Genetics, 90*(1), 7–24.

Wang, K., Li, W-D., Zhang, C.K., Wang, Z., Glessner, J.T., Grant, S.F.A., et al. (2011). A genome-wide association study on obesity and obesity-related traits. *PLoS One, 6*(4), e18939.

Whelton, P.K., Carey, R.M., Aronow, W.S., Casey Jr, D.E., Collins, K.J., Himmelfarb, C.D., et al. (2018). 2017 ACC/AHA/AAPA/ABC/ACPM/AGS/APhA/ASH/ASPC/NMA/PCNA guideline for the prevention, detection, evaluation and management of high blood pressure in adults - a report of the American College of Cardiology/American Heart Association task force on clinical practice guidelines. *Journal of the American College of Cardiology, 71*, 19.

Wiemken, T.L., & Kelley, R.R. (2020). Machine learning in epidemiology and health outcomes research. *Annual Review of Public Health, 41*, 1.1–1.16.

Williams, R.J., & Zipser, D. (1989). A learning algorithm for continually running fully recurrent neural networks. *Neural Computation, 1*(2), 270–280.

World Health Organization (WHO). *Fact sheets: Maternal mortality*. (2019). Retrieved from: https://www.who.int/news-room/fact-sheets/detail/maternal-mortality [Online Resource] (accessed 20 July 2020).

Zaremba, W., Sutskever, I., & Vinyals, O. (2014). Recurrent neural network regularization. *arXiv preprint, arXiv*, 1409.2329.

Zhang, L., Yuan, M., An, Z., Zhao, X., Wu, H., Li, H., et al. (2020). Prediction of hypertension, hyperglycemia and dyslipidemia from retinal fundus photographs via deep learning: a cross-sectional study of chronic diseases in central China. *PLoS One, 15*(5), e0233166.

9 Genomics with Deep Learning

X. Chen
University of Kentucky

CONTENTS

9.1   INTRODUCTION: BACKGROUND AND DRIVING FORCES

Genomic research is changing and will continue to change the biomedical field. The recent deluge of high-throughput sequencing data has prompted the development of novel deep learning (DL) algorithms that can integrate large, feature-rich data sets. Scientist and researchers are able to generate more data in a day than their predecessors 20 years ago generated in their entire careers (Goodwin et al., n.d.). This rapid data explosion has created a number of challenges for biomedical researchers, since a large number of the experiments lack quantitative tools that can help to distill scientific knowledge and identify key discoveries from the vast sea of data. This chapter considers providing state-of-the-art DL for genomics, which we hope could shine a light on helping readers to be able to conduct, develop and research DL methods for genomic data.

Here are two examples. In the human genome, we have genetic variants, so one question is about genome-wide association: whether we can use this variance for health purposes is a huge research topic and has major marketing potential. Direct technology would use clustered regularly interspaced short palindromic repeats (CRISPR) to repair genome and use machine learning (ML) models such as Self-Progressing Robust Training (SPROUT) to accurately predict repair outcomes, such as the percentage of insertion/deletion, the length of insertion/deletion, and nucleotide inserted diversity (Leenay et al. 2019). Another example would be that we can now leverage DL power for rare disease diagnostics based on human genomic mutation and accurately predict cell-type-specific gene expression.

The prerequisites of this chapter are general ML, statistics and biology: we will briefly review each topic in this chapter. DL is not a single technique; instead, it is a set of related algorithms or methods and a branch of ML. It is generally divided into four paradigms: supervised learning, unsupervised/representation learning, and semi-supervised learning, with a recent fourth paradigm emerging that of self-supervised learning, which has the potential to solve a significant limitation of supervised ML, namely, the requirement for lots of labeled training samples. Self-supervised learning extracts and uses the naturally available relevant context and embedded metadata as supervisory signals.

In this chapter, we will focus on supervised and unsupervised learning and their application to genetics.

9.1.1 Genomics Primer

A simple ML algorithm is a logistic regression for binary classification (Mor-Yosef et al., n.d.). For a simple ML algorithm, the performance of the model is heavily dependent on the representation of the data, which is also known as a feature. Many definitions are applied to a genome, but here it can be referenced as the complete set of genes or genetic information present in a cell, which functions as the self-copy storage of information about how to develop and maintain an organism (Figure 9.1). Genomics is the branch that studies the structure, function, evolution and mapping of the genome. In other words, genomics is the tool for understanding the fundamentals of the genome and its applications range from medicine and pharmacy to agriculture and beyond.

Genome mapping is the process of mapping the genes to the location sequence of the DNA. Since genomes, or DNA in the cell, are forming dynamic 3-dimensional structures, scientists are also concerned about its structure. Fundamentally, we are asking about the functionality of all the DNAs in the genome, the interaction between the genes, and what causes gene to be turned on or off. The ultimate goal of genomics is to find out how genotypes relate to our health phenotypes, and whether we can differentiate healthy and diseased states at a genetic level, and, of course, what gene traits could be used to predict and defend against disease. For example, the genetic sequencing of tumors has enabled the personalized treatment of cancer and has the potential to revolutionize medicine (Yaari et al., n.d.).

9.1.1.1 High-Throughput Sequencing

The year 2013 marked the completion of the human genome project (HGP) (Lander et al. 2001). Since then, genome sequencing technologies have continue reducing the cost of sequencing and have increased the number and diversity of sequenced genomes (Figure 9.2), as genomics becomes more and more data-intense thanks to high-throughput sequencing technologies. The history of the genomic sequencing started in 1977 when Frederick Sanger and colleagues invented Sanger sequencing, a method of DNA sequencing based on the selective incorporation of chain-terminating di-deoxynucleotides by DNA polymerase during in vitro DNA replication. Later in 1987, the technology was switched to using fluorescent dye incorporated on the terminating di-deoxynucleotides as signals to produce reads. Around the mid-1990s, DNA Microarrays was the dominant technology. Since about 2007, we have reached the 2nd-generation (Next-gen) of DNA sequencing, which massively parallels and dramatically reduces the cost and time required. Now, we are in the 3rd-generation and single molecule DNA sequencing era with technologies like Oxford Nanopore (Jain et al. 2016).

Since 2015, almost all DNA sequence instruments follow one of these different principles: sequencing by synthesis/ligation, SMRT (single-molecule real-time sequencing) cell (Escalante et al. 2014) and nanopore. Sequencing by synthesis ("massively parallel sequencing") so far provides the greatest throughput and is most prevalent on the market today.

9.1.1.2 Sequencing Data: DNA, RNA and Protein

DNA is a double-stranded biopolymer: the canonical form is the right-handed double helix as shown in Figure 9.2. The primary structure of DNA is a linear sequence

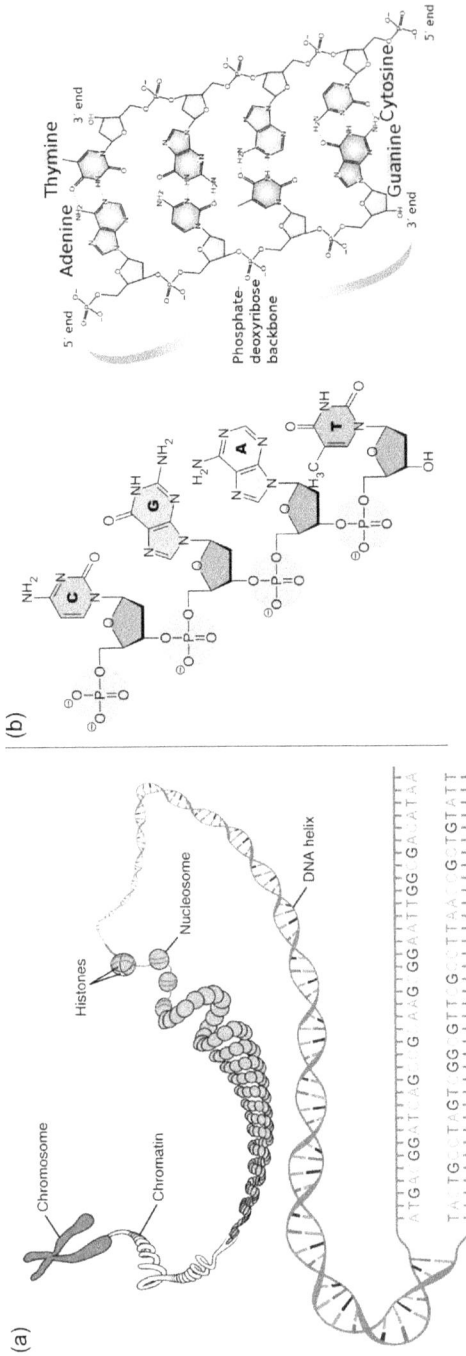

FIGURE 9.1 (a) Genetic information or DNA sequences, simple, but accurately contain instructions of cells. Genetics is a research field that helps us understand genetic code. In this figure, DNA double-helix is packed into nucleosome first, then chromatin, and eventually paired with another chromatin to form chromosome. (b) Chemical structure of DNA. Left: single-stranded DNA. Right: double-stranded DNA; hydrogen bonds are shown as dotted lines.

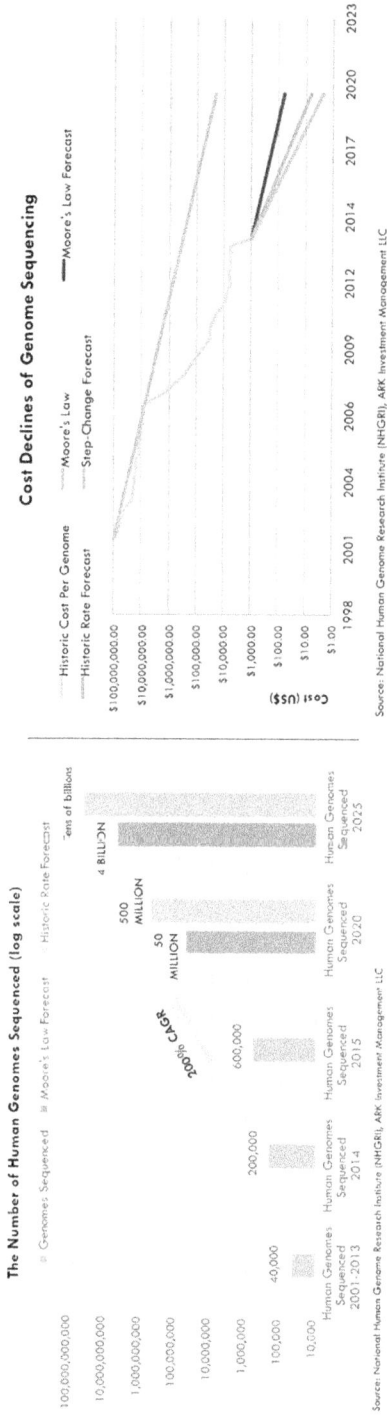

FIGURE 9.2 The exponential increase of the number of human genomes (a) and the decrease of the cost of the genome sequencing technology (b). (Source: Illumina is the Bedrock of the Genomic Revolution by Catherine Wood (Ark-Invest).)

of nucleotides that link together by a phosphodiester bind. There are four bases: Adenine (A), Guanine (G), Cytosine (C) and Thymine (T), which encode our genetic code with A pairs with T and C pairs with G (Alberts et al. 2009).

As DNA is directional and the two strands are complementary, repair is possible if one string is damaged. The weak hydrogen bonds are the main element that holds the two strands together, as shown in Figure 9.1b, which allows low-energy opening (and closing) for enzymes such as polymerase to access (and leave). The polymerase has "read" the DNA from 3' to 5', and the newly added nucleotide is extended from 5' to 3'. In a cell, the DNA strands form chromosomes instead of being free form. Humans have 23 pairs of chromosomes (diploid = 2 copies of each chromosome), with each of the pairs from our parents. Twenty-two of the 22 pairs are autosomes, and the other one is a sex chromosome pair that determines our biological sex: canonically, female is XX and male is XY. Mitochondrial DNAs are almost exclusively inherited from the female parent side: they are circular and exist with many copies per cell. The human genome consists of over 3 billion base-pairs. The functional of the gene is actually at the gene expression level, in which most of the genes are encoded for specific biomolecules, RNA or proteins. In humans, our DNA has about 20,000 protein coding genes, and many regions on the DNA encode short and long non-coding RNAs.

As Figure 9.3 shows, the ultimate goal of the information in the DNA is to produce gene products, with one major outcome being the proteins. From the simplified central dogma image, it states that DNA first undertakes a transcript to RNA, specifically messenger RNA (mRNA), then is translated into protein (Figure 9.3a). The mRNA molecules are the information medium of the DNA: they are single-stranded molecules, with backbones of ribose instead of deoxyribose sugar. In addition, one base, Uracil (U) instead of Thymine (T), is used in RNA (Figure 9.3b).

Proteins are a chain of 20 (+2) amino acids. Figure 9.4a shows the standard amino acids names, the three-letter and one-letter abbreviations, and the chemical structures: mostly we use the one-letter as the input values. The genetic codes are triples of nucleic acid (codon), which codes for amino acids. The code is redundant, e.g., both GGC and GGA code for Gly (glycine). Two additional amino acids are, in some species, coded by codons that are usually interpreted as stop codons. We have included all the DNA codons (Kimball 2010) in Figure 9.4b.

The standard format appreciated among the community is the FASTA format (Lipman and Pearson, n.d.), whose format is used to represent DNA and protein sequence reads. In Figure 9.5, we showed both DNA and the protein sequence in the FASTA format. More than often, DNA, RNA, and proteins form complex secondary and tertiary structures, and these 3-D structures are where the biochemical functionality lies (Zheng and Xie, n.d.); however, the primary sequence determines the secondary and tertiary structures as shown in Figure 9.6. The primary sequence of these biomolecules contains a tremendous amount of information, including folding instructions for their secondary and tertiary structures.

Genes are the units in the DNA sequence that program proteins, and the simplified version of the functional structure of a gene is shown in Figure 9.7. The classical textbooks in molecular biology define one gene as coding to a single protein or to a single gene product, such as a catalytic or structural RNA molecule (Alberts et al.

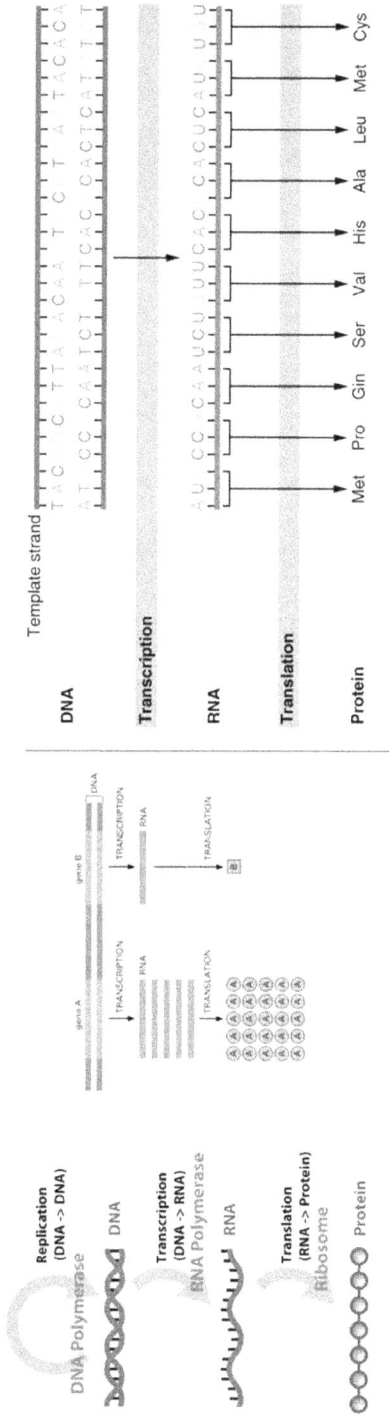

FIGURE 9.3 (a) Central dogma of molecular biology and gene expression. Left: simplified central dogma for the molecular biology. Right: different effects of the gene expression. (b) The genetic code. Information in the DNA was first transcript into RNA, and then translated into the protein. The above pinkish line is the corresponding RNA sequence of the template DNA strand.

(a)

(b)

Amino-acid biochemical properties   Nonpolar   Polar   Basic   Acidic   Termination: stop codon

Standard genetic code

1st base	T	C	A	G	3rd base
T	TTT (Phe/F) Phenylalanine	TCT (Ser/S) Serine	TAT (Tyr/Y) Tyrosine	TGT (Cys/C) Cysteine	T
	TTC	TCC	TAC	TGC	C
	TTA (Leu/L) Leucine	TCA	TAA Stop (Ochre)[R]	TGA Stop (Opal)[R]	A
	TTG[A]	TCG	TAG Stop (Amber)[R]	TGG (Trp/W) Tryptophan	G
C	CTT (Leu/L) Leucine	CCT (Pro/P) Proline	CAT (His/H) Histidine	CGT (Arg/R) Arginine	T
	CTC	CCC	CAC	CGC	C
	CTA	CCA	CAA (Gln/Q) Glutamine	CGA	A
	CTG[A]	CCG	CAG	CGG	G
A	ATT (Ile/I) Isoleucine	ACT (Thr/T) Threonine	AAT (Asn/N) Asparagine	AGT (Ser/S) Serine	T
	ATC	ACC	AAC	AGC	C
	ATA	ACA	AAA (Lys/K) Lysine	AGA (Arg/R) Arginine	A
	ATG[A] (Met/M) Methionine	ACG	AAG	AGG	G
G	GTT (Val/V) Valine	GCT (Ala/A) Alanine	GAT (Asp/D) Aspartic acid	GGT (Gly/G) Glycine	T
	GTC	GCC	GAC	GGC	C
	GTA	GCA	GAA (Glu/E) Glutamic acid	GGA	A
	GTG	GCG	GAG	GGG	G

Codon 1 — G C U
Codon 2 — A C G
Codon 3 — G A C
Codon 4 — U U C
Codon 5 — U C C
Codon 6 — G G A
Codon 7 — C U A G

RNA
Ribonucleic acid

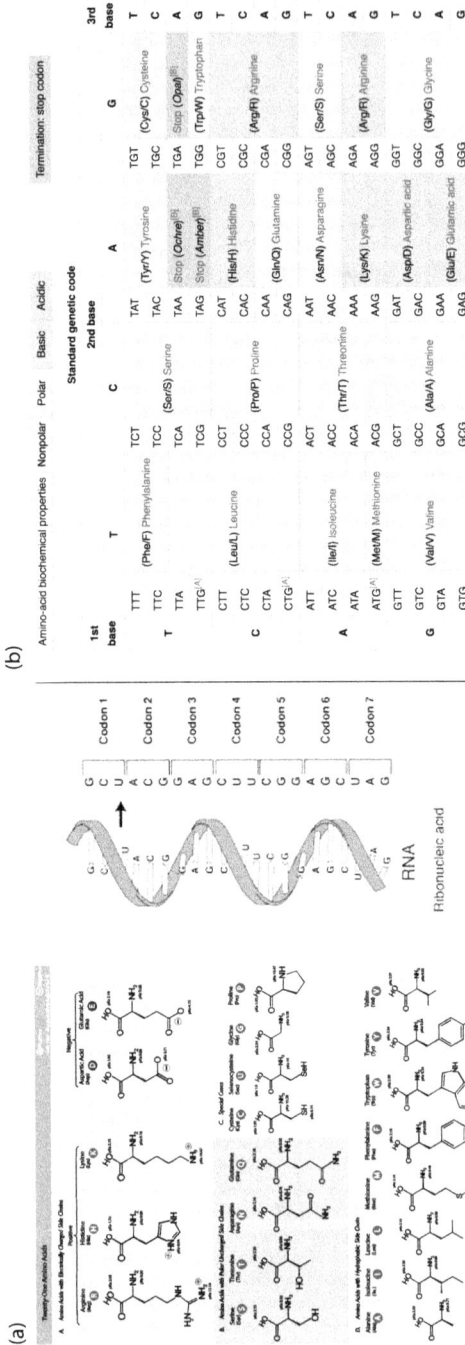

FIGURE 9.4 (a) Amino acid codes and RNA Condon. Right: A series of codons in part of a messenger RNA (mRNA) molecule. Each codon consists of three nucleotides, usually corresponding to a single amino acid. The nucleotides are abbreviated with the letters A, U, G and C. This is mRNA, which uses U (uracil). DNA uses T (thymine) instead. This mRNA molecule will instruct a ribosome to synthesize a protein according to this code. (b) DNA codon (genetic code) table. The codon ATG both codes for methionine and serves as an initiation site. The stop codons are amber, ochre and opal.

>NC_000011.10:c2160971-2159852 Homo sapiens chromosome 11, GRCh38.p13 Primary
Assembly
ATGGCCCTGTGGATGCGCCTCCTGCCCCTGCTGGCGCTGCTGGCCCTCTGGGGACCTGACCCAGCCGCAG
CCTTTGTGAACCAACACCTGTGCGGCTCACACCTGGTGGAAGCTCTCTACCTAGTGTGCGGGGAACGAGG
CTTCTTCTACACACCCAAGACCCGCCGGGAGGCAGAGGACCTGCAGGGTGAGCCAACTGCCCATTGCTGC
CCCTGGCCGCCCCCAGCCACCCCCTGCTCCTGGCGCTCCCACCCAGCATGGGCAGAAGGGGGCAGGAGGC
TGCCACCCAGCAGGGGGTCAGGTGCACTTTTTTAAAAAGAAGTTCTCTTGGTCACGTCCTAAAAGTGACC
AGCTCCCTGTGGCCCAGTCAGAATCTCAGCCTGAGGACGGTGTTGGCTTCGGCAGCCCCGAGATACATCA
GAGGGTGGGCACGCTCCTCCCTCCACTCGCCCCTCAAACAAATGCCCCGCAGCCCATTTCTCCACCCTCA
TTTGATGACCGCAGATTCAAGTGTTTTGTTAAGTAAAGTCCTGGGTGACCTGGGGTCACAGGGTGCCCCA
CGCTGCCTGCCTCTGGGCGAACACCCCATCACGCCCGGAGGAGGGCGTGGCTGCCTGCCTGAGTGGGCCA
GACCCCTGTCGCCAGGCCTCACGGCAGCTCCATAGTCAGGAGATGGGGAAGATGCTGGGGACAGGCCCTG
GGGAGAAGTACTGGGATCACCTGTTCAGGCTCCCACTGTGACGCTGCCCCGGGGCGGGGGAAGGAGGTGG
GACATGTGGGCGTTGGGGCCTGTAGGTCCACACCCAGTGTGGGTGACCCTCCCTCTAACCTGGGTCCAGC
CCGGCTGGAGATGGGTGGGAGTGCGACCTAGGGCTGGCGGGCAGGCGGGCACTGTGTCTCCCTGACTGTG
TCCTCCTGTGTCCCTCTGCCTCGCCGCTGTTCCGGAACCTGCTCTGCGCGGCACGTCCTGGCAGTGGGGC
AGGTGGAGCTGGGCGGGGGCCCTGGTGCAGGCAGCCTGCAGCCCTTGGCCCTGGAGGGGTCCCTGCAGAA
GCGTGGCATTGTGGAACAATGCTGTACCAGCATCTGCTCCCTCTACCAGCTGGAGAACTACTGCAACTAG

>NP_000198.1 insulin preproprotein [Homo sapiens]
MALWMRLLPLLALLALWGPDPAAAFVNQHLCGSHLVEALYLVCGERGFFYTPKTRREAEDLQVGQVELGG
GPGAGSLQPLALEGSLQKRGIVEQCCTSICSLYQLENYCN

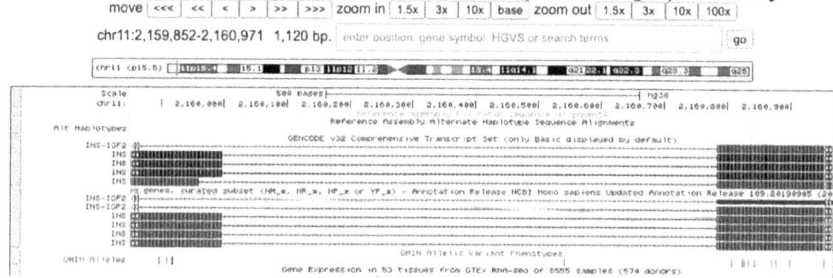

FIGURE 9.5 FAST format of the DAN and protein sequence of insulin preproprotein, a peptide hormone that plays a vital role in the regulation of carbohydrate and lipid metabolism.

2009), while a more modern defection would be a region (or regions) of sequence that include all of the elements necessary to encode a "functional transcript" (Eilbeck et al. 2005). Gene composition consists of exons and introns (slicing), and not every part of a gene is coded for protein, with the exons (coding) interrupted by the non-translated introns. Later stage of transcription will splice the intron out and the remaining mRNA will be translated into proteins. In addition, alternative splicing can take place where different exon subsets for the same gene will be translated into different protein isoforms, which creates diversity in protein structure and functionality. Non-coding RNA (ncRNS) genes will not proceed into the translation step but transcription. At the bottom of the Figure 9.5, it shows how using the UCSC Genome Browser, the insulin preproprotein appears with exons as boxes and lines as introns.

Three major DL challenges are: (a) using models to "invent" new proteins based on the characteristics of the molecule learned from the protein sequence (Greener,

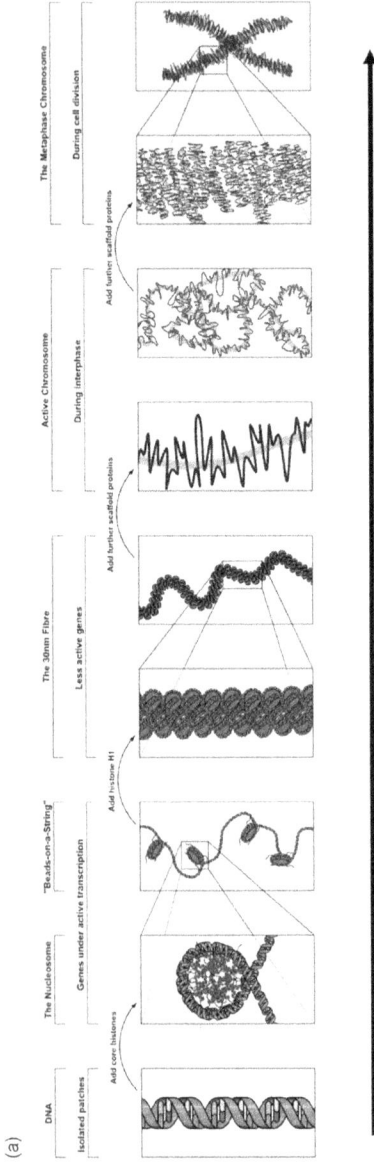

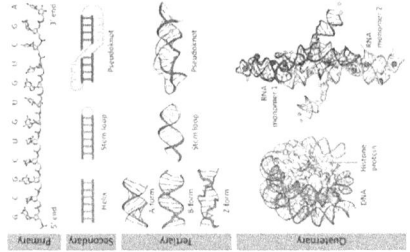

FIGURE 9.6 (a) Chromosome. DNAs are packed through multiple levels into chromosome. (b) DNA structures and RNA secondary structure. Left: primary, secondary, tertiary and quaternary structure of DNA. Right: RNA secondary structure.

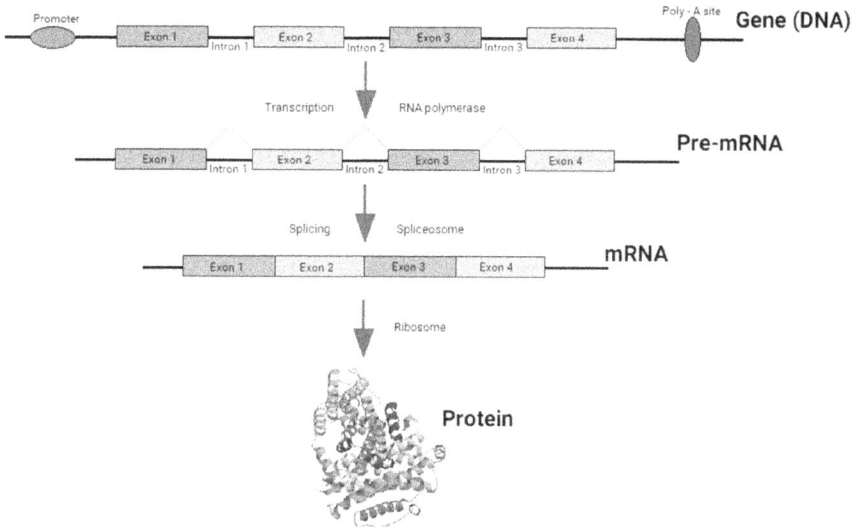

FIGURE 9.7 DNA gene product through slicing.

Moffat, and Jones 2018; Wang et al. 2018); (b) predicting the interactions between proteins, DNA, RNA, and other small molecules (Puton et al. 2012; Wen et al. 2017; Hirsch et al. 2017; Rifaioglu et al. 2018); and (c) predicting slice sites, gene isoforms and alternative splicing events, genes in the genome, and gene transcription start sites (TSS) and transcription termination sites.

9.1.1.3 DNA Regulatory

One of the most interesting DL topics in the genetic research field is learning patents in regulatory DNA sequence. All the cells in a human body have the exact same one genome, but its expression in many cell types has different effects on DNA or gene regulation through epigenomics, as shown in Figure 9.7, which dictates where and how much a gene product should be expressed. Different activation and repression of the control elements on genes define the cell types' identity and state. In general, this regulation can occur at the pre- and co-transcriptional level by controlling the level of transcripts produced. In addition, post-transcriptional regulation happens when certain biomolecules bind to the gene product and mark them for degradation before they can be used in the translation step of protein production. The large-scale data from the Encyclopedia of DNA elements (ENCODE) project (Gerstein et al. 2012) enables a systematically analysis of the regulatory scheme, especially of transcription factors (TFs). The task that DL is expected to solve is when, where and how much genes are regulated. Many schemes contribute to the gene expression regulation, and Figure 9.8 shows the overview of DNA regulation. It includes but is not limited to DNA methylation, histone and chromatin modification, and other epigenomic marking. However, at the sequence level, the regulatory mechanisms are controlled by core promoter elements as well as by distance-acting regulatory elements (REs) such as enhancers.

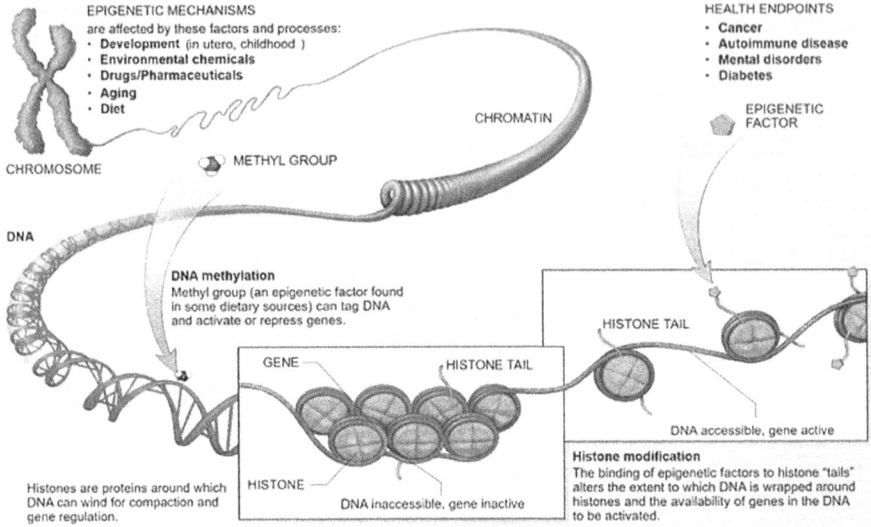

FIGURE 9.8 DNA regulatory at multiple levels.

9.1.1.3.1 Regulation by Transcription Factors through Regulatory Region

Humans have about 25,000 genes with over two million novel putative control elements. At a genomic level, the mechanisms regulating gene expression that we need to increase our understanding of in order to understand DNA transcription (gene expression) are shown in Figure 9.3. The task of transcription is carried out by the RNA polymerase enzyme, and its initiation is enabled by the existence of specific regions in the DNA sequence, called promoters. Promoters promote transcription from DNA to RNA and are commonly found upstream from the start site of transcription. Proteins that are called general TFs recognize and bind these promoters and form a pre-imitation complex. The RNA polymerases recognize these complexes and initiate the synthesis of RNAs (Hager et al., n.d.). The proteins' TFs recognize a specific DNA motif and bind on a regulatory region and regulate the downstream transcription level (rate) as shown in Figure 9.8. The major DL challenges regarding DNA or gene regulatory factors correspond to this interaction (TF / transcription factor binding preference, regulatory region concentration, and the availability of synergistic or competing TFs): (a) to predict REs and their cell type specific activity; (b) to predict which REs regulate which genes in which cell types; and (c) to predict gene expression from RE activation.

9.1.1.3.2 Regulation by Epigenetics

Epigenetics refers to gene regulation via genome construction – DNA packing and structures, other than DNA sequence. Examples are chromatin and histone modification and DNA methylation etc. DNA methylation, repeatedly adding methyl groups to cytosine of CpG (Cytosine-phosphate-Guanin) dinucleotides of high CpG regions (CpG islands) is typically associated with gene silencing/repressing, through either interfering with the TF binding on the regulation region or through the mechanism of methyl-CpG binding proteins inducing the spread of repressive chromatin domains. Other DNA modifications exist in mammalian genomes and ongoing research topics (Sood, Viner, and Hoffman 2019).

A group of eight histones are wrapped around by DNA to construct a nucleosome, then through super-coiling of the DNA and nucleosome this constructs the high-order structure of chromatin. Modification of the histones and chromatin will have a regulatory effect, both promoting and reducing gene expression (Figure 9.9). For example, modification on H3K9ac, one of the histones proteins, will active promoters and enhancers.

9.1.1.4   Genetic Variation

The diversity of the genome between individuals is due to mutation and genetic variation. In the human genome there are over 3 million base-pairs, and one contribution of the variation is the single nucleotide polymorphisms (SNPs), with about 3 million SNPs in the human population, in which one base is substituted with another one. Other contributions are short and large insertions, deletions, inversions, translocations. Mutations can be generally classified based on their effect and size. Mutation in the genome occurs due to multiple reasons all of the time, but our cells cope with this "damage" through DNA repair enzymes. Two types of mutations should be noted: germline mutation can pass the genetic alteration through the germ cells as inherited traits; and somatic mutation that can be passed to the progeny of the mutated cell in the course of cell division. The genetic variations could carry the answer to identifying the genetic disease.

We have discussed the most significant discoveries of the DNA and its regulations. Through these regulation mechanisms, the one same genome of an individual can be utilized as template across all the cell types. At a higher level, mutations in the DNA, good and bad, contribute to the diversities of the human population and they are what make us who we are.

9.1.2   Deep Learning Primer

As genetics have become a key component of modern medicine, scientists have increasingly become in need of ways to handle the various speed, scalability, energy, and cost requirements when facing large amounts of biomedical data. Rapid data generation from the biomedical and biochemical fields require a more powerful way of analyzing the data in order to be able to enable advances in genetics through allowing the identification and, hopefully, the treatment of a wide array of diseases. Many of the innovations in diagnostics and breakthroughs in instrumentation for human diseases have benefited from and will continue to be advanced by computational methods, for example, DL.

At a more granular level, in order for ML to work, we need input features, such as local DNA sequences, thermodynamics, chromatin and gene expressions. A simplified ML pipeline or model would be to take input X and predict Y′ and using the loss between the Y and Y′ to optimize the weight of the model, as shown in Figure 9.10a.

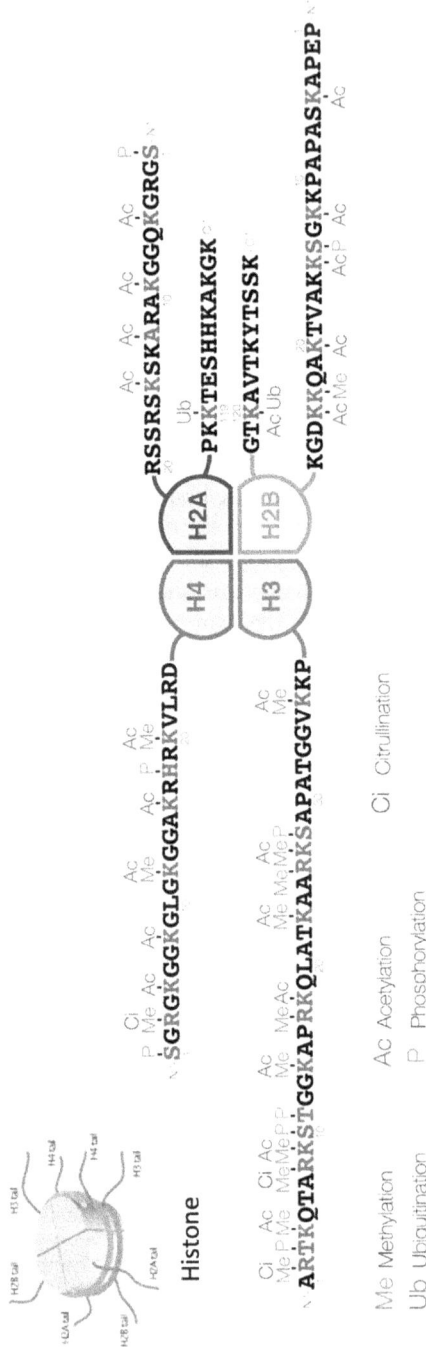

FIGURE 9.9 Common histone modification; they include histone methylation (–Me), histone phosphorylation (–P), histone acetylation (–Ac), histone citrullination (–Ci) and histone ubiquitination (–Ub).

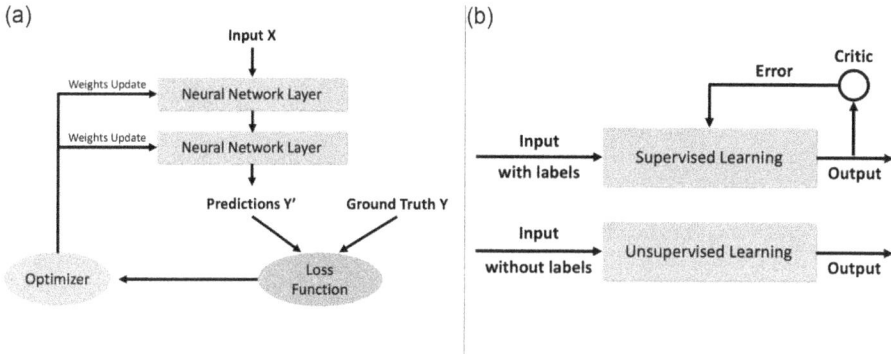

FIGURE 9.10 ML pipeline. (a) Simple ML pipeline with two layers. (b) Two major ML paradigms illustration – supervised learning vs. unsupervised learning.

In general, ML is divided into the following paradigms based on the properties of the true targets, their availability and the amount: (a) supervised learning is a task of learning a function by given input-output pairs, aka, true targets are available (Figure 9.10b); (b) unsupervised learning is learning patterns in a data set with no true targets provided; and (c) semi-supervised learning is when there is a combination of a small amount of labeled data with a large amount of unlabeled data during training. Classification is one of the most used supervised learning tasks, which aims to find a boundary to separate the labels.

The simplest representation of almost all DL architecture is the single-layer perceptron, as shown in Figure 9.11a. One important difference between lots of the statistical models, such as regression, is the non-linear activation. Here we illustrate the most common types of activations (Figure 9.11b). Other activation function will be included in the supplement. One of most related activations that originates from statistical learning is the logistic or sigmoid activation, which is part of the non-linearity of a neuron. Sigmoid function is useful for generation probability, since its output ranges between 0 and 1. For logistic regression or binary classification tasks, we can model the unknown decision boundary directly between 0 and 1, and assign a probability larger than the boundary to 1, the smaller to 0.

A dense or fully connected deep neural network (DNN) is the adding of layers of neurons together. In Figure 9.12, we show a DNN with $4 \times 5 + 5 \times 5 + 5 \times 1 = 50$ parameters, which are the weights and bias that model needs to learn. The hyper-parameters are related to the model architecture and training process, such as the number of layers, the number of neurons per layer, and what types of activation function will be used. Each set of hyper-parameters determine a different DNN. To find the best setup, there is a need to search over architectures and identify the optimal architecture by evaluating performance on a validation set.

The simplest way of ML from data is through a stochastic gradient descent (SGD). This algorithm is as following:

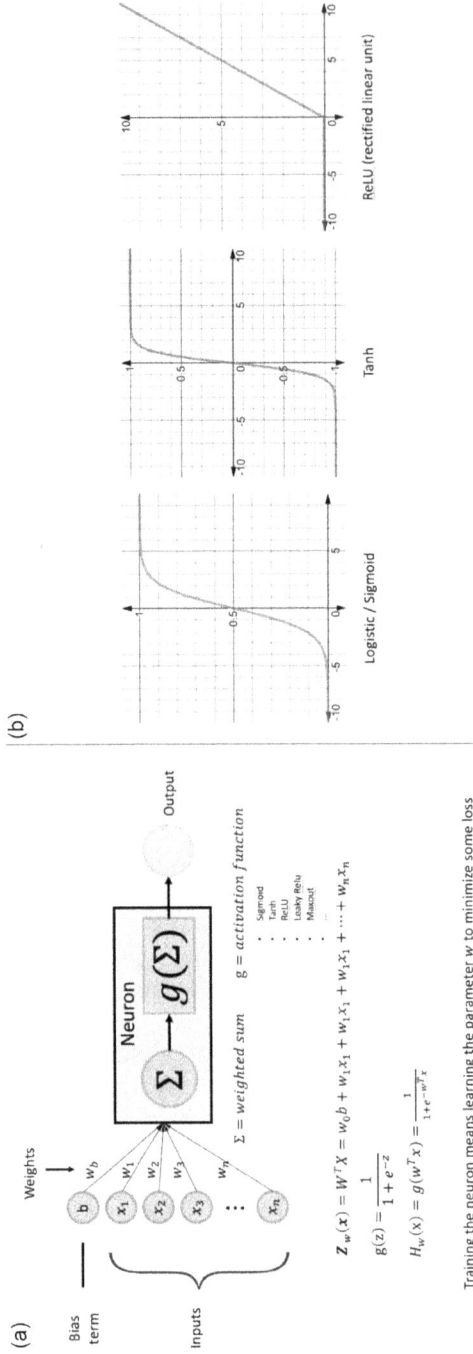

FIGURE 9.11 Non-linear activation (logistic) in perceptron or neuron. (a) The illustration of perception or neuron in a neural network. (b) Common activation functions.

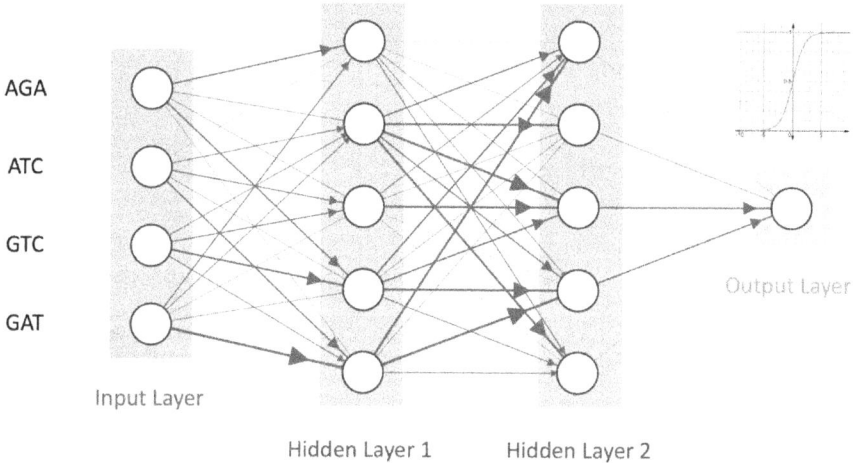

AGA

ATC

GTC

GAT

Input Layer

Hidden Layer 1   Hidden Layer 2

Output Layer

FIGURE 9.12   Dense (fully connected) deep neural networks with 2 hidden layers. The arrow lines represent the weights. Inputs of the neural network are the genetic codes for protein.

SGD Algorithm

1. **Initialize** w_0. Usually $w_0 \sim \text{Unif}[-\epsilon, +\epsilon]$.
2. **Sample** a mini batch $\{x_{(1)}, x_{(2)}, \ldots, x_{(m)}\}$ with labels $y_{(i)}$.
3. **Compute** approximate gradient $\Delta = \dfrac{1}{m}\Sigma_i \dfrac{dL\left[f\left(x_{(i)}, w\right), y_{(i)}\right]}{dw}$, where $L[*]$ is a loss function.
4. **Update** $w_{t+1} = w_t - \alpha_{t+1}\Delta$, where α_t's are the learning rates.

However, this algorithm docs nt allow the model to learn well, as it is prone to the local minimal and saddle points, so we commonly using momentum with SGD. SGD can be zig-zagging, especially when the loss landscape is ill-conditioned, while momentum will allow the new algorithm to optimize in a similar direction as the previous step. The new algorithm would be as follows:

SGD + Momentum Algorithm

1. **Initialize** w_0. Usually $w_0 \sim \text{Unif}[-\epsilon, +\epsilon]$.
2. Sample a mini batch $\{x_{(1)}, x_{(2)}, \ldots, x_{(m)}\}$ with labels $y_{(i)}$.
3. **Compute** approximate gradient $\Delta = \dfrac{1}{m}\Sigma_i \dfrac{dL\left[f\left(x_{(i)}, w\right), y_{(i)}\right]}{dw}$, where $L[*]$ is a loss function.
4. **Update** velocity: $v = 0.9v + 0.1\Delta$.
5. **Update** $w_{t+1} = w_t - \alpha_{t+1}v$, where α_t's are the learning rates.

However, the performance of the above algorithm still crucially depends on the step size: if the learning rate is too small, then it requires many steps to reach the minimal; if too large, then the gradients are no longer informative. Another optimization algorithm is RMSProp, which sets a learning rate adaptively using the history:

RMSProp Algorithm

1. **Initialize** w_0. Usually $w_0 \sim \mathrm{Unif}[-\epsilon, +\epsilon]$.
2. **Sample** a mini batch $\{x_{(1)}, x_{(2)}, \ldots, x_{(m)}\}$ with labels $y_{(i)}$.
3. **Compute** approximate gradient $\Delta = \dfrac{1}{m}\Sigma_i \dfrac{dL\left[f\left(x_{(i)}, w\right), y_{(i)}\right]}{dw}$, where $L[*]$ is a loss function.
4. **Accumulate** squared gradient: $r = \rho r + (1-\rho)\Delta \times \Delta$.
5. **Update** $w_{t+1} = w_t - \dfrac{\alpha_{t+1}}{\sqrt{r}+10^{-8}} \times \Delta$, where α_t's are the learning rates.

We can also add the momentum to the RMSProp and it is Adam optimization as follows:

Adam Algorithm

1. **Initialize** w_0. Usually $w_0 \sim \mathrm{Unif}[-\epsilon, +\epsilon]$.
2. **Sample a** mini batch $\{x_{(1)}, x_{(2)}, \ldots, x_{(m)}\}$ with labels $y_{(i)}$.
3. **Compute** approximate gradient $\Delta = \dfrac{1}{m}\Sigma_i \dfrac{dL\left[f\left(x_{(i)}, w\right), y_{(i)}\right]}{dw}$, where $L[*]$ is a loss function.
4. **Update** velocity: $v = 0.9v + 0.1\Delta$
5. **Accumulate** squared gradient: $r = \rho r + (1-\rho)\Delta \times \Delta$.
6. **Update** $w_{t+1} = w_t - \dfrac{\alpha_{t+1}}{\sqrt{r}+10^{-8}} \times v$, where α_t's are the learning rates.

When training the neural network, one aspect of concern is not to over-fit the data. DL models feed on big data, and other methods to prevent overfittings may be implemented in the weight and data level, for example, early stopping, L2 regularization transfer learning, data augmentation, and adding dropout layers. Conversely, we also need to overcome under-fitting, which can be achieved in the architecture level, for example, by SGD with momentum, RMSProp, Adam and Batch normalization.

The L2 regularization is also called weight decay. The main propose is to reduce the complexity of the function space, which adds an extra penalty of squared weight. The regularization penalty corresponds to a Bayesian prior that the weights are close to zero and restricts the complexity of the learned neural network. Here is the formula for adding the regularization penalty:

$$w^* = \mathrm{argmin}_w \left(\frac{1}{n}\sum_i L\left(f\left(x_{(i)}, w\right), y_{(i)}\right) + \frac{\lambda}{2}\theta^T\theta \right)$$

When applied to the gradient descent, the new gradient and updating function will be

$$\Delta = \frac{1}{n}\Sigma_i \frac{dL\left[f\left(x_{(i)}, w\right), y_{(i)}\right]}{dw} + \lambda\theta$$

$$w_{t+1} = w_t - \alpha_{t+1} \times \Delta$$

Another way to prevent overfitting is to include similar (the same) data set but for a different task, which "indirectly" increases the training example for the main task. One famous example is for object detection: in order to improve performance, researchers have used a multi-task learning approach (Ren et al., n.d.) by including an image segmentation task with the same data set, and a genomic related example is jointly predicting over 900 TFs and chromatin labels. In Figure 9.13, we show that the multi-task approach to improve the performance of the model utilizes data from a different task. The direct way to increase the size of the data set for data augmentation is, first, normalize the input (zero mean and unit standard deviation), then transform the input data. In Figure 9.14, we show the image augmentation methods: rotations, shifts, and adding random noise.

Last, but not least, by adding the dropout and other noise regularization algorithms, we increase the stability of the model (Goodfellow, Bengio, and Courville 2016). The general idea behind the regularization is to prevent the model memorizing the data. In

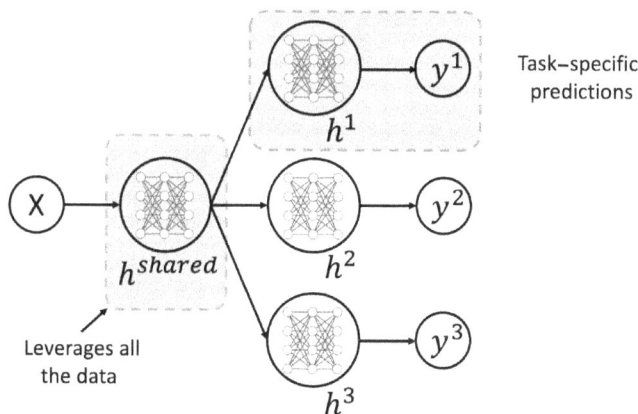

FIGURE 9.13 Multi-task learning. Multiple learning tasks are solved at the same time. By exploiting commonalities and difference among tasks, multi-task learning can improve learning efficiency and performances for some or all of the task-specific model/s.

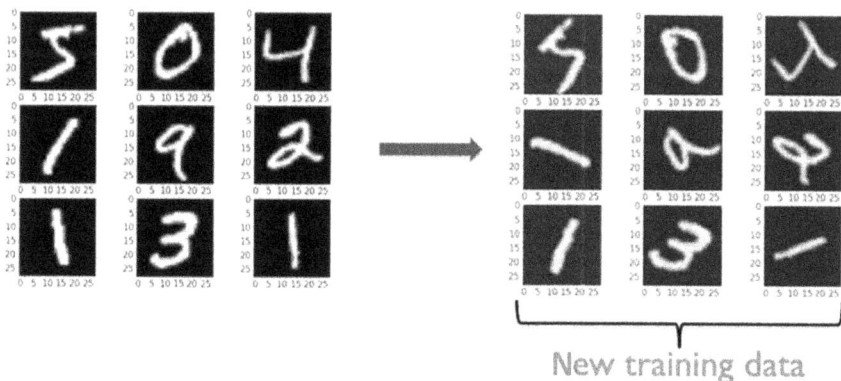

FIGURE 9.14 Data augmentation in computer vision. Through rotating, shifting and adding random noises, we can generate new training data sets.

the dropout approach, at each epoch, certain percentage of the neuron would be "shut down," which will prevent a neural network heavily depending on one or a subset of the neurons and forces all the neurons to learn, which leads to a more generalized model.

9.1.3 Classification Applications: Deciphering Syntax of a Regulatory DNA Sequence

The best way to get our hands dirty is by using an example to illustrate the DL methods that we will use. The task is to predict the regulatory code; that is, how the DNA sequence encodes regulatory information. Regulatory proteins called TFs bind to sequence patterns (motifs) in regulatory DNA with a high affinity. The regulatory sequences contain more than one binding of the same instance of TF resulting in homotypic clusters of motifs, while binding combinations of the TFs results in heterotypic clusters of motifs as shown in Figure 9.15. The key properties of a regulatory sequence is that these sequences are often organized in specific spatial and positional patterns or constraints that allow binding combinations of TFs, and result in distinct motif grammars as showing in Figure 9.16. Based on the set of aligned sequences that are bound by a particular TF, we can calculate the Position Weight Matrix (PWM), which is illustrated as a JASPAR code or PWM logo in Figures 9.15 and 9.16. We will not go over the details here of how the PWM was calculated. We can use the PWM as convolutional filter to convolve with a window of sequences, for example, if we know the motif length is 5, the window size of 5 will convolve alone the sequence. These convolutional outputs will later be passed into the neural network as shown in Figure 9.17, then by training with binary labels, whether TF binding or not, we have created a convolutional neural network (CNN) predictive model (Movva et al. 2019).

The advantages of using CNN for genetic sequence data is as follows: (a) it can capture the sparse local patterns; (b) it has a translational invariance through pooling layers, so patterns can occur at different positions in the input; (c) the CNN architecture significantly reduces the number of parameters compared to the Dense Neural Network (DNN).

9.1.4 Regression Application: Gene Expression Level Prediction

One metric to measure the regression performance is R-squared (R^2), which measures the fraction of variance explained by the regression model. For the calculation, we first compute the Residual Standard Error (RSE): $RSE = \sqrt{\dfrac{1}{n-2} RSS} = \sqrt{\dfrac{1}{n-2} \Sigma_{i=i}^{n} \left(y_i - \widehat{y}_i \right)^2}$, where RSS is residual sum of squares $RSS = \Sigma_{i=i}^{n} \left(y_i - \widehat{y}_i \right)^2$ and $R^2 = \dfrac{TSS - RSS}{TSS} = 1 - \dfrac{RSS}{TSS}$, where TSS stands for total sum of squares $TSS = \Sigma_{i=i}^{n} \left(y_i - \overline{y}_i \right)^2$. The R^2 is the square of the correlation between X and Y, and can be shown as following:

$$r = \frac{\Sigma_{i=i}^{n} \left(x_i - \overline{x}_i \right)\left(y_i - \overline{y}_i \right)}{\sqrt{\Sigma_{i=i}^{n} \left(x_i - \overline{x}_i \right)^2} \sqrt{\Sigma_{i=i}^{n} \left(y_i - \overline{y}_i \right)^2}}$$

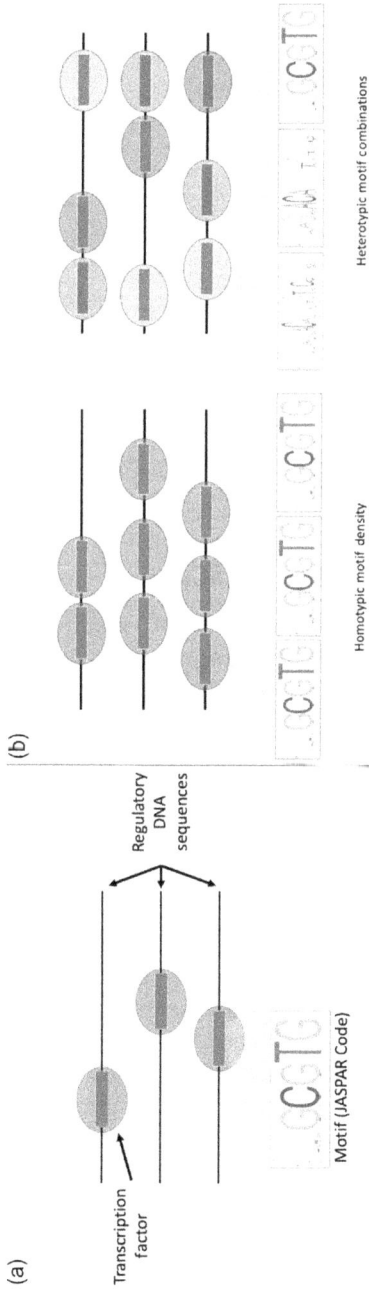

FIGURE 9.15 TFs. (a) TFs are binding regulatory motif of DNA sequences. (b) Homotypic motif density vs. heterotypic motif combinations.

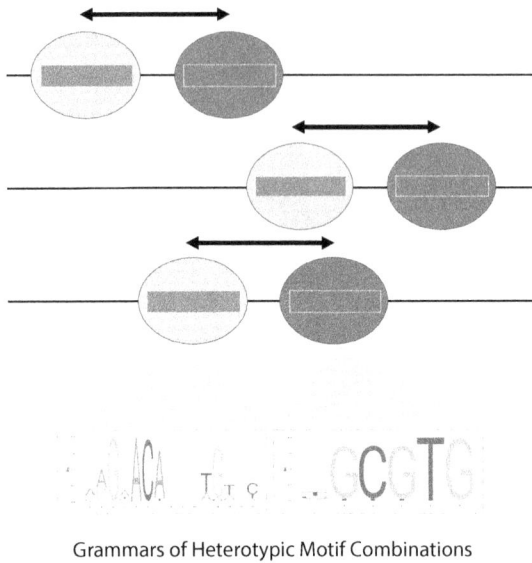

Grammars of Heterotypic Motif Combinations

FIGURE 9.16   Grammars of heterotypic motif combinations.

9.2   GENOMIC DEEP LEARNING SETUP

Genomic data analysis endeavors, including DL, require multi-domain knowledge and tools. Regardless of the research topics and tasks, the pipeline of the analysis follows a common pattern. Here we present the general setup for DL research and aim to familiarize readers with the data processes and analytical steps in the context of genomics. The common steps include data collection, data quality checks, cleaning, processing, modelling (DL or other analysis), visualization and reporting. As can be seen, a genomic DL engineer or researcher spends a lot of time on data compared to the actual building and training models.

9.2.1   DATA COLLECTION

Data collection could be from any resource, public or private. The most famous publicly available genetic DNA data repos are the ENCODE Project, the Roadmap Epigenomics Project, The Cancer Genome Atlas (TCGA), the 1000 genomes project, the USCS genome browser, GENBANK, ENSEMBL and UNIPROT. Private data can be collected from your own labs. One important question for DL is how much data and what type of data should be collected. The answer depends on the question we are trying to answer, the technical capability, and biological variability of the research.

The **ENCODE Project** was a follow-up to the HGP. The HGP sequenced the whole human genome, while the ENCODE project seeks to identify and interpret the functional elements in the human (and mouse) genomes, through studying a broader diversity of biological samples (Qu et al., n.d.). The **Roadmap Epigenomics Project**, on the other hand, focuses on the human epigenomic regulatory mechanism. This

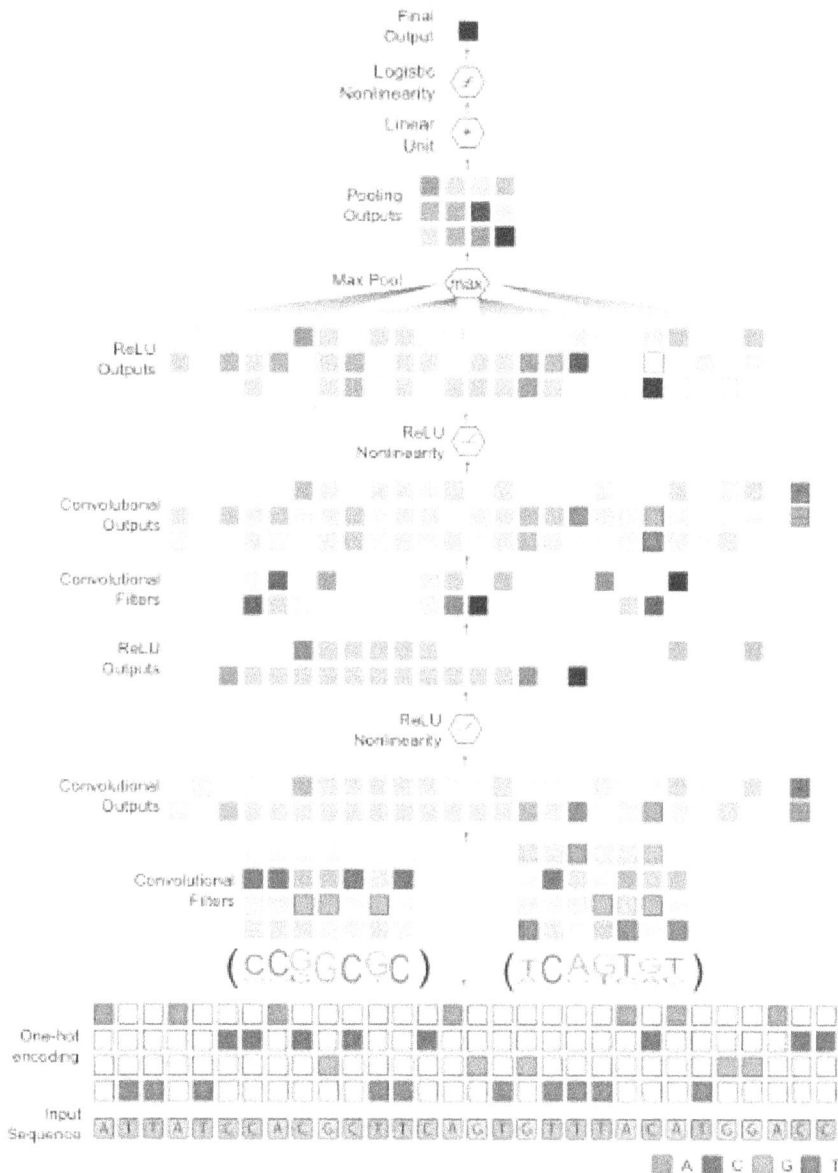

FIGURE 9.17 DragoNN library DL illustration. (Source: How to Train Your DragoNN Israeli et al. 2016.)

project contains genome-wide maps of several key histone modifications, chromatin accessibility, DNA methylation and mRNA expression across hundreds of human cell types and tissues (Meissner et al. 2008; Mullard 2015). The purpose of **TCGA** is to accelerate our understanding of the molecular basis of cancer through the application of genome analysis. This repository contains a collection of over 20,000 primary cancers with matched normal samples across 33 cancer types. The **1000 genomes project** contains human genetic variations to support medical research studies on identifying the genetic regions that are associated with common human diseases. These data include SNPs and structural variants and their haplotype contexts from 1,000 unidentified individuals from around the world (Clarke et al., n.d.).

The **USCS genome browser** (Karolchik et al., n.d.) and **ENSEMBL** (Zerbino et al., n.d.) initially were graphic viewing tools, but, in recent years, these websites have grown into a broad collection of organism assemblies and annotations, along with a large suite of tools for viewing, analyzing and downloading data. **GENBANK** is the NIH genetic sequence database. It contains all the publicly available DNA sequences with annotations. Data that accompanied public-funded research would be found in this repository (Benson et al., n.d.). **UNIPROT** is a database that contains a comprehensive, high-quality protein sequence and functional information (The UniProt Consortium, n.d.).

9.2.2 DATA QUALITY CONTROL

In real-world applications, we inevitably face low quality data. The most common data issues would be that the data set has missing values or contains noise, such as errors. Most of the data in genomics were produced through high-throughput assays, which could bring technical biases (i.e., systematic error) into the data, such as under- or overestimation of measurements: concrete examples could be batch-effect and edge-effect (Caraus et al. 2015). The best scenario is that we can "correct" or remove these errors and provide high-quality data for the downstream steps.

9.2.3 DATA CLEANING

ML is derived from statistical learning: many data cleaning methods are borrowed from statistics. The simplest statistical learning algorithm is linear regression, which was invented when computation was done by hand back in the 1800s, but continues to work well for large data sets. Therefore, isn't a surprise that both ML and DL face a similar data "problem." In linear regression, the prediction is a weighted sum of inputs: $\hat{y} = w_0 x_0 + w_1 x_1 + \cdots$ or we can write using vector representation $\hat{y} = Xw$. The typical loss for linear regression is a mean squared error $L = \|y - Xw\|^2$ for finding the best w parameters for the data. Linear regression does have a closed form solution, which can be calculated through the normal equation, but it is not practical for large data sets. The formula for calculating w is $w = \left(X^T X\right)^{-1} X^T y$. There are a lot of issues with the inversion. One of the assumptions is non-singular, meaning that all the columns of the data X (feature) matrix are linearly independent, but in real-world data sets duplications or near duplications do happen. In addition, the inversion also has a time complexity of $O\left(N^3\right)$, using the naïve algorithm but it still doesn't get much better using fancy algorithms. This is the reason why the gradient descent optimization algorithm is the most popular alternative: (a) it is less expensive computationally in both time and or memory; (b) it is more amenable to mild generalization; and (c) it is generic enough to work on most problems. However, in many ML problems the data are in a high-dimension spatial world. Since this is a gradient descent (minimization along the gradient), and not an ascent (maximization), we want to traverse the last hyper surface, searching for the global minimum. In other words, we hope to find the lowest valley, regardless of where we start on the hyper surface. However, the algorithm tends to underperform, and data suffers (multi-)collinearity issues etc. Collinearity is traditionally measured using tolerance and the variance inflation factor (VIF) (Miles 2014).

At the data cleaning steps, we need make decisions such as whether to remove NA observation and collinearity. If the data set is big enough and the observations are not unique, when facing NA data points, we can remove them either row-wise or column-wise. When we remove row-wise, we essentially remove the observations, and when we remove column-wise, we remove feature from the data. One thing worth noticing is that in some old data systems use "-9999" to represent NA. Another way to handle these NAs is imputation, which replaces missing data or uncommon values with substituted values. Imputation is commonly applied in a column-wise direction. The simplest imputation would be using a mean value of the rest of the data from a feature (column) to substitute the missing value. Other approaches could be to use a medium or mode value. When imputing the categorical data, we can easily assign the missing values to a new category: this method is called unique value imputation. Other more complicated methods are imputation with predicted value imputation (PVI) and distribution-based imputation. When we have a good understanding of the data, especially the intra-relationship among the features, we can appropriately predict the missing data based on the value of other features for the instances where data is found to be missing (Duricki, Soleman, and Moon 2016). However, the PVI approach was criticized for adding collinearity to the data, which we will talk about next. Alternatively, without relying on other features to provide information, we can use the distribution over the non-missing value of the feature to estimate the expected distribution of the target variable (weighting the possible assignments of the missing values) (Yasui et al. 2003).

Collincarity is more seen column-wise. If two or multiple features have a collinearity issue, the best practice is to keep the most informative one using domain knowledge. The duplication example of the measurement of distance could be the Manhattan distance vs the Euclidean distance: in some circumstances they measure the same thing; however, data cleaning should be processed case by case.

Another cleaning step is to correct the native data types in the raw data. For example, in almost all the modern languages, there is a differentiation between numerical and categorical data. Other data types include, but are not limited to: date, floating point, string, geolocation, etc. In many scenarios, researchers might also need to "bin" the feature/label or map a continuous feature/label into categorical one. For example, on expression data, we might need to convert to categories such as low, medium and high expressions depending on the task.

9.2.4 DATA PROCESSING

The data we have might not be immediately suitable for exploratory analysis or DL modelling even after we have cleaned and corrected them. Simply put, depending on the DL architecture and the library it builds on, it might require further data processing – such as converting it into other formats by transforming data. Examples include log transforming, normalizing, etc. Another process could be to subset the data based on the innate properties: for example, you might subset the gene expression data between cancer and non-cancer tissue types. In genomics, the data processing includes multiple steps. Commonly after the sequence steps, reads need to be aligned to the reference and quantified over genes or regions of interest, aka 'reads counting'. High-throughput screening (HTS) data are commonly generated by the robotic equipment and consist of a number of experimental steps, including incubating, rising and adding reagents to the culture of interest. Then these cultural plates, after the incubating period is over, are scanned and the measures of the biological activity obtained. Therefore, these data obtained after cleaning (as mentioned in Section 9.2.3) normally contain systematic and random bias that will affect down-the-line analysis.

One way to elevate the bias is to normalize the data. Data normalization consists of data transformation that allows data comparability across different batches (plats for HTC) of the same experiment. The common normalization schemes are: **Standardization** uses mean and standard deviation to transform the data $X_{transformed} = \dfrac{X - \mu}{\sigma}$, where μ is the mean and σ is the standard deviation of the data. Standardization does not change the type of the distribution of the original data; **Min-max Normalization** rescales the range of the data to $[0,1]$, $X_{transformed} = \dfrac{X - X_{min}}{X_{max} - X_{min}}$; while **Unit Vector Normalization** scales to unit length by shrinking/stretching the data to a unit range $X_{transformed} = \dfrac{X}{\|X\|}$. When it is applied on the entire data set, the transformed data can be visualized as a bunch of vectors with different directions on the D-dimensional unit sphere.

The goal of the normalization is to improve the model and numerical stability without affect the output or accuracy. In many cases, standardization might also speed up the training process.

Another way that helps eliminate bias is data transformation. The most common transformation is log transformation, which $X_{transformed} = \log X$. A base of 10, 2 and natural log ln are often used. This transformation compresses the value and constrains the data to a bell-shaped (or "normal-ish") distribution. Due to the fact that many of the DL algorithms have a normality assumption, log transformation is commonly the go-to transformation. In addition, log transformation also de-emphasizes the outliers.

9.2.5   DEEP LEARNING RESOURCES (PLATFORM), INFRASTRUCTURE, AND LIBRARIES

Recent advances in DL algorithms have been driven by the development in graphical processing unit (GPU) and tensor processing unit (TPU) using high-performance computing technologies. These technologies can significantly shrink the training time, which allows the possibility of training large data sets or big data using large DL architectures. To make computing resources more accessible, major cloud-computing platforms provide online training experiences: for example, Amazon Web Services, Google Cloud Platform (GCP) and Microsoft Azure are the major players in the cloud learning ecosystem, and provide flexible and on-demand GPU and TPU access. Configure-free cloud platforms, such as FloydHub, Valohai, Weights & Biases and Google CloudML provide easy "plug-and-play" access to the DL resources.

Much DL (or ML) software is open source. The most commonly used two with big community support are TensorFlow (Google) and PyTorch (Facebook). Other famous ones include Torch, Caffe, Theano, MXNet (Amazon), DMTK, fast.ai, XGBoost (DMLC), LightGBM (Microsoft) etc. And these frameworks were written in C++, Lua, Python, Matlab, Julia and Java. There are several advantages to using libraries like TensorFlow, as they're designed to perform computations efficiently with hardware like CPUs, GPUs and even TPUs. They allow you to easily perform parallel computing by running gear models on multiple machines or courses simultaneously. They keep a record of all the algebraic operations on your neural net in the order of computation. Therefore, they are able to compute the gradients of your model automatically (Figure 9.18).

Library	Rank	Overall	Github	Stack Overflow	Google Results
tensorflow	1	10.87	4.25	4.37	2.24
keras	2	1.93	0.61	0.83	0.48
caffe	3	1.86	1.00	0.30	0.55
theano	4	0.76	-0.16	0.36	0.55
pytorch	5	0.48	-0.20	-0.30	0.98
sonnet	6	0.43	-0.33	-0.36	1.12
mxnet	7	0.10	0.12	-0.31	0.28
torch	8	0.01	-0.15	-0.01	0.17
cntk	9	-0.02	0.10	-0.28	0.17
dlib	10	-0.60	-0.40	-0.22	0.02
caffe2	11	-0.67	-0.27	-0.36	-0.04
chainer	12	-0.70	-0.40	-0.23	-0.07
paddlepaddle	13	-0.83	-0.27	-0.37	-0.20
deeplearning4j	14	-0.89	-0.06	-0.32	-0.51
lasagne	15	-1.11	-0.38	-0.29	-0.44
bigdl	16	-1.13	-0.46	-0.37	-0.30
dynet	17	-1.25	-0.47	-0.37	-0.42
apache singa	18	-1.34	-0.50	-0.37	-0.47
nvidia digits	19	-1.39	-0.41	-0.35	-0.64
matconvnet	20	-1.41	-0.49	-0.35	-0.58
tflearn	21	-1.45	-0.23	-0.28	-0.94
nervana neon	22	-1.65	-0.39	-0.37	-0.89
opennn	23	-1.97	-0.53	-0.37	-1.07

FIGURE 9.18 The ranking of 23 open-source DL libraries that are useful for Data Science, based on Github and Stack Overflow activity, as well as Google search results. The table shows standardized scores, where a value of 1 means one standard deviation above average (average = score of 0).

Recently, many other high-level DL wrapper libraries that were built from the frameworks mentioned above have been developed to support genomics: examples are Kipoi, DeepChem, and DragoNN. The DragoNN is a toolkit to teach and learn about DL for genomics, which includes a command-line interface and tools for running models on cloud CPU or GPU. The DragoNN package also provides web-based Jupyter notebooks that allow an interactive learning experience. The DeepChem libraries provide a toolchain for democratizing the DL in drug discovery. And the Kipoi is a repository that contains out-of-the-box pre-trained models in genomics. This repo or model zoo currently contains 2,031 different models and covers canonical predictive tasks in transcriptional and post-transcriptional gene regulation (Eraslan et al. 2019).

9.2.6 DEEP MODELLING FROM A GENOMIC PERSPECTIVE

One of the most commonly used architectures is the DNN. Different DL algorithms have their own particular advantages for a specific type of task. So far, we have seen that most genomic data are sequence data, which are similar to many data in language tasks; therefore, recurrent neural networks (RNN) are quite often used. Another property of most genomic data is high dimensionality, or in other words a very long sequence, which invites problems such as the Curse of Dimensionality. To overcome this issue, many researchers using a dimension reduction approach to embed the data into a smaller dimension space then apply the DL algorithms and achieve a quite good performance. One particular dimension reduction approach in ML is autoencoder (AE), which is popular for denoising and pre-processing the input data. 1-D and 2-D CNNs have both been used for automatic feature capture in sequence and image data. When designing DL models, researchers should take advantage of the merits these architectures provide and use performance metrics (Section 9.3.3) to decide what are the best models for extracting reliable features and reasonable biological representations and for being able to generalize to new data for a particular genomic question.

9.2.6.1 Convolutional Neural Network

CNNs are the most successful DL architecture for extracting spatial information especially for image data (Krizhevsky, Sutskever, and Hinton 2017). Early adaptation still revolves around 2-D data, such as images or data matrices, and recently a convolutional layer has been applied to learn meaningful recurring patterns in the genomic sequence motifs, which allow the CNN model to be a suitable architecture for identifying motif and predicting its binding locations (Lanchantin et al. 2016). Although CNNs have demonstrated superiority over other methods in many research areas, including genomics, researchers still need to have an in-depth understanding of the CNNs and master model selection, i.e., match the right CNN architecture to a particular given task (Zeng et al., n.d.). In many cases, the performance of the CNNs depends on hyper-parameters. Through a hyper-parameter search, researchers can examine the performance of the variants of CNNs from different hyper-parameter settings.

One important aspect worth mentioning is that DL models, such as CNN, do not need to be deep in order to achieve high performance, but they need to be appropriately designed. Simply increasing the depth of the CNN mode might not result in improvement in model performance, since DL models are always over-parameterized; instead researchers should pay more attention to the fundamental underlying algorithm parameters, such as the kernel size and the number of the convolutional layer, the design of the pooling layer, the inclusion of batch-normalization and the choice of activation functions.

9.2.6.2   Recurrent Neural Networks

RNNs (Rumelhart et al., n.d.) are a family of neural networks that have the capability to process sequential data. RNNs have showed an impressive performance on challenging natural language tasks such as language translation, sematic prediction, speech recognition, etc. Unlike the CNNs mentioned earlier, RNNs share parameters at each step across the sequence and this very capability allows RNNs to retain "memory" of long-range information. One variant of the RNNs are bidirectional recurrent neural networks (BRNNs) that are able to learn the dependency from both sequential and intra-directions (Schuster and Paliwal, n.d.). When the input data sequence becomes longer, RNNs will suffer from a gradient vanishing issue. To resolve this problem, Long Short-Term Memory (LSTM) (Hochreiter and Schmidhuber 1997) and Gated Recurrent Units (Cho et al. 2014) have been proposed, which contain a mechanism of gates that allow the retaining and removing of learned information (memory).

Genomics data, such DNA, RNA and Protein data, are typically sequential, so RNNs are more often the most feasible model in many scenarios. For example, ProLanGo, an LSTM-based language translation DL model, was able to predict the protein function based on the protein sequence (Cao et al., n.d.; Boža, Brejová, and Vinař 2017). Other RNN models, such as DeepNano, were developed for base calling in minion nanopore reads (Boža, Brejová, and Vinař 2017) and DanQ to quantify the function of DNA sequence (Quang and Xie, n.d.). The more complicated models, such as the convolutional LSTM networks, can predict protein subcellular localization from protein sequences (Sønderby et al. 2015), and the sequence-to-sequence RNN models can predict the protein secondary structure based on previously predicted labels (Busia, Collins, and Jaitly 2016).

9.2.6.3   Autoencoders

Conventionally AEs were used for dimensionality reduction or feature learning, but recently applications such as stacked AEs, denoising autoencoders (DAEs), and contractive autoencoders are used as data pre-processing methods (Bengio 2011; Bengio, Courville, and Vincent, n.d.; Ravi et al. 2017). Using traditional AEs, researchers have been able to reduce the dimensionality of the large data sets such as gene expression data through learning a smaller subset feature representation to reconstructing input using AE (Chen, Xie, and Yuan 2018), where the AE was trained in a unsupervised learning manner; the learned latent feature was the input of supervised prediction of cancer types (Chen, Xie, and Yuan 2018). Another application used DAEs, learning from gene expression data, for gene clustering (Gupta, Wang, and Ganapathiraju, n.d.). One caveat of AEs is that a high reconstruction accuracy does not suggest a superior model or an improvement in training (Rampasek et al. 2017)

Instead of optimizing the architecture weights to achieve a better latent feature representation from the data, variational autoencoders (VAEs) learn the parameters of a probability distribution to represent the data. In essence, VAEs learn to model the data in the encoder part, then decoder samples from the distribution, and generate new input data samples (Kingma and Welling 2013). This is very similar to the generative model in the core. The VAEs can be used as a generative model to learn the data interdependencies in gene states before and after drug application(Rampasek et al. 2017), which is a similar approach to that mentioned above (Chen, Xie, and Yuan 2018) for training the VAE, then extend it to the final semi-supervised prediction.

9.2.6.4   Emergent Architectures

Deep Spatio-Temporal Neural Networks (DST-NNs) were implemented for protein structure prediction. Protein structure is a progressive folding (refinement) process; by including a temporal dimension, DST-NNs were able to capture this fact (Lena, Nagata, and Baldi 2012). The Model consists of a three dimensional stack of neural networks $NN_{i,j}^k$, where i and j are the spatial coordinates of the contact and k of temporal information that was gradually altered during the folding process (Lena, Nagata, and Baldi 2012). DST-NNs are able to automatically capture the correlations of the data in both spatial and temporal dimensions (Guo et al., n.d.).

Fusion Architecture is commonly implemented by combining together two or more models for different tasks. One example is the DeepCpG model, which uses two CNN models to learn different tasks: the CpG model for learning correlations between CpG sites within and across cells; and the DNA model for identify the motifs pattern (Angermueller et al. 2016). Later, by integrating the outputs from the two models and passing in the fusion model, the fusion model can learn higher level features derived from the two CNN models and predict methylation states of the DNA sequence (Angermueller et al. 2016).

Hybrid Architecture is the algorithm that combines the strengths of different types of DNN. Different to the fusion architecture, which is normally in a parallel manner, hybrid architecture is commonly implemented as sequentially, as output from an earlier model will be passed as the input for the next model, although these models may learn different tasks. For example, RNN-DNN hybrid architecture can use an RNN model to learn feature representation from the gene expression data (dimensionality reduction) and the DNN model for predicting cancer disease states (Chen, Xie, and Yuan 2018). Another example would be DanQ, which models the properties and function of a non-coding DNA sequence using a hybrid CNN and bi-directional LSTM recurrent neural network (BiLSTM) (Quang and Xie, n.d.). The performance from these architectures suggest that hybrid architecture often outperforms solo model architecture in many genomic tasks, so it is no surprise that their popularity is increasing in recent research.

9.2.7   TRANSFER LEARNING

Transfer learning, unlike the traditional ML method, is a framework to use previously-acquired knowledge from the auxiliary domain to facilitate modelling consisting of different data patterns in the current relevant domain more efficiently (Zhang et al. 2017). Transfer learning was adopted to tackle the imbalanced data problem and overcome the problem of limited data, especially genomic data, which is costly to obtain. Since it is usually time-consuming to train and tune a DL model, transfer learning was also applied to speed up the training.

Many fields, such as computer vision and language models, have benefited from transfer learning, and recent works have also shown promise in genomic DL. For example, the CNN model pre-trained on ImageNet was able to extract feature representation from the general image data, and then, when fine-tuned on gene expression images, was able to improve the performance on capture CV term-specific discriminative information. The model that was first pre-trained on data derived from different cell type/line/tissue in an unsupervised manner can later iteratively fine-tune the model on a subsequent cell type/tissue for supervised prediction and identify TFs (Cohn, Zuk, and Kaplan 2018; Qin and Feng 2017).

9.2.8 MULTI-TASK AND MULTI-VIEW LEARNING

Multi-task learning is an approach that can train shared architectures (models) for multiple relevant learning tasks in a parallel manner via joint optimization, which achieves an improved learning efficiency and performance when compared to training the models separately (Moeskops et al. 2016; Caruana 1997; Hatakeyama-Sato and Oyaizu 2020). Training a multi-task learning architecture consists of a supervised classification model from labeled data and semi-supervised auxiliary tasks on partially labeled data. The architecture was successfully applied for protein-protein interactions prediction (Qi et al. 2010). A DeepSEA framework using a multi-task learning approach was used for predicting the non-coding-variant effect from a DNA sequence (Zhou and Troyanskaya 2015).

Multi-view learning is another ML approach that aims to improve generalization performance through heterogenous data from multi-platform or multi-view (aka data fusion or data integration from multiple sources) (Zhao et al. 2017). The iDeep model used a hybrid framework of CNN and deep belief networks, and trained on cross-source data that contained motif, CLIP on-binding, structure, region type and sequence information to achieve the state-of-the-art performance (Pan and Shen 2017). Another DL framework used data of the RNA primary sequence, and (predicted) secondary and tertiary structural features to predict RNA-binding proteins target sites (Zhang et al. 2016).

9.3 DEEP LEARNING EFFECTIVELY ON GENOMIC DATA

Most biomedical research scientists have limited experience with DL and generally fall into one of the following two categories: either they haven't a clear idea of what to do with DL, what guidance should be taken, and what the ultimate goal is, or they already have a research project they are excited about and possibly already working on. Here we provide some general guidance for how to effectively apply DL on genomic data.

No matter the area of focus, the first thing is to find a few relevant research papers for your research topic, and, of course, to find out whether you have enough data and what kind of data this is. Next, you should think about how you hope to use or adapt ideas from these papers and how you plan to extend or improve it in your research work. The following elements are needed for any DL research: a research/project plan, relevant existing literature, the kind(s) model you will use or explore, the data you will use (how do you plan to obtain it), and what are the metrics for success. Keep in mind, it is always a good approach to start with implementing an existing model. Most research projects follow one of the four approach statements below:

1. Apply an existing neural network model to a topic/task/application of interest and explore how to solve it effectively;
2. Implement a complex DL architecture and demonstrate its performance on existing data that is to hand;
3. Transfer learning with a new or variant of a neural network model and explore its performance;
4. An analysis project to analyze the behavior of a model or review and compare existing models for a set of particular tasks.

The online proceedings of major ML conferences, such as NeurIPS (Neural Information Processing Systems), ICML (International Conference on Machine Learning) and ICLR (International Conference on Learning Representations), are good resources for finding useful research literature. Most ML researchers choose online preprint servers, especially https://arxiv.org, for exposure.

For pre-trained and existing state-of-the-art architectures, one good website would be https://paperswithcode.com/sota. This repository includes codes that correspond to the literature; however, the codes there might need to be selected and cleaned up before they can be actually used. One huge concern, however, relates to the library dependency as many of the codes are aimed for portability, so more than often they only run on a certain type of infrastructure with an explicit developing environment.

The must-have of every project is data. For a feasible task, researchers need to have suitable data. In the biomedical field, we commonly encounter the situation of $p \gg n$ (feature dimension p is much bigger than the sample size n), which states we have limited observations, but a very large number of features. As genomic technology such as DNA sequencing becomes more accessible, the number of observations might no longer be an issue for certain tasks, but the number of feature dimensions will remain huge. Last, but not least, is the evaluation of the DL model. Generally, automatic metrics, such as accuracy and precision, allow for a rapid development and evaluation cycle at the development phase; however, more than often these types of metrics could be misleading due to the innate properties of the data such as an unbalanced data set. Another method of evaluation would be to manually score the results, which is common for applications involving a clinical setup with experts to evaluate the output of the DL model.

Now, let us look at some good practices that will help.

9.3.1 STRICT DATA SET HYGIENE

After defining a task, researchers should define the data set. If the data of your project is from an academic source, it normally already has baselines, and at least the training and test data set are already separated for you. Right at the beginning of any DL project, data should be separated off, with DevTest and test splits; this is quite important, since without this separation, the later reported performances of the models will not be reliable and could even be wrong.

Many publicly available data sets are released with a structure of train/dev/test. In the field, we are all on the honor system to do test-set runs only when development is complete: this means your models have never seen test data sets in the development phase. However, this structure applies to a fairly large data set; if you have a much smaller data set, as is common in the biomedical field, you cannot include the dev data set, which is often the tuning hyper-parameter, instead of splitting the training data with size/usefulness against the reduction in train-set size. Having a fixed test set ensures that all the experiments are assessed against the same gold-standard data, only if the test set does not have unusual properties that is drastically different from the training data set.

9.3.2 Always Be Close to Your Data!

This applies to the development phase training (validation) data set, not for the final test set. One of the most important aspects of DL is not only to focus on the model perdition, but also to be able to understand the data. Without understanding the data, all the effort could be in vain. You need to look over the data in many ways; it is always good to visualize the data set to understand what is important in it, what you might be able to take advantage of, and what problems you need to avoid. In this way, you will have a better idea of how to improve the models that would be able to be used to undertake this. In addition, this also helps you analyze how the different hyper-parameters affect performance though graphing, such as loss plot and AUC (Area under the ROC Curve) plot.

One important insight for success in building a model, regardless of the statistical or DL model, is dependent on the understanding of the data. The model itself is no magic wand: in essence, it is a tool to help us use data to solve a task. But DL can only go as deep as the data leads, so being close to the data is useful advice for all levels of researchers and engineers.

Another important application of DL, or ML in general, is to understand which predictor variables are important, besides predicting the outcome based on genomic data. This could offer some insights into the biological understanding for a given task. For example, by investigating feature space gene expression data through analyzing the weights assigned correspondingly or variable importance metrics, researchers could understand which genes play an important role for a given disease state.

9.3.3 Define Metrics and Establish a Baseline Model

There is no way to compares models or evaluate the DL system at any stage without using metrics (commonly automatic evaluation). For a certain DL task, the standard metrics should already be well established, but it is not unreasonable to compute them for ourselves. Human evaluations, for some tasks, are still much better than the automatic metrics. If possible, a small-scale human evaluation is preferable. The base line is for a sanity check. Implement the simplest model first, and often a logistic regression is a good baseline for many research projects. It is useful to try these on the task, see how they work, and see what kinds of things are already right and what kind of things are wrong. The metrics should be computed on both training and dev data sets. Although the baseline model ultimately won't be the final model, it is still insightful for the purpose of analyzing the errors and metrics, and to shine light on what to do next. One possible outcome of the baseline for a very simple model is that it is performing very well, which suggests either the task is too simple or there is some caveat that needs to be examined. One of the most common pitfalls is the unbalanced data set.

9.3.4   Start Small, Iteratively Add Complexity

The goal of this practice is to create a well-designed and implemented experimental setup; in this way, you can easily turn around experiments when you wish to try several models and model variants in the time available. When training, models over-fit to that on which you are training: that is, the model has a high accuracy on the data on which it is trained, but just because this pattern is recognized by the model from the data doesn't necessary mean it is general enough to apply to new data. One common cause is that the model is too complex, and it is able to "memorize" the data it trained on. In the old days, we saw over-fitting as evil, but now we don't see it that way, because all good DL models should be able to over-fit the data. The way to monitor and avoid problematic overfitting is to use independent validation and test sets. As development goes on, the model should be iteratively more complex. One reason is that through this progress, inevitably you will encounter a situation where the model does not learn well, since there many factors that prevent a model fitting well to the data. Progressively increasing the complexity will help you in debugging and make your life easier.

9.4   A COLLECTION STATE-OF-THE-ART MODELS AND THEIR GENOMIC APPLICATIONS

Many articles have already surveyed the most recent applications. A more comprehensive list can be found at this reference (Yue and Wang 2018). Later, we will also provide an in-depth description of a few of the most recent significant models in the field.

9.4.1   SPROUT: CRISPR Outcome Prediction

As mentioned early, being able to repair our genes by using CRISPR could be an efficient way to battle genetic diseases. *Streptococcus pyogenes* Cas9 (SpCas9) can be used to edit the human genome through using guided RNAs (gRNAs) as searching template to find an editing location. For example, genetically edited T cells can be reintroduced to a patient's body as a therapeutic treatment (Fischbach, Bluestone, and Lim 2013). However, the repair outcomes across target sites vary due to the sequence variation near the cut site (van Overbeek et al. 2016; Brinkman et al. 2018;

Lemos et al. 2018). There are 1,656 unique target locations within 559 genes in the primary CD4+ T cells, with an average of 98 discrete repair outcomes per target site. In order to predict the repair outcomes beforehand, an ML model, SPROUT, was developed. It takes nucleotide sequences around the target site and a protospacer adjacent motif (PAM), and it utilizes gradient boosting to train an ensemble of decision trees (Leenay et al. 2019). The authors reported that the most important prediction power came mostly from the area located around the 3 nucleotides before and after the target site. The SPROUT can accurately predict the length, probability and sequence of nucleotide insertions and deletions. In addition, SPROUT can also be used for gRNA design (Leenay et al. 2019).

9.4.2   DEEP LEARNING FOR RARE DISEASE DIAGNOSTICS

DL can be used to predict healthy/disease status or disease subtypes using genomic data. The importance of classifying cancer patients into subgroups either based on the level of risk or subtype of cancers would provide valuable information for the down-the-line treatments, and many methods have been developed (Zhu et al. 2020; Silva and Rohr 2020; Chen, Xie, and Yuan 2018; Calp 2020). Using genetic data, which are easy to acquire, researchers have been develop DL models for early diagnosis and prognosis of a cancer type (Cruz and Wishart 2006; Cicchetti 2019; Cochran 1997; Kourou et al. 2015; Park et al. 2013; Sun et al. 2007). Most of the earlier works rely on feature selection algorithms and focus on identifying informative factors that are utilized afterwards in a classification task. In other words, the models were not "deep" enough to utilize all the features, since the resources were not available to develop complicated models. The new generation of DL models has already overcome this technique bottleneck. For example, a DL model was successfully applied to predict the clinical impact based on human genomic mutation (Sundaram et al. 2018). This model consists of six residual blocks (He et al. 2015) with the input of secondary structures, solvent accessibility, and a 51-length amino acid sequence centered at the variant of interest with the missense variant substituted in at the central position. By using common variants, this model was able to identify pathogenic mutations in a rare disease with 88% accuracy and was able to discover 14 novel candidate genes for an intellectual disability. Another example is to using gene expression data to predict cancer types through a fusion approach: applying an AE for feature representation learning first, then later predicting the classification using these features for classification (Chen, Xie, and Yuan 2018). This model achieved 98% accuracy in cancer detection, with false negative and false positive rates below 1.7% (Chen, Xie, and Yuan 2018).

9.4.3   GENERATIVE MODELS

The unsupervised learning models lead us to the last application: generative models. The models mentioned above are mostly supervised learning models: they are discriminative models. The difference between these two classes of the model is that the discriminative model focuses on predicting an output after learning the labelled data or $P(y \mid x)$, while a generative model models the distribution of data $P(x, y)$ and later generates new data from this distribution. Figure 9.20 illustrates the difference between the two classes.

In the real-world, a probability distribution of the task (P_r) could be very complex, but we can use Gaussian distributions $z \sim N(0,I)$ to generate a distribution P_θ that mimics P_r. A transformation function $g(z;\theta)$ can then be used to generate a new sample x {Murphy:2012uq}. The algorithm that minimizes the difference between the two distributions of P_θ and P_r can be achieved by one of the follow methods: L_1 distance $\delta(P_r, P_\theta) = \frac{1}{2} \int |P_r(x) - P_\theta(x)| \, dx$, KL-divergence $\text{KL}(P_r \| P_\theta) = E\left[\log \frac{P_r}{P_\theta}\right]$, Earth mover's distance $W(P_r, P_\theta) \approx \max_w \; E_{X \sim P_r}\left[f_w(X)\right] - E_{Z \sim N(0,I)}\left[f_w(g(Z;\theta))\right]$, where f_w is the discriminator (Lipshitz function) (Levina, and Bickel, n.d.), etc.

9.4.3.1 Deep RNN Can be Used for Molecule Design

The DL model RNN can be used to generate a sequence of small molecules, protein, and even DNA, based on certain criteria. This is especially relevant to novel drugs design. Traditionally the synthesis of small organic molecules uses a retrosynthetic model, building a search tree, and working backwards recursively to find the simpler precursor molecules with functional groups (patterns of atoms and bonds) from the target product (Anderson 2003). However, in the lab, the chemist executes this process forwards, and this approach demands a broad knowledge and deep understanding of the chemicals. It is hard to apply the computing power to simplify and fast-track the design-make-test process. Computer-aided retrosynthesis would provide a better and faster solution for the molecular design-synthesis cycle(Todd, n.d.; Law et al. 2009) and combining DL power would allow the model to gain "chemical intelligence," allowing it to mimic the expert's intuition and decision making (Neil et al. 2018; Segler and Waller 2017; Segler, Preuss, and Waller 2017). A molecular graph or chemical structure can be represented as the strings using the SMILES notation (Figure 9.19). These letter strings correspond to element symbols and will be the input for training an RNN model (Figure 9.20). Two questions are how to validate the generative model if we have no ground truth and how to validate the resulting molecule if we don't have the access to the lab to synthesize the results. The answer is to measure the similarity between the known and the generated molecules (Figure 9.21).

9.4.3.2 Deep Learning for Generate Anti-Microbial Peptide

Antimicrobial peptides (AMPs), also known as host defense peptides, are innate antibiotics. These short peptides have demonstrated therapeutic potentials (Mahlapuu et al. 2016). A DL approach to design novel effect AMPs, especially for cationic AMPs (CAMPs), has shown promise in speeding up development (Veltri et al. n.d.; Meher et al. n.d.). By using a CNN to perform the combination of classification and regression tasks on peptide sequences to quantitatively AMP activity against E. Coli, researchers were able to design AMPs with a low predicted minimum inhibitory concentration (MIC), which is the standard measurement of antibiotic activity, with a lower MIC suggesting that a lower drug concentration is required to inhibit bacterial growth (Witten and Witten 2019).

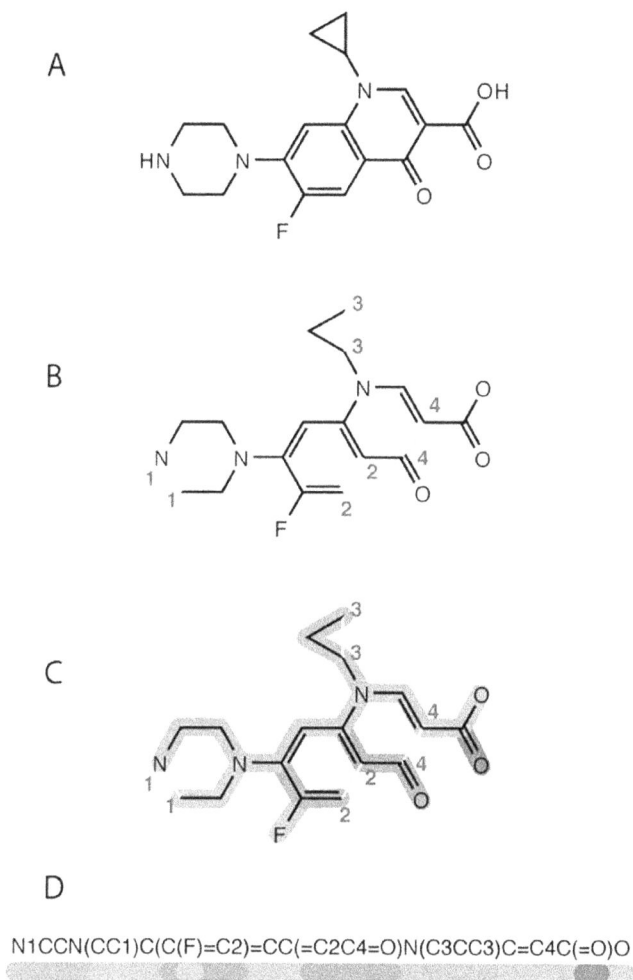

FIGURE 9.19 SMILES generation algorithm for Ciprofloxacin: break cycles, then write as branches off a main backbone.

FIGURE 9.20 Difference between discriminative mode and generative model.

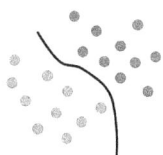

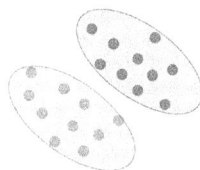

$$W(P_r, P_\theta) \approx \max_{w} \underbrace{\mathbb{E}_{X \sim P_r}[f_w(X)]}_{} - \underbrace{\mathbb{E}_{Z \sim N(0,I)}[f_w(g(Z;\theta))]}_{}$$

Discriminator score   Discriminator score on
on real examples   generated examples

FIGURE 9.21 Earth mover's distance function, which is commonly used to discriminate between real examples and generated example in the generative models.

9.4.3.3 GAN for DNA Optimizes Protein Function

At the beginning of Section 9.4.3, we mentioned the Earth mover's distance function (Levina and Bickel, n.d.): the general idea of this function is illustrated in Figure 9.21. The first term of the function calculates the discriminator score on the real examples and the second term on generated examples. This function was used in the Generative Adversarial Network (GAN) models (Goodfellow 2016) with some modifications. The GAN is composed of two DL models, one for generating examples (generator) and the other for discriminating the real example from the example generated from the generator (Figure 9.22). The improved version of the GAN, Wasserstein GAN (WGAN), is more stable at training and provides a loss function that correlates with the quality of generated data (Arjovsky and Bottou 2017). The adaptations were: first, a linear activation function was used at the output layer of the discriminator model instead of a sigmoid function; second, the labeling scheme was changed from 1 for the real image and 0 for the generated image to −1 (real) and 1 (generated); third, the Wasserstein loss was used to train the discriminator and generator models; fourth, the discriminator model weights were constrained to a limited range after each mini batch update (e.g., [−0.01,0.01]); fifth, the discriminator model was updated more frequently than the generator model in each iteration; and sixth, the RMSProp was used for the gradient descent with a small learning rate and no momentum(Arjovsky and Bottou 2017).

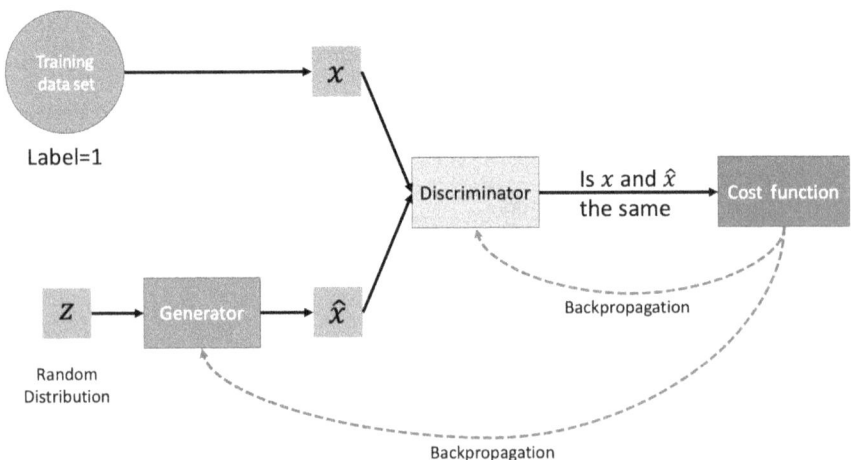

FIGURE 9.22 Generative adversarial network models.

Thus far, GANs have been used to generate realistic gene, protein, drugs, and images in the biology and medical fields (Goldsborough et al. 2017; Ghahramani, Watt, and Luscombe 2018; Osokin et al. 2017; Zhu and Bento 2017; Killoran et al. 2017). One particular application has been to use feedback from a GAN to optimize the synthetic gene sequences for the desirable properties of the gene product, such as proteins (Gupta and Zou 2019). The generator was from a WGAN architecture, and the discriminator could be any black-box discriminative neural network that takes in a gene and can predict the probability score. Through a suite of metrics, this application demonstrates that it is feasible to use this DL mode to generate desirable proteins (Gupta and Zou 2019).

9.5 OUTRO

We have discussed many successful applications of DL in genomics, but in this section we would like to go over some limitations. We will provide some useful resources to better understand DL and genomics where a reader can find references, textbooks, tutorials and even codes, all aiming to shed light on future developments of DL applications in genomic research.

9.5.1 CHALLENGES OF DEEP LEARNING

DL for genomics has shown promise in many applications; however, comparing it with other research fields such as computer vision or natural language processes, it still has a long way to go. One unique scenario that genomic research faces is the limitations of the data. First, it is generally much more costly to acquire genomic data, which causes the data to be less abundant than other data types such as imaging, text, etc. Cancer research is one of most studied areas, and the National Cancer Institute Genomic Data Commons has collected a large amount of genomic data from multiple projects that are publicly available for researchers. However, when compared to other fields, such as computer vision (Jensen et al. n.d.; Russakovsky et al. 2015; Deng et al. n.d.), the collection is still small.

In addition, due to the nature of the research, true labels might not be as obvious due to the requirement for sophisticated domain knowledge from the labeler or the unavailability of an automatic labelling process. Conversely, the nature of the genomic data is unbalanced due to, for example, the oversampling of disease states and under-sampling of the control state, or due to heterogeneity due to the HTS performed in many data centers. Take the epigenetic data sets, for example, there are far fewer DNA methylated region (DMR) sites than non-DMR sites (Haque, Skinner, and Holder 2014). Or, the example of functional genomics, where the imbalance ration of non-slice site to slice site, is over a thousand (Yoon and Kwek 2007). Many solutions have proposed, such as over-sampling, under-sampling and partitioning, while ensemble approaches that apply a voting scheme using multiple learning algorithms (Opitz, and Maclin n.d.; Polikar n.d.; West et al. 2018) appear to be powerful. Another way to improve the discriminating power of the model is to include various types of data as model inputs.

9.5.2 Deep Learning Resources

There are many resources available online about DL. Here we will summarize a few that we believe would be of most benefit for readers. First, online classes. The most renowned entry-level online class with certification is the ML course taught by Stanford Professor Andrew Ng (Coursera, https://www.coursera.org/specializations/deep-learning/). Dr. Ng also teaches another series of five DL courses that focus on using Python. Google also provides some entry courses focusing on using GCP: one of them that is particularly useful is called ML with TensorFlow on GCP. This course is also taught on Coursera.

For an introductory book about DL, we would suggest "Deep Learning" (Goodfellow, Bengio, and Courville 2016). This book is an introduction to a broad range of topics in DL, covering the fundamental math and background needed for understanding and implementing DL architectures. To learn ML (DL) tools, such as Scikit-Learning, TensorFlow, and Pytorch, O'Reilly Media has published a series of books. To learn the math theories behind many ML algorithms, we suggest 'The Elements of Statistical Learning', which describes the important original ideas.

Another good resource that allows hands-on experience is provided by the Nvidia Deep Learning Institute (DLI, www.nvidia.com/dli). DLI has designed a online education platform that provides developers and engineers with knowledge and resources to solve real-world problems (Chen, Gutmann, and Bungo 2018). It covers a range of topics from DL to accelerated computing, and the best part is that students need to actually program in order to obtain a certificate.

9.5.3 Outlook

Genomics is fundamental to human biology, but it contains a lot of unknowns. Just as the microscope revolutionized biology in the 1600s, DL will be the next tool that helps us understand the mechanisms behind human genomics. Recent breakthroughs in genomics through DL have surpassed many previous state-of-the-art that scientists have taken centuries to achieve. However, due to many factors, such as the sparsity of the genomic data, a watershed in genomics has been hindered. Many new DL methods are constantly being proposed, and through carefully selection of data sources and features, with the appropriate design of architecture structures, DL can help to advance and revolutionize the course of genomics.

REFERENCES

Alberts, Bruce, Alexander Johnson, Julian Lewis, Keith Roberts, and Martin Raff. 2009. Molecular biology of the cell. Garland Pub. Garland Pub. ISBN-10: 0-8153-3218-1ISBN-10: 0-8153-4072-9.

Anderson, Amy C. 2003. "The process of structure-based drug design." *Chemistry & Biology* 10 (9): 787–97. Doi: 10.1016/j.chembiol.2003.09.002.

Angermueller, Christof, Heather J Lee, Wolf Reik, and Oliver Stegle. 2016. "Accurate prediction of single-Cell DNA methylation states using deep learning." *BioRxiv* 11 (May): 055715. Doi: 10.1101/055715.

Arjovsky, Martin, and Léon Bottou. 2017, January. "Towards principled methods for training generative adversarial networks." arXiv preprint arXiv:1701.04862.

Bengio, Yoshua. 2011, January. "Contractive auto-encoders: Explicit invariance during feature extraction." In *In International Conference on Machine Learning*, Bellevue, Washington, DC.

Bengio, Y, A Courville, and P Vincent. n.d. "Representation learning: A review and new perspectives." *IEEE Transactions on Pattern Analysis and Machine Intelligence* 35 (8): 1798–1828. Doi: 10.1109/tpami.2013.50.

Benson, D A, I Karsch-Mizrachi, DJ Lipman. n.d., 2005 "Nucleic acids." GenBank. Academic. Oup.Com.

Boža, Vladimír, Broňa Brejová, and Tomáš Vinař. 2017. "DeepNano: Deep recurrent neural networks for base calling in MinION nanopore reads." Edited by Degui Zhi. *PloS One* 12 (6): e0178751. Doi: 10.1371/journal.pone.0178751.

Brinkman, Eva K., Tao Chen, Marcel de Haas, Hanna A. Holland, Waseem Akhtar, and Bas van Steensel. 2018. "Kinetics and fidelity of the repair of Cas9-induced double-strand DNA breaks." *Molecular Cell* 70 (5): 801–813.e6. Doi:10.1016/j.molcel.2018.04.016.

Busia, Akosua, Jasmine Collins, and Navdeep Jaitly. 2016, November. "Protein secondary structure prediction using deep multi-scale convolutional neural networks and next-step conditioning." arXiv preprint arXiv:1611.01503.

Calp, M. Hanefi. 2020. *"Deep Learning for Cancer Diagnosis,"* 249–67. Doi: 10.1007/978–981-15–6321–8_15.

Cao, R, C Freitas, L Chan, M Sun, H Jiang, Z Chen Molecules, and n.d, 2017. "ProLanGO: protein function prediction using neural machine translation based on a recurrent neural network." Mdpi.Com.

Caruana, Rich. 1997. "Multitask learning." *Machine Learning* 28 (1): 41–75.

Caraus, I, A A Alsuwailem, R Nadon, and V Makarenkov. 2015. "Detecting and overcoming systematic bias in high-throughput screening technologies: A comprehensive review of practical issues and methodological solutions." *Briefings in Bioinformatics* 16 (6): 974–86. Doi: 10.1093/bib/bbv004.

Chen, Xi, Gregory S Gutmann, and Joe Bungo. 2018, December. "Deep learning by doing: The NVIDIA deep learning institute and university ambassador program " arXiv preprint arXiv:1812.08671.

Chen, Xi, Jin Xie, and Qingcong Yuan. 2018, December. "A method to facilitate cancer detection and type classification from gene expression data using a deep autoencoder and neural network." arXiv preprint arXiv:1812.08674.

Cho, Kyunghyun, Bart van Merrienboer, Caglar Gulcehre, Dzmitry Bahdanau, Fethi Bougares, Holger Schwenk, and Yoshua Bengio. 2014, June. "Learning phrase representations using RNN encoder-decoder for statistical machine translation." arXiv preprint arXiv:1406.1078.

Cicchetti, Domenic V. 2019. "Neural networks and diagnosis in the clinical laboratory: State of the art." *Clinical Chemistry* 38 (1): 9–10. Doi: 10.1093/clinchem/38.1.9.

Clarke, L, X Zheng-Bradley, R Smith, E Kulesha Nature, n.d., 2012. "The 1000 genomes project: Data management and community access." Nature.Com.

Cochran, Alistair J. 1997. "Prediction of outcome for patients with cutaneous melanoma." *Pigment Cell Research* 10 (3): 162–67. Doi: 10.1111/j.1600–0749.1997.tb00479.x.

Cohn, Dikla, Or Zuk, and Tommy Kaplan. 2018. "Enhancer identification using transfer and adversarial deep learning of DNA sequences." *BioRxiv* 107 (50): 264200. Doi: 10.1101/264200.

Cruz, Joseph A., and David S. Wishart. 2006. "Applications of machine learning in cancer prediction and prognosis." *Cancer Informatics* 2: 117693510600200030. Doi: 10.1177/117693510600200030.

Deng, J, W Dong, R Socher, L J Li, K Li n.d., 2009 "Imagenet: A large-scale hierarchical image database." *IEEE Conference*, Ieeexplore.Ieee.Org.

Duricki, Denise A, Sara Soleman, and Lawrence DF Moon. 2016. "Analysis of longitudinal data from animals with missing values using SPSS." *Nature Protocols* 11 (6): 1112–29. Doi: 10.1038/nprot.2016.048.

Eilbeck, Karen, Suzanna E Lewis, Christopher J Mungall, Mark Yandell, Lincoln Stein, Richard Durbin, and Michael Ashburner. 2005. "The sequence ontology: A tool for the unification of genome annotations." *Genome Biology* 6 (5): R44. Doi: 10.1186/gb-2005-6-5-r44.

Eraslan, Gökcen, Žiga Avsec, Julien Gagneur, and Fabian J Theis. 2019. "Deep learning: New computational modelling techniques for genomics." *Nature Reviews Genetics* 20 (7): 389–403. Doi: 10.1038/s41576-019-0122-6.

Escalante, Ana E., Lev Jardón Barbolla, Santiago Ramírez-Barahona, and Luis E. Eguiarte. 2014. "The study of biodiversity in the era of massive sequencing." *Revista Mexicana de Biodiversidad* 85 (4): 1249–64. Doi: 10.7550/rmb.43498.

Fischbach, Michael A., Jeffrey A. Bluestone, and Wendell A. Lim. 2013. "Cell-based therapeutics: The next pillar of medicine." *Science Translational Medicine* 5 (179): 179ps7–179ps7. Doi: 10.1126/scitranslmed.3005568.

Gerstein, Mark B, Anshul Kundaje, Manoj Hariharan, Stephen G Landt, Koon-Kiu Yan, Chao Cheng, Xinmeng Jasmine Mu, et al. 2012. "Architecture of the human regulatory network derived from ENCODE data." *Nature* 489 (7414): 91–100. Doi: 10.1038/nature11245.

Ghahramani, Arsham, Fiona M Watt, and Nicholas M Luscombe. 2018. "Generative adversarial networks uncover epidermal regulators and predict single cell perturbations." *BioRxiv* 3 (February): 262501. Doi: 10.1101/262501.

Goldsborough, Peter, Nick Pawlowski, Juan C Caicedo, Shantanu Singh, and Anne E Carpenter. 2017. "CytoGAN: Generative modeling of cell images." *BioRxiv* 9 (7): 227645. Doi: 10.1101/227645.

Goodfellow, Ian. 2016. "NIPS 2016 tutorial: Generative adversarial networks." Arxiv.Org, December. arxiv.org.

Goodfellow, I, Y Bengio, and A Courville. 2016. "Deep learning.", Cambridge: MIT Press.

Goodwin, S, J D McPherson. WR McCombie. n.d., 2016 "Coming of age: Ten years of next-generation sequencing technologies." *Nature Reviews Genetics*. Nature.Com.

Greener, Joe G, Lewis Moffat, and David T Jones. 2018. "Design of metalloproteins and novel protein folds using variational autoencoders." *Scientific Reports* 8 (1): 16189. Doi: 10.1038/s41598-018-34533-1.

Guo, Shengnan, Youfang Lin, Shijie Li, Zhaoming Chen, and Huaiyu Wan. n.d. "Deep spatial–temporal 3D convolutional neural networks for traffic data forecasting." *IEEE Transactions on Intelligent Transportation Systems* 20 (10): 3913–26. Doi: 10.1109/tits.2019.2906365.

Gupta, A, H Wang, and M Ganapathiraju. n.d. "Learning structure in gene expression data using deep architectures, with an application to gene clustering." In *2015 IEEE International Conference on Bioinformatics and Biomedicine (BIBM)*, 1328–35, Washington, DC.

Gupta, Anvita, and James Zou. 2019. "Feedback GAN for DNA optimizes protein functions." *Nature Machine Intelligence* 1 (2): 105–11. Doi: 10.1038/s42256-019-0017-4.

Hager, G L, J G McNally, T Misteli. n.d., 2009. "Transcription dynamics." *Molecular Cell*, 35 (6), 741–53. Elsevier.

Haque, M Muksitul, Michael K Skinner, and Lawrence B Holder. 2014. "Imbalanced class learning in epigenetics." *Journal of Computational Biology* 21 (7): 492–507. Doi: 10.1089/cmb.2014.0008.

Hatakeyama-Sato, Kan, and Kenichi Oyaizu. 2020. "Integrating multiple materials science projects in a single neural network." *Communications Materials* 1 (1): 1–10. Doi: 10.1038/s43246-020-00052-8.

He, K, X Zhang, S Ren, and J Sun. 2015. Deep residual learning for image recognition. CoRR Abs/1512.03385.

Hirsch, Tad, Kritzia Merced, Shrikanth Narayanan, Zac E Imel, and David C Atkins. 2017. "Designing contestability: Interaction design, machine learning, and mental health." *DIS. Designing Interactive Systems (Conference)* 2017 (June): 95–99. Doi: 10.1145/3064663.3064703.

Hochreiter, Sepp, and Jürgen Schmidhuber. 1997. "Long short-term memory." *Neural Computation* 9 (8): 1735–80. Doi: 10.1162/neco.1997.9.8.1735.

Israeli, Johnny, Anshul Kundaje, Anna Scherbina, and Chuan Sheng Foo. 2016, June 9. "How to train your Dragonn." https://drive.google.com/file/d/0B4Yo77Kh_QeeaXZK QUtZWjNrWkE/view.

Jain, Miten, Hugh E Olsen, Benedict Paten, and Mark Akeson. 2016. "The Oxford nanopore MinION: Delivery of nanopore sequencing to the genomics community." *Genome Biology* 17 (1): 1–11. Doi: 10.1186/s13059-016-1103-0.

Jensen, M A, V Ferretti, R L Grossman, LM Staudt. n.d., 2017. "The NCI genomic data commons as an engine for precision medicine." *Blood*. Ashpublications.Org.

Karolchik, D, R Baertsch, M Diekhans. n.d., 2003. "The UCSC genome browser database." *Nucleic Acids Research*. Academic.Oup.Com.

Killoran, Nathan, Leo J Lee, Andrew Delong, David Duvenaud, and Brendan J Frey. 2017, December. "Generating and designing DNA with deep generative models." arXiv preprint arXiv:1712.06148.

Kimball, J. 2010. "The genetic code." *Cold Spring Harbor Symposia on Quantitative Biology* 3, 238–248.

Kingma, Diederik P, and Max Welling. 2013, December. "Auto-encoding variational bayes." arXiv preprint arXiv:1312.6114.

Kourou, Konstantina, Themis P. Exarchos, Konstantinos P. Exarchos, Michalis V. Karamouzis, and Dimitrios I. Fotiadis. 2015. "Machine learning applications in cancer prognosis and prediction." *Computational and Structural Biotechnology Journal* 13: 8–17. Doi: 10.1016/j.csbj.2014.11.005.

Krizhevsky, Alex, Ilya Sutskever, and Geoffrey E Hinton. 2017. "ImageNet classification with deep convolutional neural networks." *Communications of the ACM* 60 (6): 84–90. Doi: 10.1145/3065386.

Lanchantin, Jack, Ritambhara Singh, Zeming Lin, and Yanjun Qi. 2016, May. "Deep motif: Visualizing genomic sequence classifications." arXiv preprint arXiv:1605.01133.

Lander, E S, L M Linton, B Birren, C Nusbaum, and M C Zody. 2001. "Initial sequencing and analysis of the human genome." *Nature* 409(6822): 860–921.

Law, James, Zsolt Zsoldos, Aniko Simon, Darryl Reid, Yang Liu, Sing Yoong Khew, A Peter Johnson, Sarah Major, Robert A Wade, and Howard Y Ando. 2009. "Route designer: A retrosynthetic analysis tool utilizing automated retrosynthetic rule generation." *Journal of Chemical Information and Modeling* 49 (3): 593–602. Doi: 10.1021/ci800228y.

Leenay, R T, A Aghazadeh, J Hiatt, D Tse, TL Roth, and 2019. "Large dataset enables prediction of repair after CRISPR–Cas9 editing in primary T cells." *Nature Biotechnology* Nature.Com 37 (9). Doi: 10.1038/s41587-019-0203-2.

Lemos, Brenda R., Adam C. Kaplan, Ji Eun Bae, Alexander E. Ferrazzoli, James Kuo, Ranjith P. Anand, David P. Waterman, and James E. Haber. 2018. "CRISPR/Cas9 cleavages in budding yeast reveal templated insertions and strand-specific insertion/deletion profiles." *Proceedings of the National Academy of Sciences* 115 (9): 201716855. Doi: 10.1073/pnas.1716855115.

Lena, Pietro D, Ken Nagata, and Pierre F Baldi. 2012. "Deep Spatio-temporal architectures and learning for protein structure prediction." In, edited by F Pereira, C J C Burges, L Bottou, and K Q Weinberger, 512–20. *Advances in Neural Information Processing Systems* 25. Curran Associates, Inc.

Levina, E, P Bickel. n.d., 2001. "The earth mover's distance is the mallows distance: Some insights from statistics." *Proceedings Eighth IEEE International Conference on Computer Vision.* Ieeexplore.Ieee.Org.

Lipman, D J, WR Pearson. n.d., 1985. "Rapid and sensitive protein similarity searches." *Science.* Sciencemag.Org.

Mahlapuu, Margit, Joakim Håkansson, Lovisa Ringstad, and Camilla Björn. 2016. "Antimicrobial peptides: An emerging category of therapeutic agents." Frontiers in Cellular and Infection Microbiology 6 (December): 239. Doi: 10.3389/fcimb.2016.00194.

Meher, P K, T K Sahu, V Saini, AR Rao. n.d., 2017. "Predicting antimicrobial peptides with improved accuracy by incorporating the compositional, physico-chemical and structural features into chou's general ...." *Scientific Reports.* Nature.Com.

Meissner, Alexander, Tarjei S Mikkelsen, Hongcang Gu, Marius Wernig, Jacob Hanna, Andrey Sivachenko, Xiaolan Zhang, et al. 2008. "Genome-scale DNA methylation maps of pluripotent and differentiated cells." *Nature* 454 (7205): 766–70. Doi: 10.1038/nature07107.

Miles, Jeremy. 2014. *Tolerance and Variance Inflation Factor.* John Wiley & Sons, Ltd. Doi: 10.1002/9781118445112.stat06593.

Moeskops, Pim, Jelmer M Wolterink, Bas HM van der Velden, Kenneth GA Gilhuijs, Tim Leiner, Max A Viergever, and Ivana Išgum. 2016. Deep learning for multi-task medical image segmentation in multiple modalities. In *Medical Image Computing and Computer-Assisted Intervention – MICCAI 2016*, Vol. 9901, Springer International Publishing. Doi: 10.1007/978-3-319-46723-8_55.

Mor-Yosef, S, A Samueloff, B Modan. n.d., 1990 "Ranking the risk factors for cesarean: Logistic regression analysis of a nationwide study." *Obstetrics and Gynecology* Journals.Lww.Com.

Movva, Rajiv, Peyton Greenside, Georgi K. Marinov, Surag Nair, Avanti Shrikumar, and Anshul Kundaje. 2019. "Deciphering regulatory DNA sequences and noncoding genetic variants using neural network models of massively parallel reporter assays." *PLOS One* 14 (6): e0218073. doi:10.1371/journal.pone.0218073.

Mullard, A. 2015. "The roadmap epigenomics project opens new drug development avenues."

Neil, Daniel, Marwin Segler, Laura Guasch, Mohamed Ahmed, Dean Plumbley, Matthew Sellwood, and Nathan Brown. 2018, February. "Exploring deep recurrent models with reinforcement learning for molecule design."

Opitz, D, and Maclin, R, n.d., 1999. "Popular ensemble methods: An empirical study." *Journal of Artificial Intelligence Research.* Jair.Org.

Osokin, Anton, Anatole Chessel, Rafael E Carazo Salas, and Federico Vaggi. 2017. "GANs for biological image synthesis." 2233–42.

Pan, Xiaoyong, and Hong-Bin Shen. 2017. "RNA-protein binding motifs mining with a new hybrid deep learning based cross-domain knowledge integration approach." BMC *Bioinformatics* 18 (1): 1–14. Doi: 10.1186/s12859-017-1561-8.

Park, Kanghee, Amna Ali, Dokyoon Kim, Yeolwoo An, Minkoo Kim, and Hyunjung Shin. 2013. "Robust predictive model for evaluating breast cancer survivability." *Engineering Applications of Artificial Intelligence* 26 (9): 2194–2205. doi:10.1016/j. engappai.2013.06.013.

Polikar R. n.d., 2006 "Ensemble based systems in decision making." *IEEE Circuits and Systems, Magazine* Ieeexplore.Ieee.Org.

Puton, Tomasz, Lukasz Kozlowski, Irina Tuszynska, Kristian Rother, and Janusz M. Bujnicki. 2012. "Computational methods for prediction of protein–RNA interactions." *Journal of Structural Biology* 179 (3): 261–68. Doi: 10.1016/j.jsb.2011.10.001.

Qi, Y, O Tastan, J G Carbonell, J Klein-Seetharaman, and J Weston. 2010. "Semi-supervised multi-task learning for predicting interactions between HIV-1 and human proteins." *Bioinformatics (Oxford, England)* 26 (18): i645–52. Doi: 10.1093/bioinformatics/btq394.

Qin, Qian, and Jianxing Feng. 2017. "Imputation for transcription factor binding predictions based on deep learning." Edited by Ilya Ioshikhes. *PLoS Computational Biology* 13 (2): e1005403. Doi: 10.1371/journal.pcbi.1005403.

Qu, H, and X Fang. n.d., 2013. "A brief review on the human encyclopedia of DNA elements (ENCODE) project." *Genomics, Proteomics Bioinformatics* 11: 135–141. Elsevier.

Quang, D, and X Xie. n.d., 2016. "DanQ: A hybrid convolutional and recurrent deep neural network for quantifying the function of DNA sequences." *Nucleic Acids Research* 44 (11): e107–e107 Academic.Oup.Com.

Rampasek, Ladislav, Daniel Hidru, Petr Smirnov, Benjamin Haibe-Kains, and Anna Goldenberg. 2017, June. "Dr.VAE: Drug response variational autoencoder." arXiv preprint arXiv:1706.08203.

Ravi, Daniele, Charence Wong, Fani Deligianni, Melissa Berthelot, Javier Andreu-Perez, Benny Lo, and Guang-Zhong Yang. 2017. "Deep learning for health informatics." *IEEE Journal of Biomedical and Health Informatics* 21 (1): 4–21. Doi: 10.1109/jbhi.2016.2636665.

Ren, Shaoqing, Kaiming He, Ross Girshick, and Jian Sun. n.d. "Faster R-CNN: Towards real-time object detection with region proposal networks." *IEEE Transactions on Pattern Analysis and Machine Intelligence* 39 (6): 1137–49. Doi: 10.1109/tpami.2016.2577031.

Rifaioglu, Ahmet Sureyya, Heval Atas, Maria Jesus Martin, Rengul Cetin-Atalay, Volkan Atalay, and Tunca Doğan. 2018. "Recent applications of deep learning and machine intelligence on in silico drug discovery: Methods, tools and databases." *Briefings in Bioinformatics* 20 (5): 1878–1912. Doi: 10.1093/bib/bby061.

Rumelhart, D E, P Smolensky, and JL McClelland n.d, 1986. "Sequential thought processes in PDP models." *Parallel Distributed Processing: Explorations in the Microstructures of Cognition*, 2: 3–57. Cs.Toronto.Edu.

Russakovsky, Olga, Jia Deng, Hao Su, Jonathan Krause, Sanjeev Satheesh, Sean Ma, Zhiheng Huang, et al. 2015. "ImageNet large scale visual recognition challenge." *International Journal of Computer Vision*, 115 (3): 211–52. Doi: 10.1007/s11263-015-0816-y.

Schuster, M, and KK Paliwal n.d., 1997. "Bidirectional recurrent neural networks." *IEEE Transactions on Signal Processing*, 45 (11), 2673–2681. Ieeexplore.Ieee.Org.

Segler, Marwin H S, Mike Preuss, and Mark P Waller. 2017. "Learning to plan chemical syntheses." *Nature* 555 (7698): 604–10. Doi: 10.1038/nature25978.

Segler, Marwin H S, and Mark P Waller. 2017. "Neural-symbolic machine learning for retrosynthesis and reaction prediction." *Chemistry - A European Journal* 23 (25): 5966–71. Doi: 10.1002/chem.201605499.

Silva, Luís A. Vale, and Karl Rohr. 2020. "Pan-cancer prognosis prediction using multimodal deep learning." *2020 IEEE 17th International Symposium on Biomedical Imaging (ISBI)*, 568–71. Doi: 10.1109/isbi45749.2020.9098665.

Sønderby, Søren Kaae, Casper Kaae Sønderby, Henrik Nielsen, and Ole Winther. 2015. "Convolutional LSTM networks for subcellular localization of proteins." *Computer Vision – ECCV 2014*, 9199: 68–80. Springer International Publishing. Doi: 10.1007/978-3-319-21233-3_6.

Sood, Ankur Jai, Coby Viner, and Michael M Hoffman. 2019. "DNAmod: The DNA modification database." *Journal of Cheminformatics* 11 (1): 75. Doi: 10.1186/s13321-019-0349-4.

Sun, Yijun, Steve Goodison, Jian Li, Li Liu, and William Farmerie. 2007. "Improved breast cancer prognosis through the combination of clinical and genetic markers." *Bioinformatics* 23 (1): 30–37. Doi: 10.1093/bioinformatics/btl543.

Sundaram, Laksshman, Hong Gao, Samskruthi Reddy Padigepati, Jeremy F. McRae, Yanjun Li, Jack A. Kosmicki, Nondas Fritzilas, et al. 2018. "Predicting the clinical impact of human mutation with deep neural networks." *Nature Genetics* 50 (8): 1161–70. Doi: 10.1038/s41588-018-0167-z.

The UniProt Consortium. n.d., 2017. "UniProt: The universal protein knowledgebase." *Nucleic Acids Research*, 45: D158–D169. Academic.Oup.Com.

Todd, MH. n.d, 2005. "Computer-aided organic synthesis." *Chemical Society Reviews*, 34, 247–266. Pubs.Rsc.Org.

van Overbeek, Megan, Daniel Capurso, Matthew M. Carter, Matthew S. Thompson, Elizabeth Frias, Carsten Russ, John S. Reece-Hoyes, et al. 2016. "DNA repair profiling reveals nonrandom outcomes at Cas9-mediated breaks." *Molecular Cell* 63 (4): 633–46. Doi: 10.1016/j.molcel.2016.06.037.

Veltri, D, U Kamath, and A Shehu. n.d., 2018. "Deep learning improves antimicrobial peptide recognition." *Bioinformatics* 34: 2740–2747. Academic.Oup.Com.

Wang, Jingxue, Huali Cao, John Z. H. Zhang, and Yifei Qi. 2018. "Computational protein design with deep learning neural networks." *Scientific Reports* 8 (1): 6349. Doi: 10.1038/s41598-018-24760-x.

Wen, Ming, Zhimin Zhang, Shaoyu Niu, Haozhi Sha, Ruihan Yang, Yonghuan Yun, and Hongmei Lu. 2017. "Deep learning-based drug-target interaction prediction." *Journal of Proteome Research* 16 (4): acs.jproteome.6b00618–1409. Doi: 10.1021/acs.jproteome.6b00618.

West, Michael D, Ivan Labat, Hal Sternberg, Dana Larocca, Igor Nasonkin, Karen B Chapman, Ratnesh Singh, et al. 2018. "Use of deep neural network ensembles to identify embryonic-fetal transition markers: Repression of COX7A1 in embryonic and cancer cells." *Oncotarget* 9 (8): 7796–7811. Doi: 10.18632/oncotarget.23748.

Witten, Jacob, and Zack Witten. 2019. "Deep learning regression model for antimicrobial peptide design." *BioRxiv* 6 (July): 692681. Doi: 10.1101/692681.

Yaari, Z, D Da Silva, A Zinger, E Goldman, Kajal, A, Tshuva, R, Barak, E, Dahan, N, Hershkovitz, D, Goldfeder, M, and Roitman, JS n.d., 2016. "Theranostic barcoded nanoparticles for personalized cancer medicine." *Nature Communications*, 7 (1): 1–10. Nature.Com.

Yasui, Yutaka, Margaret Pepe, Mary Lou Thompson, Bao-Ling Adam, George L. Wright, Yinsheng Qu, John D. Potter, Marcy Winget, Mark Thornquist, and Ziding Feng. 2003. "A Data-analytic strategy for protein biomarker discovery: Profiling of high-dimensional proteomic data for cancer detection." *Biostatistics* 4 (3): 449–63. Doi: 10.1093/biostatistics/4.3.449.

Yoon, Kihoon, and Stephen Kwek. 2007. "A data reduction approach for resolving the imbalanced data issue in functional genomics." *Neural Computing and Applications* 16 (3): 295–306. Doi: 10.1007/s00521-007-0089-7.

Yue, Tianwei, and Haohan Wang. 2018, February. "Deep learning for genomics: A concise overview."

Zeng, H, M D Edwards, G Liu, and DK Gifford. n.d., 2016 "convolutional neural network architectures for predicting DNA–protein binding." *Bioinformatics*, 32 (12): i121–i127. Academic.Oup.Com.

Zerbino, D R, P Achuthan, and W Akanni, n.d, 2018. "Ensembl 2018." *Nucleic Acids Research* 46, D754–D761. Academic.Oup.Com.

Zhang, Lu, Jianjun Tan, Dan Han, and Hao Zhu. 2017. "From machine learning to deep learning: Progress in machine intelligence for rational drug discovery." *Drug Discovery Today* 22 (11): 1680–85. Doi: 10.1016/j.drudis.2017.08.010.

Zhang, Sai, Jingtian Zhou, Hailin Hu, Haipeng Gong, Ligong Chen, Chao Cheng, and Jianyang Zeng. 2016. "A deep learning framework for modeling structural features of RNA-binding protein targets." *Nucleic Acids Research* 44 (4): e32–e32. Doi: 10.1093/nar/gkv1025.

Zhao, Jing, Xijiong Xie, Xin Xu, and Shiliang Sun. 2017. "Multi-view learning overview: recent progress and new challenges." *Information Fusion* 38 (November): 43–54. Doi: 10.1016/j.inffus.2017.02.007.

Zheng, H, and W Xie. n.d., 2019. "The role of 3D genome organization in development and cell differentiation." *Nature Reviews Molecular Cell Biology*, 20 (9): 535–550. Nature.Com.

Zhou, Jian, and Olga G Troyanskaya. 2015. "Predicting effects of noncoding variants with deep learning–based sequence model." *Nature Methods* 12 (10): 931–34. Doi: 10.1038/nmeth.3547.

Zhu, Jia-Jie, and José Bento. 2017, February. "Generative adversarial active learning." arXiv preprint arXiv:1702.07956.

Zhu, Wan, Longxiang Xie, Jianye Han, and Xiangqian Guo. 2020. "The Application of Deep Learning in Cancer Prognosis Prediction." *Cancers* 12 (3): 603. Doi: 10.3390/cancers12030603.

10 A Review of Deep Learning-Based Methods for Cancer Detection and Classification

Kusum Lata and Sandeep Saini
The LNM Institute of Information Technology

CONTENTS

10.1 INTRODUCTION

Presently, cancer is the world's second most deadly illness. In 2018, 9.6 million people lost their lives because of various types of cancers globally. Early cancer diagnosis will cure the disease, so accurate cancer detection and classification is a very critical aspect of cancer. In the medical field, a disease can be diagnosed by invasive (Adami et al., 1994) as well as noninvasive methods (Kang et al., 2017; Samria et al., 2014). The recent trends in diagnosis are more inclined towards non-invasive methods. Cancer can be detected by lab tests, imaging tests, and biopsy. In this work, we focus on imaging tests. The images can be taken by various types of machines and observed by experts as well as machines to detect the cancer cells.

Deep learning is a sub-field of Artificial intelligence and it is emerging as a very robust universal solution for most of the problems that are dependent on classification. Deep learning has established itself as the most advanced technique for such problems and the current phase of deep learning has started in 2012. Cancer detection from various types of images is a simple classification problem in the deep learning field. Around six decades ago, the notion of deep learning was presented and it has slowly emerged as a potential contender for solving real-world problems. The approaches need high computational facilities for training large-sized neural networks. The lack of such a computing facility was the bottleneck in the development of such approaches. In 2012, with the introduction of AlexNet (Krizhevsky et al., 2012) model and availability of high-power graphical processing units (GPUs) around the globe, the field has started to grow at an exponential pace. A lot of state-of-the-art models and architectures have emerged in this duration that solve almost every real-world problem.

In this chapter, we have reviewed deep learning-based methods for cancer detection and classification. Initially, we have compiled the types of cancers for our study. We have considered different types of cancer that can be detected by deep learning-based image processing methods. We have provided the details about the existing work on these types of cancers and their detection methods. Then we have provided the details of various deep learning models that are used for object detection and classification on medical images. We have listed over 20 latest deep learning-based model in our study. These models are listed in the order of their introduction year. We have explained the basic architecture and model parameters for the same. A very basic requirement for any deep learning-based model is the availability of a good amount of relevant data set. The data set should be prepared under standard conditions and labeled properly. We have compiled a list of more than 15 publically available data sets for various types of cancers. In the end, we have provided a comprehensive study of the performance of deep learning architectures in cancer detection and classification. The work will help the research community in deciding the appropriate model to carry forward research in this field.

10.2 TYPES OF CANCER

Different types of cancers which are reported in the literature for their identification and classification using Deep Learning approaches are discussed here. Various research articles are published which discuss and show that deep learning techniques are quite useful in identifying and helping doctors to diagnosis cancer at the early stage.

10.2.1 BRAIN CANCER

Brain cancer is the most dangerous cancer for people of all ages. Brain cancer is an abnormal growth in the cells in and around the brain structure (Abdelaziz Ismael et al., 2020). Table 10.1 summarizes the recently published work for detecting brain cancer using deep learning methods.

10.2.2 BREAST CANCER

In developed and developing countries, breast cancer is the most common form of cancer in women and the second most common cancer overall (Azamjah et al., 2019). A lot of papers are published recently which emphasize the application of deep learning for detection and classifying breast cancer with various applications. Table 10.2 summarizes reported work in the literature.

TABLE 10.1

Description of the Identification and Classification of Brain Cancer Using Deep Learning Methods

Application	Modality	Reference
BraTS	Magnetic resonance images	Sajid et al. (2019), Iqbal et al. (2019)
Brain cancer classification	Magnetic resonance images	Abdelaziz Ismael et al. (2020), Muhammad et al. (2020)
Survival prediction	Magnetic resonance images	Sun et al. (2019), Feng et al. (2020)
Glioblastoma	Magnetic resonance images	Tang et al. (2020), Wong et al. (2019)

TABLE 10.2

Description of the Identification and Classification of Breast Cancer Using Deep Learning Methods

Application	Modality	Reference
Mass detection and classification	Mammographic	Agarwal et al. (2020), Dhungel et al. (2015a)
Mitosis detection	Histopathology images	Sebai et al. (2020a, b)
Lesion recognition and classification	Mammographic	Swiderski et al. (2017), Wei et al. (2019)
Mass segmentation	CT imaging	Caballo et al. (2020)
Breast cancer classification	CT imaging	Murtaza et al. (2020), Gour et al. (2020)

10.2.3 COLON CANCER

Colon cancer is one of the top-most cancers that has become the major mortality cause of the global population including men and women.[1] Table 10.3 summarizes the several studies conducted to detect and analyze with the help of several deep learning methods.

10.2.4 LUNG CANCER

Deep learning-based methods are becoming popular in detecting and classifying the lung cancer (Katiyar & Singh, 2020). Recently various research papers have reported their results on lung cancer detection, their classification, lung cancer patient survival analysis and survival prediction, etc. Table 10.4 summarizes the published literature.

TABLE 10.3

Description of the Identification and Classification of Colon Cancer Using Deep Learning Methods

Application	Modality	Reference
Polyp detection in colonoscopy videos	Colonoscopy	Poon et al. (2020), Lee et al. (2020), Mohammadi (2020)
Colonic polyp classification	Colonoscopy	Wang et al. (2020a), Azer (2019) "Comparative Analysis and Proposal of Deep Learning-Based Colorectal Cancer Polyps Classification Technique," (2020)
Grade classification in colon cancer	Histopathology	Vuong et al. (2020), Chowdhury et al. (2017)
Detection and classification of nuclei	Histopathology	Sirinukunwattana et al. (2016)
Cell nuclei segmentation	Histopathology	Mandloi et al. (2019)

TABLE 10.4

Description of the Identification and Classification of Lung Cancer Using Deep Learning Methods

Application	Modality	Reference
Pulmonary nodule detection and classification	Volumetric computed tomography	Hua et al. (2015), Dou et al. (2017), Setio et al. (2016), Wang et al. (2017), Rahman et al. (2019), Katiyar and Singh (2020), Riquelme and Akhloufi (2020)
Survival analysis	Pathology report	Zhu et al. (2016)
Nodule characterization	Volumetric computed tomography	Hussein et al. (2017)
Survival prediction	Computed tomography	Paul et al. (2016)
Extraction of ground glass opacity candidate region	Computed tomography	Hirayama et al. (2016)

10.2.5　PROSTATE CANCER

Prostate cancer is the most frequent cancer after lung cancer in men, which may be asymptomatic at the early stage and might require minimal or no treatment (Rawla, 2019). Deep learning methods are being used for prostate detection and classification. Table 10.5 summarizes the research articles published for detecting and classifying prostate cancer.

10.2.6　SKIN CANCER

Skin cancer is one of the most common types of cancer, which is typically identified with the help of dermoscopic images (Afza et al., 2019). Several studies report the

TABLE 10.5

Description of the Identification and Classification of Prostate Cancer Using Deep Learning Methods

Application	Modality	Reference
Prostate cancer classification	Magnetic resonance image	Schelb et al. (2019)
Prostate cancer detection and segmentation	Magnetic resonance image	Arif et al. (2020)
Prediction of prostate cancer	Magnetic resonance image	Takeuchi et al. (2019)
Prostate cancer detection	Contrast-enhanced ultrasound imaging	Feng et al. (2019)
Prostate cancer detection	Temporal-enhanced ultrasound imaging	Azizi et al. (2018)
Prostate segmentation	3D Transrectal ultrasound	Orlando et al. (2020)
Prostate segmentation	Magnetic resonance image	Zavala-Romero et al. (2020)

TABLE 10.6
Description of the Identification and Classification of Skin Cancer Using Deep Learning Methods

Application	Modality	Reference
Skin lesion detection and classification	Dermoscopy images	Gessert et al. (2020), Aishwarya et al. (2020)
Skin cancer detection	Dermoscopy images	Wei et al. (2020a)
Melanoma detection	Dermatology image	Zunair and Ben Hamza (2020)
Skin lesion segmentation	Dermoscopy images	Hasan et al. (2020)
Melanoma segmentation and classification	Whole slide images	Van Zon et al. (2020)
Border detection of melanoma lesions	Dermoscopy images	Jadhav et al. (2019)

detection and classification of skin cancer using deep learning techniques. Table 10.6 summarizes the various published research papers which discuss deep learning techniques that are quite useful in identifying and helping doctors to diagnosis cancer at the early stage.

10.3 DEEP LEARNING ARCHITECTURES AND MODELS FOR CANCER DETECTION AND CLASSIFICATION

Deep learning has emerged as an universal learning that applies to almost every area of research. The major difference between Machine Learning (ML) and Deep Learning (DL) approaches is the process of feature extraction. In ML we have more human intervention in extracting the features, tagging data and eventually learning. While in Deep learning, the features are learned by the architecture itself and stored in hierarchical order. Artificial intelligence (AI), ML and DL are closely related and the relation is shown in Figure 10.1.

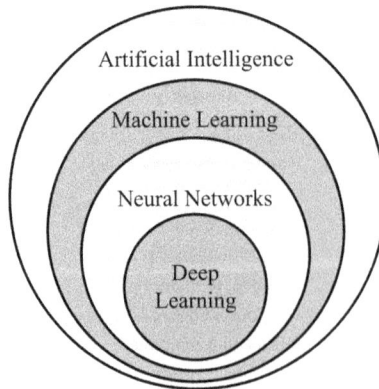

FIGURE 10.1 Hierarchy of AI, ML and DL.

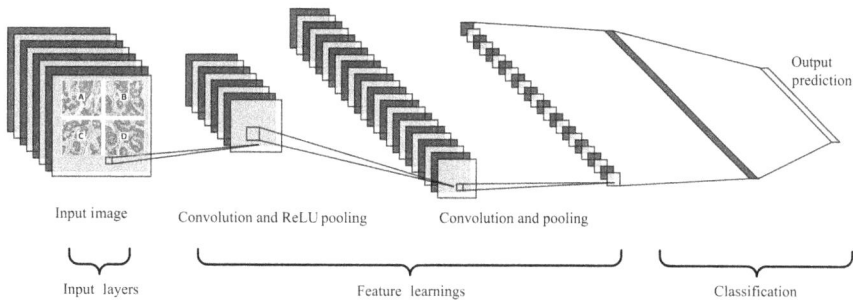

FIGURE 10.2 A CNN-based architecture for cancer detection and classification.

Deep learning is better applicable under the following circumstances:

a. Human expertise is limited in a field.
b. Human expertise task is time-consuming.
c. Errors are more with human involvement.
d. Solutions need to adapt itself to particular aspects over time.
e. The problem size is very vast and manual processing is not possible.

Thus, for cancer detection and classification for a large variety of cancers with high accuracy, deep learning approaches are the best candidate.

The current state-of-the-art Deep Learning architectures and model development started with the introduction of AlexNet (Krizhevsky et al., 2012) in 2012. Krizhevsky et al. proposed this model and trained on the ImageNet data set[2] for the ImageNet Large-Scale Visual Recognition Challenge (ILSVRC)[3] competition. Convolutional Neural Networks (CNNs) were used before AlexNet and it is also based on CNN. There are a total of eight layers in AlexNet. Five layers are convolutional layers and three are fully connected network layers. The authors used Rectified Linear Units instead of tanh function as the activation function. This approach resulted in six times faster results as compared to conventional CNN models. AlexNet achieved an error rate of 16.4%, compared to the 2nd place result of 26.1%. CNN-based deep learning models are used not only for images but also for video applications (Wang et al., 2020b) and (Pan et al., 2019). A CNN-based architecture for cancer detections is shown in Figure 10.2. The stages involved are almost the same in every network and the convolutional and pooling layers are changed for experimenting to get better results.

After AlexNet, a lot of similar models and architectures are developed. The most popular ones are ZFNet (Zeiler & Fergus, 2014), Overfeat (Sermanet et al., 2013), Oxford's VGG (Simonyan & Zisserman, 2014), GoogleNet (Szegedy et al., n.d.), ResNet (He et al., 2016), and Xception (Chollet, 2017). With the availability of fast GPUs, developing highly dense networks and training them with expansive computational costs were no longer a hindrance in the process. Thus, there is an exponential growth in the quality of image classification using Deep Learning-based models. Deep Neural Network and Transfer-based models are among the most popular models for cancer detection. Figures 10.3 and 10.4 show DNN and Transfer learning-based architecture. We provided the details of such models developed over these years in an orderly manner.

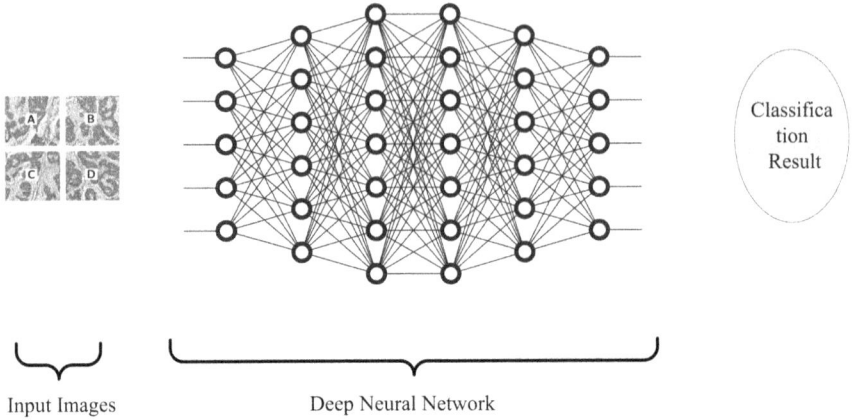

FIGURE 10.3 A deep neural network-based architecture for cancer detection and classification.

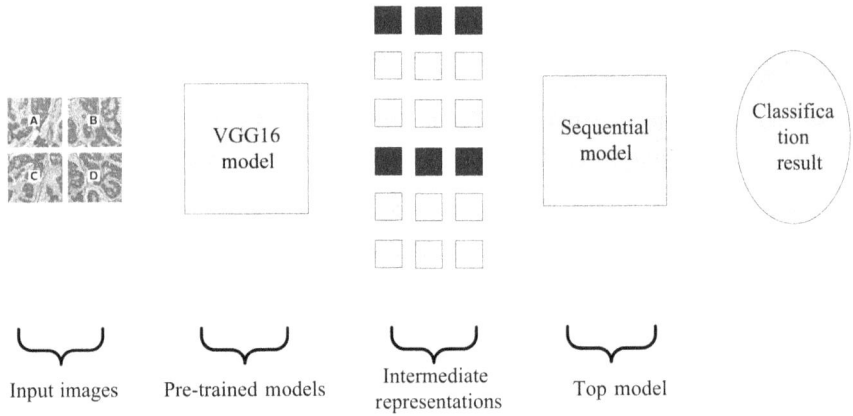

FIGURE 10.4 A transfer learning-based model for image classification.

There has been a significant amount of development and we have chosen the most popular and revolutionizing models for this review. The list of these models along with their key features is given in Table 10.7. These models are proposed for any sort of image classification task and the majority of these are used for cancer detection as well.

10.4 DATA SETS FOR CANCER DETECTION AND CLASSIFICATION USING DEEP LEARNING METHODS

Machine learning and deep learning algorithms require an annotated data set of suitable images for training and testing of the system. Thus, the availability of a suitable data set is the foremost requirement for testing a system. In this section, we have listed publically available data sets for different types of cancer detection and classifications.

TABLE 10.7
Deep Learning-Based Model and Architectures for Image Classification

Model Name	Year of Introduction	Basic Architecture and Functions	Activation Function	Type of Learning and Special Features
LeNet (LeCun et al., 1998, 1999),	1998	CNN-based with 60,000 parameters	Tanh and Sigmoid	Transfer Learning
Alexnet (Krizhevsky et al., 2012)	2012	CNN-based with 60 million parameters	ReLU	AlexNet was the first breakthrough model in the revolutionizing the current Deep Learning approaches. The model was designed with eight layers.
Overfeat (Sermanet et al., 2013)	2013	145 million parameters	Tanh	SGD and the model was the winner of the ILSVRC 2013 challenge as well.
ZfNet (Zeiler & Fergus, 2014)	2013	Fully Supervised CNN-based 8-layered model trained on 1.3 million images.	ReLU and Softmax	One-shot learning
AlexNetOWTBn (Krizhevsky, 2014)	2014	SGD-based parallel NN	ReLU	This model is a "One Weird Trick (OWT)" variation of the AlexNet in which the authors adopted batch normalization (Bn) at the end of each convolutional layer.
NiN (Lin et al., 2013)	2014	CNN- and MLP-based model	Tanh	Transfer learning
VGG (Simonyan & Zisserman, 2014)	2014	140 million parameters trained on 1.3 million images.	ReLU	Visual Geometry Group (VGG) at Oxford university proposed this model as their entry for the ILSVRC 2014 challenge. Transfer learning-based.

(Continued)

TABLE 10.7 (*Continued*)
Deep Learning-Based Model and Architectures for Image Classification

Model Name	Year of Introduction	Basic Architecture and Functions	Activation Function	Type of Learning and Special Features
FCN (Long et al., 2015)	2014	SGD-based end-to-end, pixels-to-pixels trained network.	ReLU and Tanh	End-to-end learning
GoogleNet (Szegedy et al., 2015)	2014	22-layer deep CNN-based model with 60 million parameters.	Tanh	The model was the official entry from Google for ILSVRS 2014 and the winner of the challenge. The model is based on Transfer learning.
ResNet (He et al., 2016)	2015	VGG-based model trained on 25.5 million parameters.	ReLU	Transfer learning
SegNet (Badrinarayanan et al., 2017)	2015	SGD-based classifier	Tanh and sigmoid	Transfer learning
U-Net (Ronneberger et al., 2015)	2015	ReLU with 2x2 max pooling	ReLU	Transfer learning. The proposed model won the ISBI cell tracking challenge 2015.
YOLO (Redmon et al., 2016)	2016	CNN-based 24 layers architectures	Tanh and sigmoid	You Only Look Once (YOLO) detects multiple objects in a single image by considering it as a regression problem
SqueezeNet (Iandola et al., 2016)	2016	Replace large filters with smaller and uses the same activation as CNN.	Tanh and Sigmoid	This is based on AlexNet but with 50 times fewer parameters. The model applies a singular value decomposition (SVD) to a pre-trained CNN model for compression.

(*Continued*)

TABLE 10.7 (Continued)
Deep Learning-Based Model and Architectures for Image Classification

Model Name	Year of Introduction	Basic Architecture and Functions	Activation Function	Type of Learning and Special Features
CapsuleNet (Sabour et al., 2017)	2017	256, 9×9 convolution kernels	ReLU	Transfer learning.
DenseNet (Huang et al., 2017)	2017	250 layers with 25 million parameters	ReLU	End-to-end learning
Fast RCNN (Girshick, 2015)	2017	Softmax classifier-based model for fast training and testing.	Softmax	Transfer learning
MobileNet (Howard et al., 2017)	2017	MobileNet use both batchnorm and ReLU nonlinearities	ReLU	MobileNet is designed by focusing on Mobile and Embedded systems-based applications. End-to-End learning.
DeepLab (Chen et al., 2017)	2018	SegNet-based model	ReLU	Transfer Learning
Xception (Chollet, 2017)	2018	Trained on 350 million images and 17,000 classes.	ReLU	Xception is a deep network proposed by Google for large image classifications.
PataNET (Islam et al., 2019)	2019	Using CNN with Adam Optimizer	ReLU and softmax	Transfer learning
IRRCNN (Alom et al., 2020)	2020	The hybrid model trained on 3.5 million parameters.	SGD and ReLU	End-to-End learning
MDFC–ResNet (Hu et al., 2020)	2020	ResNet-based network. 2 million parameters.	ReLU	Transfer learning

10.4.1 MITOS-ATYPIA Data Set

The data set is made available as a part of the MITOS-ATYPIA challenge. The challenge was held in 2012 and 2014. The latest data set is available for 2014[4] for breast cancer detection and classification. There were two main tasks associated with the challenge, i.e., detection of mitosis on the one hand and evaluation of nuclear atypia score on the other hand. The data set contains 284 frames at $\times 20$ magnification and 1,136 frames at $\times 40$ magnification. The frames are RGB bitmap images in the TIFF format. For $\times 20$ magnification frames, the authors have provided the nuclear atypia score as a number: 1, 2 or 3. Score 1 denotes low-grade atypia, score 2 a moderate grade atypia, and score 3 a high-grade atypia. This score has been given independently by two different senior pathologists.

For the $\times 40$ magnification frames, the authors have provided a list of mitosis given by two different pathologists. The pathologists have annotated mitosis as true mitosis, probably mitosis, or not mitosis. Six criteria are given by three junior pathologists to evaluate the nuclear atypia. The criteria for nuclear atypia are provided as a number: 1, 2 or 3. Sample images from the data set are shown in Figure 10.5.

10.4.2 BreakHis Data Set

The Breast Cancer Histopathological Image Classification (BreakHis) is created by the Department of Informatics and Graduate Program in Computer Science of UFPR, Brazil. There are an aggregate of 7,909 minute pictures of bosom tumor tissue. These pictures are gathered from 82 patients utilizing diverse amplifying factors. Each picture size is 700×460 pixels, 3-channel RGB, 8-bit profundity in each channel, and put away in PNG design. The data set subtleties are as per the following (Table 10.8).

10.4.3 INbreast Database

The INbreast information base is a mammographic data set, with pictures procured at a Breast Cancer Center, situated in a University (Hospital de São João, Breast Center, Porto, Portugal). The data set contains an aggregate of 115 cases and 410 pictures. Of these 90, female cases have both bosom pictures (four pictures for each case) and

(a)

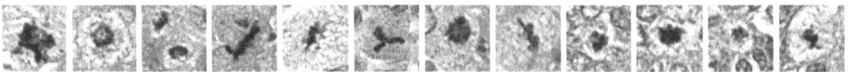

Examples of mitosis.

(b)

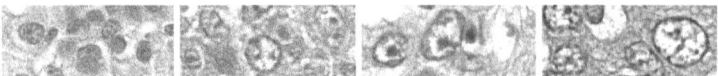

Examples of various degrees of nuclear atypia.

FIGURE 10.5   Sample images from the MITOS-ATYPIA data set.

TABLE 10.8
Details of the BreakHis Data Set Images

Magnification	Benign	Malignant	Total
40×	652	1,370	1,995
100×	644	1,437	2,081
200×	623	1,390	2,013
400×	588	1,232	1,820
Total no. of images	2,480	5,429	**7,909**

25 cases have just two pictures for every case. In the explanations, a few sorts of injuries, for example, calcifications, masses, asymmetries and bends are incorporated.

10.4.4 CBIS-DDSM DATA SET

Curated Breast Imaging Subset of DDSM (CBIS-DDSM) is an updated and standardized version of the previous Digital Database for Screening Mammography (DDSM) that was released in 1997. The latest data set is released in 2017. This data set contains 2,620 scanned film mammography studies. The data set focuses on breast cancer images only. The images contain normal, benign and malignant cases with verified pathology information (Lee et al., 2017). The data set is available for the public at Cancer Imaging Archive.[5]

10.4.5 LIDC-IDRI DATA SET

The Lung Image Database Consortium image collection (LIDC-IDRI) is released in 2015 and it consists of diagnostic and lung cancer screening thoracic CT scans (Armato III et al., n.d.). The data set is available for the public at Cancer Imaging Archive.[6] The data set consists of 244,617 images contributed by 1,010 patients. The data set is developed by the collaboration of eight medical imaging companies. The data set contains CT (computed tomography), SEG (DICOM segmentation), DX (digital radiography) and CR (computed radiography) modalities. The total data set size is 125 GB.

10.4.6 LUNA DATA SET

The LUng Nodule Analysis 2016 (LUNA 2016) challenge was an open challenge for Lung Cancer detection and classification at the International Symposium on Biomedical Imaging ISBI 2016. The challenge is having two tasks, i.e., nodule detection (NDET) using raw CT scans and false positive reduction (FPRED). The available data set for this challenge contains 888 CT scans.[7] The data set is partially derived from the LIDC-IDRI data set by excluding the slices of thickness more than 2.5 mm. The entire data set is split into ten subsets to use for the 10-fold cross-validation process. All subsets come as compressed zip files.

10.4.7   DLCST DATA SET

Danish Lung Cancer Screening Trial (DLCST) was initially released in 2007 as a collaborative output of the Danish Lung Cancer Group and Ministry of the Interior and Health, Denmark. The data set contains CT scans of 4,104 participants for a period of 10 years.[8] The experiment is a parallel randomized controlled experiment that either compares an annual low-dose CT scan or no screening. Four-thousand one-hundred and four smokers and former smokers participated in the study.

10.4.8   JSTR DATA SET

Japanese Society of Radiological Technology (JSRT) in cooperation with the Japanese Radiological Society (JRS) released the Lung cancer Chest X-ray image data set in 1998. The data set contains a total of 247 images, of which 154 are nodule and 93 nonnodule images. Each image resolution is $2,048 \times 2,048$ matrix size with a 0.175 mm pixel size. A registered user can download the data set from the official website[9] or Kaggle.[10]

10.4.9   HAM10000 DATA SET

Human Against Machine with 10,000 (HAM10000) is a large dataset for skin cancer-related images (Tschandl et al., 2018). The data set consists of 10,015 dermatoscopic images that are published as a training set for academic machine learning purposes and are accessible publicly through the International Skin Imaging Collaboration (ISIC) archive. The data set was initially provided for ISIC 2018: Skin Lesion Analysis towards Melanoma Detection challenge. The challenge had three main tasks, namely, Lesion Segmentation, Lesion Attribute Detection and Disease Classification.

10.4.10   MED-NODE DATA SET

MED-NODE is a medical assistance system that takes non-dermoscopic digital images of lesions from which it automatically extracts the lesion regions and then computes descriptors regarding the color and texture (Giotis et al., 2015). The data set used in this system consists of 70 melanoma and 100 naevus images. The data set was released in 2015 at the digital image archive of the Department of Dermatology of the University Medical Center Groningen.

10.4.11   PROMISE12 DATA SET

As a part of the Medical Image Computing and Computer-Assisted Intervention (MICCAI), 2012 conference, PROstate MR Image SEgmentation (PROMISE) 2012 contest was held. In this contest, a data set of 1,200 images of 2D MRI slides was provided for the classification and detection of prostate cancer. Registered users can access the data from the official website.[11] The data include patients with benign disease and prostate cancer. The data set is prepared from multiple centers and multiple MRI vendors.

10.4.12   PROSTATE MRI DATA SET

This data set was obtained with an endorectal and phased array surface coil at 3T. The data were generated at the National Cancer Institute, Bethesda, Maryland, the USA, between 2008 and 2010 (Clark et al., 2013) and made publically available at Cancer Imaging Archive.[12] The data set contains 22,036 images from 26 participants and the total size is 3.2 GB.

10.4.13   PROSTATE MR IMAGE DATABASE

The national center for Image-guided Therapy has released a data set of 1,150 images of prostate cancer.[13] The data set is collected for around 3 years on 230 patients. The data set is publically available for researchers.

10.4.14   BRATS DATA SET

As part of MICCAI's Brain Tumor Segmentation (BraTS) challenge, the BraTS data set is released since 2016. The data set volumes are arranged into T1, T2, Flair and T1Ce sequences. Each of these volumes contains 155 slices that are MRI images. The total number of images is more than 200,000. The data set is updated every year and available on request.[14]

10.4.15   BRAIN-TUMOR-PROGRESSION DATA SET

The data set contains images from 20 newly diagnosed primary glioblastoma subjects who were treated with surgery and regular concomitant chemoradiation therapy, followed by adjuvant chemotherapy. The data set contains a total of 8,798 images from 20 patients in 383 series within 90 days. All image sets are in DICOM format and include T1w, FLAIR, T2w, ADC, normalized cerebral blood flow, uniform relative cerebral blood volume and binary tumor masks. Following a preload of contrast, the perfusion images were created from dynamic susceptibility contrast images. The data set is available at the Cancer Imaging Archive.[15]

10.5   PERFORMANCE OF DEEP LEARNING-BASED MODELS FOR CANCER DETECTION AND CLASSIFICATION

Deep learning-based models and architecture are proposed as potential solutions for cancer detection and classification. Any such tasks must be quantified and its performance must be measured. All the approaches mentioned in the above sections of this chapter fall under the classification-related tasks for a deep learning model. This category of tasks can be measured with the following metrics.

10.5.1   CONFUSION MATRIX

This is not a performance measuring metric but one of the basic concepts to understand the other metrics. Let us consider a classification task for binary classification

TABLE 10.9

A Sample Confusion Matrix for Binary Classification Tasks of 2,200 Leaf Images

		Actual Class	
		Leaf	Non-leaf
Predicted class	Leaf	180	120
	Nonleaf	20	1880

to classify leaf images in a particular image data set. If our data set contains a total of 2,200 images which contain only 200 leaf images and the remaining 2,000 nonleaf images. Then a sample confusion matrix after the training is shown in Table 10.9.

The model predicts 180 correct leaf images from actual 200 leaf images and incorrectly predicts 120 nonleaf images as leaf images. Thus, we can say that the true positive prediction is 180/200=90% and 20 samples are predicted as false negatives. Similarly, for nonleaf images, 120 images are classified as false positives and 1,880 images as true negatives. These parameters help us in formulating other evaluation metrics.

10.5.2 CLASSIFICATION ACCURACY

This is one of the simplest and one of the most common metrics to comprehend the performance of a deep learning model. The accuracy of the model on its predictions is defined as the ratio of the number of correct predictions to the total number of predictions made by the model. The number will always be in the range of 0–1 and it can be multiplied by 100 to obtain percentage accuracy. In the example given above the classification accuracy is calculated as (180+1,880)/2,200=0.9363 or 93.63%.

10.5.3 PRECISION

Classification accuracy is an easy metric but not always a good way to measure the performance of the model. If we have imbalanced classes in our data set (i.e., there are more data values for one class than others), then if the system predicts more values belonging to this class, the accuracy will be high which should not be the case for a true classifier. To overcome such issues, we use the precision metric. Precision is defined as

$$\text{Precision} = \text{True\_Positive}/\left(\text{True\_Positive} + \text{False\_Positive}\right) \qquad (10.1)$$

The consideration of true and false predictions makes this metric a better alternative to the accuracy alone. Thus, for the above given example, the values of precision are calculated for the leaf as well as nonleaf classification.

$$\text{Precision\_leaf} = 180/(180+120) = 60\%$$

$$\text{Precision\_non-leaf} = 1880/1900 = 98.9\%.$$

Thus we can comprehend that for this imbalanced example, the precision values are also highly varying for each class while accuracy was not able to provide such information.

10.5.4 RECALL

The recall is another important metric which is defined as the fraction of samples that are correctly predicted by the deep learning model.

$$Recall = True\_Positive/ \left(True\_Positive+ False\_Negative\right) \qquad (10.2)$$

In the given example, the recall values for two classes are as follows:

$$Recall\_leaf = 180/200 = 90\%$$

$$Recall\_non\text{-}leaf = 1880/2000 = 94\%.$$

10.5.5 F1 SCORE

F1 score or simply F score is a measurement metric that is derived from the precision and recall metrics. F score is defined as

$$F1 \text{ score}= 2*Recall*Precision/\left(Recall + Precision\right) \qquad (10.3)$$

F1 score is also in the range of 0–1 and can be multiplied by 100 to obtain the percentage value.

For our given example the values of F scores for both the classes are

$$F-score\_leaf = 2*0.6*0.9(0.6+0.9) = 0.72$$

$$F-score\_non\text{-}leaf = 2*0.\ 94*0.989/(0.94+0.989) = 0.9638$$

10.5.6 SENSITIVITY AND SPECIFICITY

Sensitivity and specificity are the two most common metrics used in the biomedical field. Sensitivity is equal to the recall value of the classification task and specificity is defined as the true negative rate which is expressed as

$$Specificity = True\_Negative/\left(True\_Negative + False\ Positive\right) \qquad (10.4)$$

It can be comprehended that the performance of a model on a particular data set is dependent on various parameters. The same model will perform in different ways on different data sets and under different training conditions. A particular model can perform in a different way for different feature classification of the same data set. This also helps us in deciding which features are better suited for a particular classification task. In Table 10.10, we have compiled the performances of various deep learning-based models for different types of cancers.

TABLE 10.10

Performance Measures of Different Deep Learning-Based Model and Architectures for Detection and Classification of Tasks Related to Different Types of Cancer

Model/Authors	Type of Cancer	Task	Accuracy	Precision	Recall	F Score
CNN-based model (Albayrak & Bilgin, 2016)	Breast cancer	Mitosis detection	0.968	0.98	0.94	0.969
CNN-based model (Spanhol et al., 2016)	Breast cancer	Histopathological image classification	0.89	0.84	0.85	0.848
CNN-based skin cancer detection (Cruz-Roa et al., 2013)	Skin cancer	Image representation, visual interpretability	0.921	0.901	0.887	0.894
RNN-based model (Shakeel, Burhanuddin, et al., 2019)	Lung cancer	Lung image segmentation	0.945	0.94	0.968	0.954
Propagation neural network-based model (Shakeel, Tobely, et al., 2019)	Brain cancer	Brain tumor classification	0.97	0.94	0.98	0.97
CNN-based model (Setio et al., 2016)	Lung cancer	Pulmonary nodule detection	0.891	0.93	0.857	0.89
CNN-based model (Gao et al., 2017)	Brain cancer	Classification of CT brain images	0.876	0.863	0.85	0.86
FCN-based model (Chen et al., 2016)	Breast Cancer	Mitosis detection	0.886	0.804	0.772	0.778
FCN-based model (Liu et al., 2017)	Prostate cancer	Prostate cancer diagnosis	0.83	0.872	0.86	0.868
Deep auto encoder-based model (Sabbaghi et al., 2016)	Skin cancer	Classification of melanomas in dermoscopy images	0.95	0.939	0.949	0.943
SVM-based model (Dhungel et al., 2015b)	Breast cancer	Mass segmentation from mammograms	0.88	0.90	0.93	0.916
FCN-based model (Wei et al., 2020b)	Skin cancer	Skin lesion segmentation	0.962	0.923	0.867	0.912

It is evident from the values of performance metrics in Table 10.10 that computer-aided deep learning-based models for cancer detection are highly accurate and provide more than 95% accuracy on an average. This is quite satisfactory considering the amount of time and human efforts they save in the process. With the availability of high-power computational facilities and pre-trained models, the process of cancer detection and classification is much easier now compared to the human verification process.

10.6 CONCLUSION

In this chapter, we have reviewed and compiled the latest deep learning-based models and architectures for various cancer detection and classification. The models work on the principle of classification of various features extracted from the images of cancer patients. The availability of efficient and fast models has enabled highly accurate and fast detection for all types of cancers by reducing human efforts in this field. In this study, we have focused on breast cancer, lung cancer, skin cancer, prostate cancer, brain cancer and other cancers as well. One of the major requirements for training a deep learning-based model is the availability of a suitable data set. We have also compiled the list of publically available data sets in this chapter. We have shown the performances of various architectures for different cancer detection and conclude that the performance of each such system is highly satisfactory. The work will help the research community to take future directions in the field.

NOTES

1 https://www.cancer.org/cancer/colon-rectal-cancer/about/key-statistics.html.
2 http://www.image-net.org/.
3 http://image-net.org/challenges/LSVRC/2012/index.
4 https://mitos-atypia-14.grand-challenge.org/Dataset/.
5 https://wiki.cancerimagingarchive.net/display/Public/CBIS-DDSM.
6 https://wiki.cancerimagingarchive.net/display/Public/LIDC-IDRI.
7 https://luna16.grand-challenge.org/data/.
8 https://clinicaltrials.gov/ct2/show/study/NCT00496977.
9 http://db.jsrt.or.jp/eng.php.
10 https://www.kaggle.com/raddar/nodules-in-chest-xrays-jsrt.
11 https://promise12.grand-challenge.org/Home/.
12 https://wiki.cancerimagingarchive.net/display/Public/PROSTATE-MRI.
13 http://prostatemrimagedatabase.com/Database/index.html.
14 https://www.med.upenn.edu/cbica/brats2020/data.html.
15 https://wiki.cancerimagingarchive.net/display/Public/Brain-Tumor-Progression.

REFERENCES

Abdelaziz Ismael, S. A., Mohammed, A., & Hefny, H. (2020). An enhanced deep learning approach for brain cancer MRI images classification using residual networks. *Artificial Intelligence in Medicine*, *102*, 101779. Doi: 10.1016/j.artmed.2019.101779.

Adami, H.-O., Pontén, J., Sparén, P. Ä. R., Bergström, R., Gustafsson, L., & Friberg, L.-G. (1994). Survival trend after invasive cervical cancer diagnosis in Sweden before and after cytologic screening. 1960--1984. *Cancer*, *73*(1), 140–147.

Afza, F., Khan, M. A., Sharif, M., & Rehman, A. (2019). Microscopic skin laceration segmentation and classification: A framework of statistical normal distribution and optimal feature selection. *Microscopy Research and Technique*, *82*(9), 1471–1488. Doi: 10.1002/jemt.23301.

Agarwal, R., Díaz, O., Yap, M. H., Lladó, X., & Martí, R. (2020). Deep learning for mass detection in full field digital mammograms. *Computers in Biology and Medicine*, *121*. Doi: 10.1016/j.compbiomed.2020.103774.

Aishwarya, U., Daniel, I. J., & Raghul, R. (2020). Convolutional neural network based skin lesion classification and identification. *Proceedings of the 5th International Conference on Inventive Computation Technologies, ICICT 2020*, 264–270. Doi: 10.1109/ICICT48043.2020.9112485.

Albayrak, A., & Bilgin, G. (2016). Mitosis detection using convolutional neural network based features. *2016 IEEE 17th International Symposium on Computational Intelligence and Informatics (CINTI)*, 335–340, Budapest.

Alom, M. Z., Hasan, M., Yakopcic, C., Taha, T. M., & Asari, V. K. (2020). Improved inception-residual convolutional neural network for object recognition. *Neural Computing and Applications*, *32*(1), 279–293.

Arif, M., Schoots, I. G., Castillo Tovar, J., Bangma, C. H., Krestin, G. P., Roobol, M. J., Niessen, W., & Veenland, J. F. (2020). Clinically significant prostate cancer detection and segmentation in low-risk patients using a convolutional neural network on multiparametric MRI. *European Radiology*. Doi: 10.1007/s00330-020-07008-z.

Armato III, S. G., McLennan, G., Bidaut, L., McNitt-Gray, M. F., Meyer, C. R., Reeves, A. P., & Clarke, L. P. (n.d.). Data from LIDC-IDRI. The cancer imaging archive. 2015.

Azamjah, N., Soltan-Zadeh, Y., & Zayeri, F. (2019). Global trend of breast cancer mortality rate: A 25-year study. *Asian Pacific Journal of Cancer Prevention*, *20*(7), 2015–2020. Doi: 10.31557/APJCP.2019.20.7.2015.

Azer, S. A. (2019). Challenges facing the detection of colonic polyps: What can deep learning do? *Medicina (Lithuania)*, *55*(8). Doi: 10.3390/medicina55080473.

Azizi, S., Bayat, S., Yan, P., Tahmasebi, A., Kwak, J. T., Xu, S., Turkbey, B., Choyke, P., Pinto, P., Wood, B., Mousavi, P., & Abolmaesumi, P. (2018). Deep recurrent neural networks for prostate cancer detection: Analysis of temporal enhanced ultrasound. *IEEE Transactions on Medical Imaging*, 37(12), 2695–2703. Doi: 10.1109/TMI.2018.2849959.

Badrinarayanan, V., Kendall, A., & Cipolla, R. (2017). Segnet: A deep convolutional encoder-decoder architecture for image segmentation. *IEEE Transactions on Pattern Analysis and Machine Intelligence*, *39*(12), 2481–2495.

Caballo, M., Pangallo, D. R., Mann, R. M., & Sechopoulos, I. (2020). Deep learning-based segmentation of breast masses in dedicated breast CT imaging: Radiomic feature stability between radiologists and artificial intelligence. *Computers in Biology and Medicine*, *118*, 103629. Doi: 10.1016/j.compbiomed.2020.103629.

Chen, H., Dou, Q., Wang, X., Qin, J., & Heng, P. A. (2016). Mitosis detection in breast cancer histology images via deep cascaded networks. *Proceedings of the AAAI Conference on Artificial Intelligence (Vol. 30, No. 1)*, (pp. 1160–1166), Phoenix, AZ.

Chen, L.-C., Papandreou, G., Kokkinos, I., Murphy, K., & Yuille, A. L. (2017). Deeplab: Semantic image segmentation with deep convolutional nets, atrous convolution, and fully connected crfs. *IEEE Transactions on Pattern Analysis and Machine Intelligence*, *40*(4), 834–848.

Chollet, F. (2017). Xception: Deep learning with depthwise separable convolutions. *Proceedings of the IEEE Conference on Computer Vision and Pattern Recognition*, 1251–1258.

Chowdhury, A., Sevinsky, C. J., Santamaria-Pang, A., & Yener, B. (2017). A computational study on convolutional feature combination strategies for grade classification in colon cancer using fluorescence microscopy data. In M. N. Gurcan & J. E. Tomaszewski (Eds.), *Medical Imaging 2017: Digital Pathology* (Vol. 10140, pp. 183–187). SPIE. Doi: 10.1117/12.2255687.

Clark, K., Vendt, B., Smith, K., Freymann, J., Kirby, J., Koppel, P., Moore, S., Phillips, S., Maffitt, D., Pringle, M., & Tarbox L. (2013). The Cancer Imaging Archive (TCIA): maintaining and operating a public information repository. *Journal of Digital Imaging*, *26*(6), 1045–1057.

Tanwar, S., & Vijayalakshmi, S. (2020). Comparative analysis and proposal of deep learning based colorectal cancer polyps classification technique. *Journal of Computational and Theoretical Nanoscience*, *17*(5), 2354–2362.

Cruz-Roa, A. A., Ovalle, J. E. A., Madabhushi, A., & Osorio, F. A. G. (2013). A deep learning architecture for image representation, visual interpretability and automated basal-cell carcinoma cancer detection. *International Conference on Medical Image Computing and Computer-Assisted Intervention*, 403–410.

Dhungel, N, Carneiro, G., & Bradley, A. P. (2015a). Automated mass detection in mammograms using cascaded deep learning and random forests. *2015 International Conference on Digital Image Computing: Techniques and Applications (DICTA)*, 1–8.

Dhungel, N., Carneiro, G., & Bradley, A. P. (2015b). Deep structured learning for mass segmentation from mammograms. *2015 IEEE International Conference on Image Processing (ICIP)*, 2950–2954.

Dou, Q., Chen, H., Yu, L., Qin, J., & Heng, P. (2017). Multilevel contextual 3-D CNNs for false positive reduction in pulmonary nodule detection. *IEEE Transactions on Biomedical Engineering*, *64*(7), 1558–1567.

Feng, X., Tustison, N. J., Patel, S. H., & Meyer, C. H. (2020). Brain tumor segmentation using an ensemble of 3D U-nets and overall survival prediction using radiomic features. *Frontiers in Computational Neuroscience*, *14*. Doi: 10.3389/fncom.2020.00025.

Feng, Y., Yang, F., Zhou, X., Guo, Y., Tang, F., Ren, F., Guo, J., & Ji, S. (2019). A Deep Learning approach for targeted contrast-enhanced ultrasound based prostate cancer detection. *IEEE/ACM Transactions on Computational Biology and Bioinformatics*, *16*(6), 1794–1801. Doi: 10.1109/TCBB.2018.2835444.

Gao, X. W., Hui, R., & Tian, Z. (2017). Classification of CT brain images based on deep learning networks. *Computer Methods and Programs in Biomedicine*, *138*, 49–56.

Gessert, N., Sentker, T., Madesta, F., Schmitz, R., Kniep, H., Baltruschat, I., Werner, R., & Schlaefer, A. (2020). Skin lesion classification using CNNs with patch-based attention and diagnosis-guided loss weighting. *IEEE Transactions on Biomedical Engineering*, *67*(2), 495–503. Doi: 10.1109/TBME.2019.2915839.

Giotis, I., Molders, N., Land, S., Biehl, M., Jonkman, M. F., & Petkov, N. (2015). MED-NODE: a computer-assisted melanoma diagnosis system using non-dermoscopic images. *Expert Systems with Applications*, *42*(19), 6578–6585.

Girshick, R. (2015). Fast r-cnn. *Proceedings of the IEEE International Conference on Computer Vision*, 1440–1448.

Gour, M., Jain, S., & Sunil Kumar, T. (2020). Residual learning based CNN for breast cancer histopathological image classification. *International Journal of Imaging Systems and Technology*, *30*(3), 621–635. Doi: 10.1002/ima.22403.

Hasan, M. K., Dahal, L., Samarakoon, P. N., Tushar, F. I., & Martí, R. (2020). DSNet: Automatic dermoscopic skin lesion segmentation. *Computers in Biology and Medicine*, *120*. Doi: 10.1016/j.compbiomed.2020.103738.

He, K., Zhang, X., Ren, S., & Sun, J. (2016). Deep residual learning for image recognition. *Proceedings of the IEEE Conference on Computer Vision and Pattern Recognition*, 770–778.

Hirayama, K., Tan, J. K., & Kim, H. (2016). Extraction of GGO candidate regions from the LIDC database using deep learning. *2016 16th International Conference on Control, Automation and Systems (ICCAS)*, 724–727.

Howard, A. G., Zhu, M., Chen, B., Kalenichenko, D., Wang, W., Weyand, T., Andreetto, M., & Adam, H. (2017). Mobilenets: Efficient convolutional neural networks for mobile vision applications. *ArXiv Preprint ArXiv:1704.04861*.

Hu, W.-J., Fan, J., Du, Y.-X., Li, B.-S., Xiong, N., & Bekkering, E. (2020). MDFC--ResNet: An agricultural IoT system to accurately recognize crop diseases. *IEEE Access, 8,* 115287–115298.

Hua, K.-L., Hsu, C.-H., Hidayati, S. C., Cheng, W.-H., & Chen, Y.-J. (2015). Computer-aided classification of lung nodules on computed tomography images via deep learning technique. *OncoTargets and Therapy, 8,* 2015–2022. Doi: 10.2147/ott.s80733.

Huang, G., Liu, Z., Van Der Maaten, L., & Weinberger, K. Q. (2017). Densely connected convolutional networks. *Proceedings of the IEEE Conference on Computer Vision and Pattern Recognition,* 4700–4708, Honolulu, HI.

Hussein, S., Gillies, R., Cao, K., Song, Q., & Bagci, U. (2017). TumorNet: Lung nodule characterization using multi-view convolutional neural network with Gaussian process. *2017 IEEE 14th International Symposium on Biomedical Imaging (ISBI 2017),* 1007–1010, Melbourne.

Iandola, F. N., Han, S., Moskewicz, M. W., Ashraf, K., Dally, W. J., & Keutzer, K. (2016). SqueezeNet: AlexNet-level accuracy with 50x fewer parameters and< 0.5 MB model size. *ArXiv Preprint ArXiv:1602.07360.*

Iqbal, S., Ghani Khan, M. U., Saba, T., Mehmood, Z., Javaid, N., Rehman, A., & Abbasi, R. (2019). Deep learning model integrating features and novel classifiers fusion for brain tumor segmentation. *Microscopy Research and Technique, 82*(8), 1302–1315. Doi: 10.1002/jemt.23281

Islam, M. M., Rabby, A. K. M. S. A., Arfin, M. H. R., & Hossain, S. A. (2019). PataNET: A convolutional neural networks to identify plant from leaf images. *2019 10th International Conference on Computing, Communication and Networking Technologies (ICCCNT),* 1–6.

Jadhav, A. R., Ghontale, A. G., & Shrivastava, V. K. (2019). Segmentation and border detection of melanoma lesions using convolutional neural network and SVM. *Advances in Intelligent Systems and Computing, 798.* Doi: 10.1007/978-981-13-1132-1_8.

Kang, S., Li, Q., Chen, Q., Zhou, Y., Park, S., Lee, G., Grimes, B., Krysan, K., Yu, M., Wang, W., & others. (2017). CancerLocator: non-invasive cancer diagnosis and tissue-of-origin prediction using methylation profiles of cell-free DNA. *Genome Biology, 18*(1), 1–12.

Katiyar, P., & Singh, K. (2020). A comparative study of lung cancer detection and classification approaches in CT images. *2020 7th International Conference on Signal Processing and Integrated Networks (SPIN),* 135–142.

Krizhevsky, A. (2014). *One weird trick for parallelizing convolutional neural networks.* http://arxiv.org/abs/1404.5997.

Krizhevsky, A., Sutskever, I., & Hinton, G. E. (2012). Imagenet classification with deep convolutional neural networks. *Advances in Neural Information Processing Systems,* 1097–1105.

LeCun, Y., Bottou, L., Bengio, Y., & Haffner, P. (1998). Gradient-based learning applied to document recognition. *Proceedings of the IEEE, 86*(11), 2278–2324.

LeCun, Y., Haffner, P., Bottou, L., & Bengio, Y. (1999). Object recognition with gradient-based learning. In *Shape, Contour and Grouping in Computer Vision* (pp. 319–345). Springer.

Lee, J. Y., Jeong, J., Song, E. M., Ha, C., Lee, H. J., Koo, J. E., Yang, D.-H., Kim, N., & Byeon, J.-S. (2020). Real-time detection of colon polyps during colonoscopy using deep learning: systematic validation with four independent datasets. *Scientific Reports, 10*(1). Doi: 10.1038/s41598-020-65387-1.

Lee, R. S., Gimenez, F., Hoogi, A., Miyake, K. K., Gorovoy, M., & Rubin, D. L. (2017). A curated mammography data set for use in computer-aided detection and diagnosis research. *Scientific Data, 4,* 170177.

Lin, M., Chen, Q., & Yan, S. (2013). Network in network. *ArXiv Preprint ArXiv:1312.4400.*

Liu, S., Zheng, H., Feng, Y., & Li, W. (2017). Prostate cancer diagnosis using deep learning with 3D multiparametric MRI. *Medical Imaging 2017: Computer-Aided Diagnosis, 10134*, 1013428.

Long, J., Shelhamer, E., & Darrell, T. (2015). Fully convolutional networks for semantic segmentation. *Proceedings of the IEEE Conference on Computer Vision and Pattern Recognition*, 3431–3440, Boston, MA.

Mandloi, A., Daripa, U., Sharma, M., & Bhattacharya, M. (2019). An automatic cell nuclei segmentation based on deep learning strategies. *2019 IEEE Conference on Information and Communication Technology, CICT 2019*. Doi: 10.1109/CICT48419.2019.9066259.

Mohammadi, H. M. (2020). Polyp detection using CNNs in colonoscopy video. *IET Computer Vision*, *14*(5), 241–247(6). https://digital-library.theiet.org/content/journals/10.1049/iet-cvi.2019.0300

Muhammad, K., Khan, S., Ser, J. D., & de Albuquerque, V. H. C. (2020). Deep learning for multigrade brain tumor classification in smart healthcare systems: A prospective survey. *IEEE Transactions on Neural Networks and Learning Systems*, *32*(2), 1–16.

Murtaza, G., Shuib, L., Abdul Wahab, A. W., Mujtaba, G., Mujtaba, G., Nweke, H. F., Al-garadi, M. A., Zulfiqar, F., Raza, G., & Azmi, N. A. (2020). Deep learning-based breast cancer classification through medical imaging modalities: state of the art and research challenges. *Artificial Intelligence Review*, *53*(3), 1655–1720. Doi: 10.1007/s10462-019-09716-5.

Orlando, N., Gillies, D. J., Gyacskov, I., & Fenster, A. (2020). Deep learning-based automatic prostate segmentation in 3D transrectal ultrasound images from multiple acquisition geometries and systems. *Proceedings of SPIE - The International Society for Optical Engineering*, *11315*. Doi: 10.1117/12.2549804.

Pan, X., Zhang, S., Guo, W., Zhao, X., Chuang, Y., Chen, Y., & Zhang, H. (2019). Video-based facial expression recognition using deep temporal–spatial networks. *IETE Technical Review*, 1–8. Doi: 10.1080/02564602.2019.1645620.

Paul, R., Hawkins, S. H., Hall, L. O., Goldgof, D. B., & Gillies, R. J. (2016). Combining deep neural network and traditional image features to improve survival prediction accuracy for lung cancer patients from diagnostic CT. *2016 IEEE International Conference on Systems, Man, and Cybernetics (SMC)*, 2570–2575.

Poon, C. C. Y., Jiang, Y., Zhang, R., Lo, W. W. Y., Cheung, M. S. H., Yu, R., Zheng, Y., Wong, J. C. T., Liu, Q., Wong, S. H., Mak, T. W. C., & Lau, J. Y. W. (2020). AI-doscopist: a real-time deep-learning-based algorithm for localising polyps in colonoscopy videos with edge computing devices. *NPJ Digital Medicine*, *3*(1). Doi: 10.1038/s41746-020-0281-z.

Rahman, M. S., Shill, P. C., & Homayra, Z. (2019). A new method for lung nodule detection using deep neural networks for CT images. *2019 International Conference on Electrical, Computer and Communication Engineering (ECCE)*, 1–6.

Rawla, P. (2019). Epidemiology of prostate cancer. *World Journal of Oncology*, *10*(2), 63–89. Doi: 10.14740/wjon1191.

Redmon, J., Divvala, S., Girshick, R., & Farhadi, A. (2016). You only look once: Unified, real-time object detection. *Proceedings of the IEEE Conference on Computer Vision and Pattern Recognition*, 779–788, Las Vegas, NV.

Riquelme, D., & Akhloufi, M. A. (2020). Deep learning for lung cancer nodules detection and classification in CT scans. *AI*, *1*(1), 28–67. Doi: 10.3390/ai1010003.

Ronneberger, O., Fischer, P., & Brox, T. (2015). U-net: Convolutional networks for biomedical image segmentation. *International Conference on Medical Image Computing and Computer-Assisted Intervention*, 234–241.

Sabbaghi, S., Aldeen, M., & Garnavi, R. (2016). A deep bag-of-features model for the classification of melanomas in dermoscopy images. *2016 38th Annual International Conference of the IEEE Engineering in Medicine and Biology Society (EMBC)*, 1369–1372.

Sabour, S., Frosst, N., & Hinton, G. E. (2017). Dynamic routing between capsules. *Advances in Neural Information Processing Systems*, 3856–3866.

Sajid, S., Hussain, S., & Sarwar, A. (2019). Brain tumor detection and segmentation in MR images using deep learning. *Arabian Journal for Science and Engineering*, *44*(11), 9249–9261. Doi: 10.1007/s13369-019-03967-8.

Samria, R., Jain, R., Jha, A., Saini, S., & Chowdhury, S. R. (2014). Noninvasive cuff'less estimation of blood pressure using Photoplethysmography without electrocardiograph measurement. *2014 IEEE Region 10 Symposium*, 254–257.

Schelb, P., Kohl, S., Radtke, J. P., Wiesenfarth, M., Kickingereder, P., Bickelhaupt, S., Kuder, T. A., Stenzinger, A., Hohenfellner, M., Schlemmer, H.-P., Maier-Hein, K. H., & Bonekamp, D. (2019). Classification of cancer at prostate MRI: Deep learning versus clinical PI-RADS assessment. *Radiology*, *293*(3), 607–617. Doi: 10.1148/radiol.2019190938.

Sebai, M, Wang, T., & Al-Fadhli, S. A. (2020a). PartMitosis: A partially supervised deep learning framework for mitosis detection in breast cancer histopathology images. *IEEE Access*, *8*, 45133–45147.

Sebai, M., Wang, X., & Wang, T. (2020b). MaskMitosis: A deep learning framework for fully supervised, weakly supervised, and unsupervised mitosis detection in histopathology images. *Medical & Biological Engineering & Computing*, *58*(7), 1603–1623. Doi: 10.1007/s11517-020-02175-z.

Sermanet, P., Eigen, D., Zhang, X., Mathieu, M., Fergus, R., & LeCun, Y. (2013). Overfeat: Integrated recognition, localization and detection using convolutional networks. *ArXiv Preprint ArXiv:1312.6229*.

Setio, A. A. A., Ciompi, F., Litjens, G., Gerke, P., Jacobs, C., van Riel, S. J., Wille, M. M. W., Naqibullah, M., Sánchez, C. I., & van Ginneken, B. (2016). Pulmonary nodule detection in CT images: False positive reduction using multi-view convolutional networks. *IEEE Transactions on Medical Imaging*, *35*(5), 1160–1169.

Shakeel, P. M., Burhanuddin, M. A., & Desa, M. I. (2019). Lung cancer detection from CT image using improved profuse clustering and deep learning instantaneously trained neural networks. *Measurement*, *145*, 702–712.

Shakeel, P. M., Tobely, T. E. El, Al-Feel, H., Manogaran, G., & Baskar, S. (2019). Neural network based brain tumor detection using wireless infrared imaging sensor. *IEEE Access*, *7*, 5577–5588.

Simonyan, K., & Zisserman, A. (2014). Very deep convolutional networks for large-scale image recognition. *ArXiv Preprint ArXiv:1409.1556*.

Sirinukunwattana, K., Raza, S. E. A., Tsang, Y., Snead, D. R. J., Cree, I. A., & Rajpoot, N. M. (2016). Locality sensitive deep learning for detection and classification of nuclei in routine colon cancer histology images. *IEEE Transactions on Medical Imaging*, *35*(5), 1196–1206.

Spanhol, F. A., Oliveira, L. S., Petitjean, C., & Heutte, L. (2016). Breast cancer histopathological image classification using convolutional neural networks. *2016 International Joint Conference on Neural Networks (IJCNN)*, 2560–2567.

Sun, L., Zhang, S., Chen, H., & Luo, L. (2019). Brain tumor segmentation and survival prediction using multimodal MRI scans with deep learning. *Frontiers in Neuroscience*, *13*, 810. Doi: 10.3389/fnins.2019.00810.

Swiderski, B., Kurek, J., Osowski, S., Kruk, M., & Barhoumi, W. (2017). Deep learning and non-negative matrix factorization in recognition of mammograms. In Y. Wang, T. D. Pham, V. Vozenilek, D. Zhang, & Y. Xie (Eds.), *Eighth International Conference on Graphic and Image Processing (ICGIP 2016)* (Vol. 10225, pp. 53–59). SPIE. Doi: 10.1117/12.2266335.

Szegedy, C., Liu, W., Jia, Y., Sermanet, P., Reed, S., Anguelov, D., Erhan, D., Vanhoucke, V., & Rabinovich, A. (n.d.). Going deeper with convolutions.

Szegedy, C., Liu, W., Jia, Y., Sermanet, P., Reed, S., Anguelov, D., Erhan, D., Vanhoucke, V., & Rabinovich, A. (2015). Going deeper with convolutions. *Proceedings of the IEEE Conference on Computer Vision and Pattern Recognition*, 1–9.

Takeuchi, T., Hattori-Kato, M., Okuno, Y., Iwai, S., & Mikami, K. (2019). Prediction of prostate cancer by deep learning with multilayer artificial neural network. *Canadian Urological Association Journal*, *13*(5), E145–E150. Doi: 10.5489/cuaj.5526.

Tang, Z., Xu, Y., Jin, L., Aibaidula, A., Lu, J., Jiao, Z., Wu, J., Zhang, H., & Shen, D. (2020). Deep learning of imaging phenotype and genotype for predicting overall survival time of glioblastoma patients. *IEEE Transactions on Medical Imaging*, *39*(6), 2100–2109. Doi: 10.1109/TMI.2020.2964310.

Tschandl, P., Rosendahl, C., & Kittler, H. (2018). The HAM10000 dataset, a large collection of multi-source dermatoscopic images of common pigmented skin lesions. *Scientific Data*, *5*, 180161.

Van Zon, M., Stathonikos, N., Blokx, W. A. M., Komina, S., Maas, S. L. N., Pluim, J. P. W., Van Diest, P. J., & Veta, M. (2020). Segmentation and classification of melanoma and nevus in whole slide images. *Proceedings - International Symposium on Biomedical Imaging*, *2020-April*, 263–266. Doi: 10.1109/ISBI45749.2020.9098487, Iowa City, IA.

Vuong, T. L. T., Lee, D., Kwak, J. T., & Kim, K. (2020). Multi-task deep learning for colon cancer grading. *2020 International Conference on Electronics, Information, and Communication, ICEIC 2020*. Doi: 10.1109/ICEIC49074.2020.9051305, Barcelona.

Wang, C., Elazab, A., Wu, J., & Hu, Q. (2017). Lung nodule classification using deep feature fusion in chest radiography. *Computerized Medical Imaging and Graphics*, *57*, 10–18. Doi: 10.1016/j.compmedimag.2016.11.004.

Wang, W., Tian, J., Zhang, C., Luo, Y., Wang, X., & Li, J. (2020a). An improved deep learning approach and its applications on colonic polyp images detection. *BMC Medical Imaging*, *20*(1). Doi: 10.1186/s12880-020-00482-3.

Wang, X., Niu, S., & Wang, H. (2020b). Image inpainting detection based on multi-task deep learning network. *IETE Technical Review*, 1–9. Doi: 10.1080/02564602.2020.1782274.

Wei, L., Ding, K., & Hu, H. (2020a). Automatic skin cancer detection in dermoscopy images based on ensemble lightweight deep learning network. *IEEE Access*, *8*, 99633–99647. Doi: 10.1109/ACCESS.2020.2997710.

Wei, L., Ding, K., & Hu, H. (2020b). Automatic skin cancer detection in dermoscopy images based on ensemble lightweight deep learning network. *IEEE Access*, 8(2020), 99633–99647.

Wei, X., Ma, Y., & Wang, R. (2019). A new mammography lesion classification method based on convolutional neural network. *Proceedings of the 3rd International Conference on Machine Learning and Soft Computing*, 39–43. Doi: 10.1145/3310986.3311019, Da Lat.

Wong, K. K., Rostomily, R., & Wong, S. T. C. (2019). Prognostic gene discovery in glioblastoma patients using deep learning. *Cancers*, *11*(1), 53. Doi: 10.3390/cancers11010053.

Zavala-Romero, O., Breto, A. L., Xu, I. R., Chang, Y.-C. C., Gautney, N., Pra, A. D., Abramowitz, M. C., Pollack, A., & Stoyanova, R. (2020). Segmentation of prostate and prostate zones using deep learning: A multi-MRI vendor analysis. *Strahlentherapie Und Onkologie*. Doi: 10.1007/s00066-020-01607-x.

Zeiler, M. D., & Fergus, R. (2014). Visualizing and understanding convolutional networks. *European Conference on Computer Vision*, 818–833, Zurich.

Zhu, X., Yao, J., & Huang, J. (2016). Deep convolutional neural network for survival analysis with pathological images. *2016 IEEE International Conference on Bioinformatics and Biomedicine (BIBM)*, 544–547, Shenzhen.

Zunair, H., & Ben Hamza, A. (2020). Melanoma detection using adversarial training and deep transfer learning. *Physics in Medicine and Biology*, *65*(13). Doi: 10.1088/1361-6560/ab86d3.

11 Enhancing Deep Learning-Based Organ Segmentation for Diagnostic Support Systems on Chest X-rays

Gokhan Altan
Iskenderun Technical University

CONTENTS

11.1 INTRODUCTION

Medical images are diagnostic tools used primarily for the visualization and identification of pathological nodules and tissues from healthy tissue. Medical images have many types which visualize the density of organs depending on the posing of a specific dose of X-ray or photons. The X-ray is used for the elimination of the lung, and cardiac discomfort contains low-dose radiography and is often preferred since it contains low-dose radiography which is not harmful to human health and is cheaper than computed tomography. It is still used as a supportive diagnostic tool and as an indispensable tool for disorders for internal organs such as the lung, heart, bone, kidney and intestine (Litjens et al., 2017). The pathological cell in the tissue has a determining feature for advanced lung diseases due to its high density in X-ray images. Therefore, chest X-rays still stand out as the primary approach in imaging respiratory disease and early detection of a majority of pathologies. However, since chest X-ray is a noisy medical image, it incurs additional clinical tests, the workload for specialists and additional time-wasting for each case. These disadvantages can be overcome in a short time by using computer-aided diagnosis (CADx) systems to detect small pathologies that can be missed by even multiple radiologists and accelerate the patient-specific treatment process (Rajaraman et al., 2019). CADx systems come to the forefront as clinical decision support mechanisms by conducting guiding diagnosis by virtue of analysis capabilities. Correspondingly, CADx models are more prominent than traditional diagnostic and form the basis for the emergence of enhancing medical imaging technologies and diagnostic systems.

In the machine learning algorithms used to develop successful CADx models, data and feature extraction take an important place. The homogenization of the distribution in the data set, preventing over-fitting by increasing the amount of data and preparing the training and test sets independently based on the issue are among the parameters to be considered during modelling a CADx (Hooda et al., 2019). Conventional CADx systems on chest X-rays should be trained to include the features of their pathological regions. They should be included in responsible areas in learning progress to achieve high-discrimination performances. Significantly, airway situation, obstructions, damages and edema areas in lung diseases should be improved with sensitive image processing approaches for diagnosis and visualizations in the early stages (Litjens et al., 2017). In this case, instead of using whole chest X-rays, local descriptor features for enabling more successful threshold and histogram procedures can be determined by semantic segmentation of lungs.

Lung segmentation is utilized as the first stage of the above advancing techniques for image restoration. Standardized methods to be performed in the specific lung regions rather than the general features of the chest region provide advantages for CADx models on the common respiratory disease (Candemir et al., 2014). It allows CADx systems to be applied to devices that are more stable and robust with various types of specification and to identify significant pathologies with simple fine-tuning procedures. Significantly, increasing Deep Learning efficiency with transfer learning, generalization capability and extended image analysis algorithms bring forward image analysis in medical image analysis and CADx systems in recent years (Dai et al., 2018; Wang et al., 2019). For the last decades applying popular Deep Learning architectures into the medical analysis, models have contributed to advancing the prognosis and diagnosis techniques for specialized respiratory disorders. The conventional image processing approaches extracted hand-crafted landmarks on chest X-rays. Using the hand-crafted features provides advantages for recognizing different colour values of images, minimizing errors caused by different clothes, determining postures originating from different angular values, eliminating variations in illumination changes, contrast, and more (Wang et al., 2019). However, the hand-crafted analysis is insufficient due to it is quite a time consuming and the ample amount of data. Therefore, using Deep Learning models without pre-progress and feature extraction stages provides a standardized procedure for lung segmentation. Whereas semantic segmentation represents interactions between label assignments in conventional approaches, DL approaches aim to define a probabilistic framework that analyzes the relationship between pixels with conditional random field learning procedure (Chen et al., 2018).

The conventional approaches focused on hand-crafted features and analyzing them with multiple machine learning algorithms. Although extracting hand-crafted features is time-consuming and reveals limitations for CADx models, many well-accurate proposals are performing robust overlap detections. Brown et al. used the knowledge-based descriptors, including the relational vocabulary of lung anatomy, edge detection and blackboard algorithm. They defined fuzzy sets for detecting the borders of lung anatomy (Brown et al., 1998). Candemir et al. proposed a lung segmentation model using anatomical features of lung shape on non-rigid registration. They fused partial Radon transform, ranking atlas model with SIFT-flow registration and energy function of the image for a patient-based assessment using chest X-rays (Candemir et al., 2014). Chondro et al. proposed a CADx model for segmentation of lung from chest X-rays. Their proposal focused on advanced image processing techniques including ROI selection, contrast enhancement, spatial image analysis and statistical region masking, respectively. They reported the impact of the energy distribution of the medical images for the lung segmentation (Chondro et al., 2018). Hwang and Park established a network-wise training procedure on CNN for refinement of lung anatomy on chest X-rays. They applied atrous convolution using bilinear interpolation and fed the incorrect segmentation results by feeding outputs ground truth masks (Hwang & Park, 2017). Zotin et al. applied advanced image processing techniques to get hand-crafted features from chest X-rays to segment the lung regions. They applied contrast enhancement, Otsu thresholding and edge-detection algorithms to prepare the X-rays for analysis, respectively. They extracted texture features from grey-level co-occurrence matrix sets and fed them into the probabilistic neural network model (Zotin et al., 2019).

The capabilities of DL with advanced image processing and generating responsible presentations have increased the use of many DL algorithms including Generative Adversarial Networks (GAN), Convolutional Neural Networks (CNN), Deep Belief Networks (DBN), and more for semantic segmentation issues. Novel fusion models and deep generative representations provided high Intersection-over-Union rates for segmentation models with detailed analysis performances. Hooda et al. proposed a CNN architecture for semantic segmentation of lungs. They used a fusion method to precede the various representations of convolutional layers on augmented ROI features. They performed various factorization and regularization algorithms for training the fully connected layers. They reported one of the highest overlapping rates on lung regions (Hooda et al., 2019). Dai et al. used a multi-stage DL approach using CNN and GAN models, respectively. They performed a semantic segmentation on chest X-ray to identify lungs and heart regions at the first stage using convolutional layers and performed a structure correcting approach before fully connected layers. After generating fitted organ regions according to the trained Deep autoencoder representations, they achieved high-segmentation Intersection-over-Union rates on both heart and lungs (Dai et al., 2018). Zhang et al. performed a multi-organ segmentation using GAN on full-body X-rays. They analyzed chest X-ray images for the heart and lung segmentation, additionally. They extracted anatomy overlaps using flexible unsupervised learning procedure of DL algorithms to get semantic segmentation of organs (Zhang et al., 2020). Arbabshirani et al. directly focused on segmenting lungs from chest X-rays. They discussed the efficiency of extracting size, shape and texture features of the lungs from chest X-rays. They reported high enough intersection over union rates on a heterogeneous dataset using CNN architecture (Arbabshirani et al., 2017). Kalinovsky and Kovalev analyzed a limited number of chest X-rays for semantic segmentation of lungs. They adapted an encoding and decoding model for the reconstructing the segmented regions using spatial tolerance of autoencoder advances. They finalized the convolutional layers by deconvolution and up-sampling of the segmented regions on lungs (Kalinovsky & Kovalev, 2016). Ngo and Carneiro proposed a semantic segmentation model that is based on DBN using a small-scale chest X-ray dataset. Their proposal is an adaptive procedure consists of the analysis of distance regularized level set and deep structured inference (Ngo & Carneiro, 2015). Rashid et al. applied U-Net CNN architecture to the chest X-rays. The resultant segmentation on lungs was post-processed using the flood-fill algorithm and morphological opening, iteratively. By post-processing, unwanted small contours and device-based noise as probes were eliminated from the segmentation results (Rashid et al., 2018). Souza et al. performed a hybrid model using many DL algorithms step-by-step. Their proposal consists of an AlexNet based CNN for initial segmentation, ResNet-based CNN for the reconstruction of segmented lungs and a patch-based CNN with resblock architecture for an accurate semantic segmentation (Souza et al., 2019). The literature focused on small- and medium-scale chest X-ray databases for lung segmentation. Whereas high Intersection-over-Union rates were achieved using many practical DL algorithms, a majority of them comprise multi-stage DL algorithms. Considering comprehensive analysis for the training of DL algorithms, requiring high workload in training and predictions and requiring a large database to avoid overfitting, the literature has deficiency on identifying a robust and standardized lung segmentation model on chest X-rays with various specifications.

In this study, an optimized simplistic CNN-based semantic lung segmentation model was proposed. Hereby the experiments were performed using many CNN architectures with dropout and various learning procedures to determine the highest Intersection-over-Union rates for lungs. The main contribution of the work is that the proposed model is simplistic and needs a minimum workload in post-processing and segmentation with full adaptability of generative models. The paper presents analyzing the ability of the different representations, learning approaches and statistical coherence models on CNN-based models by extract low-, medium- and high-level features for semantic segmentation on a large-scale data set.

The remaining of the paper organized as an explanation of ChexNet database, CNN with learning procedures and impact of classification parameters for semantic lung segmentation in materials and methods; experimental setup and achievements depending on various CNN architectures in results; eventually the discussion and comments on the lung segmentation and enhancing the lung airway distribution on chest X-rays, main contributions and comparison of the achievements with state-of-art in the last section.

11.2 MATERIALS AND METHODS

11.2.1 CONVOLUTIONAL NEURAL NETWORKS

CNN is a popular DL algorithm with analyzing capabilities of different level features for computer vision issues. CNN generates convolution-based representations with a sequential order. The most significant advantage of CNN is that it transfers the dominant characteristic information of the relationship between pixels with advanced filters that applied consecutively in convolution layers. The depth of CNN enables extracting low-, middle- and high-level features from the input layer to the last layer (Cireşan et al., 2011). Whereas the first convolutional layers analyze low-level features, last layers can identify the relationship between low-level features and high-level features by feature learning in CNN depending on the filter specifications in convolution (Krizhevsky et al., 2017). Therefore, CNN has many classification parameters depending on the depth of the model, the number of hidden layers and a big number of neuron in supervised learning (Altan, 2019). The final form of the input after consecutive convolution processes is flattened to fed the dense layers. In short, the convolutional layers learn the low-level features and transfer the most dominant filtered values to the following layers.

The feature learning stage consists of non-ordered layers, including convolution (Conv), pooling and rectified linear unit (RELU). These layers can be established to the CNN architecture in different sequences and repetitions (Cireşan et al., 2011). After applying feature learning layers to the input image, the last representation is transferred to flattening layer for reshaping the last feature map into a vector. The flattened vector is fed into fully connected (dense) layers in supervised learning (Krizhevsky et al., 2017). In the supervised training of fully connected, various regularization, optimization and factorization techniques are utilized to minimize the loss function. In the dropout method, it excludes neurons depending on the probabilistic similarity between neurons. The softmax activation function is the most preferred output function (Altan, 2019; Krizhevsky et al., 2017).

Convolution layer comprises using various size and number of filters to represent different representations of inputs. The depth of the CNN is defined by the number of the filters in each Conv layer (Cireşan et al., 2011).

Max pooling layer is a down-sampling procedure that transfers maximum pixel value for a defined pooling size. The consecutive convolutions are applied to the down-sampled representation for transferring dominant pixels for small size images. RELU layer outputs non-negative values, zero for negative values and linear function for positive values (Cireşan et al., 2011).

U-Net and SegNet models are the most popular semantic segmentation CNN architectures excluding fully connected layers from DL approaches. These architectures consist of a stack of encoders and decoders. SegNet encodes the input image using convolutional layers and performs an enhancement in the resolution at the end of the decoding layer to make output with the same dimensions as the input image. U-Net is a more detailed model for biomedical images with contraction and expansion progresses using up-convolution.

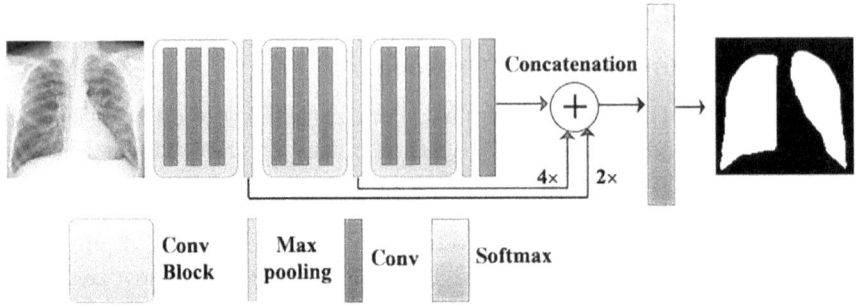

FIGURE 11.1   The proposed pruned CNN architecture for lung segmentation.

Unlike these methods, our proposal focused on pixel-wise semantic segmentation using a concatenation of feature maps after third pooling layer by up-sampling to the output dimensions. In this way, we could prevent losing significant pixel values by reserving them into the concatenation. At the last stage, we used the softmax activation function to get the probabilistic concern pf the pixels (lung, nonlung). The proposed architecture is depicted in Figure 11.1.

11.2.2   CHEST X-RAY DATABASE

Chest X-rays are the low-dose radiography images that are postured on the idea the tissues have different permeability, density and thickness specification demanding on their textures. A chestX-ray is one of the most crucial visualization tools that is used for respiratory and lung diseases, including pneumonia, COPD, asthma, infiltration, nodule, edema and more. Besides that, it is a noisy image including spatial, temporal, and contrast resolutions that make hard to diagnose the pathology at the early stages. Analyzing local discriminators for lung diseases has vital importance to assess airways, abnormal patterns, including edema, nodule and more. The aim of this study is localizing the lung regions and enabling application and analysis of local image pixels by excluding non-lung regions from the chest X-rays. Therefore, we used a large-scale chest X-ray database, chest X-ray, to segment the lungs (Rajpurkar et al., 2017).

Chest X-ray which is the largest publicly accessible database comprises 112,120 frontal-view chest X-ray images with 14 common lung diseases (Wang et al., 2019). Chest X-ray was shared by Stanford machine learning group with a pre-trained 121-layered CNN model for pneumonia detection (Rajpurkar et al., 2017). We randomly selected a total number of 1,500 images for training and a total number of 400 images for testing the proposed model. Training data set consisted of 500 chest X-rays without findings and 100 chest X-ray images for each pathology including atelectasis, cardiomegaly, effusion, infiltration, mass, nodule, pneumonia, pneumothorax, edema and fibrosis. The testing data set consisted of 200 chest X-rays without findings and 200 chest X-rays with pathology. Random chest X-rays with no finding, and thoracic pathology are depicted in Figure 11.2.

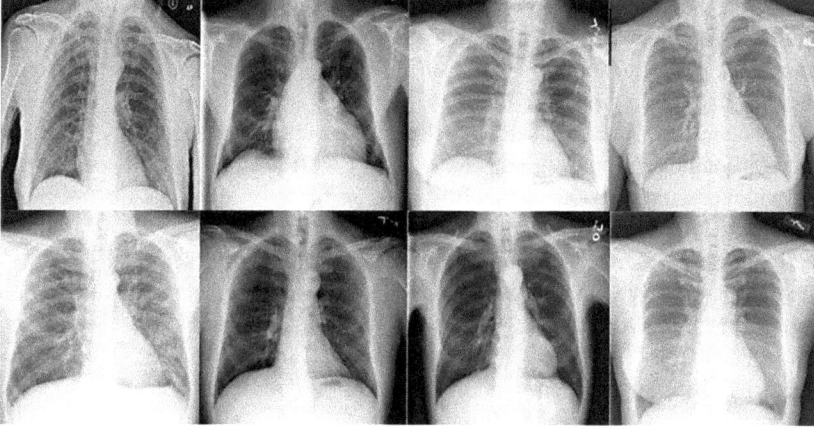

FIGURE 11.2   Randomly selected chest X-rays from Chest X-ray data set.

11.3   EXPERIMENTAL RESULTS

CADx models have increased its use demanding on self-adaptability to many medical systems, new functionality, transferring the methods to novel techniques and fusing the pre-diagnosis systems with conventional techniques. Although CT images have the ability to provide more clear visualization for lungs, chest X-rays are more harmless due to using only one scan at a specified radiology dose. Moreover, a chest X-ray is cheaper diagnostics that can be accessed for even low-budget small healthcare centres. Therefore, lung segmentation and advancing lung tissue on chest X-rays have great importance for medical image analysis researches.

The performance of the proposed models was evaluated using statistical metrics demanding on the output of the segmentation model. Using independent test characteristics is a priority to determine the reliability and validity of the models. In this study, we used sensitivity (SEN), specificity (SPE), accuracy (ACC), Dice similarity coefficient (DSC) and Intersection-over-Union rate (Jaccard similarity coefficient, Overlap, IoU) to assess the segmentation performance of proposals. The proposed models predict lung or non-lung pixels.

$$\mathrm{ACC} = (\mathrm{TP} + \mathrm{TN})/(\mathrm{TP+TN+FP+FN}) \qquad (11.1)$$

$$\mathrm{SEN} = \mathrm{TP}/(\mathrm{TP} + \mathrm{FN}) \qquad (11.2)$$

$$\mathrm{SPE} = \mathrm{TN}/(\mathrm{TN} + \mathrm{FP}) \qquad (11.3)$$

$$\mathrm{IoU} = |\ \mathrm{lung} \cap \mathrm{non-lung}\ |/|\mathrm{lung} \cup \mathrm{non-lung}| = \mathrm{TP}/(\mathrm{TP} + \mathrm{FP} + \mathrm{FN}) \qquad (11.4)$$

$$\mathrm{DSC} = 2|\mathrm{lung} \cap \mathrm{non-lung}|/|\mathrm{lung}| + |\mathrm{non-lung}| = 2\mathrm{TP}/(2\mathrm{TP} + \mathrm{FP} + \mathrm{FN}) \qquad (11.5)$$

where TP is the number of correctly identified pixels as lung; FP is the number of non-lung pixels incorrectly identified as lung; TN is the number of correctly identified non-lung pixels as non-lung pixels and FN is the number of incorrectly identified lung pixels as non-lung pixels.

A pre-check on randomly selected chest X-ray images that consists of ten types of thoracic pathology and regular chest X-rays with no findings was performed to check whether each chest X-ray has full chest vision. It is noted that the training and testing folds have none of the chest X-rays from the same patients. Classification performances for many CNN models were compared in Table 11.1.

The proposed CNN model has many segmentation parameters for feature learning stage, including the number of Conv layers, filter dimensions, number of the filters in each Conv layer, pooling size and more. Finding the highest independent characteristics for an optimum model is iteration progress. On the other hand, building deeper models extends the training time and time complexity of the applications. Therefore, in the proposed segmentation models, the CNN segmentation architectures are fixed at 3 of Conv blocks including at least one Conv and max 3 Conv blocks. The number of filters in each Conv layer was iterated as 32, 64, 96 and 128 filters, whereas the dimension of filters experimented between 2-by-2 and 10-by-10 with an increase of 1-by-1 in dimension. The Conv layer filter dimensions were iterated in brute force. Max pooling (2×2) was applied to down-sampling the representation after each Conv block in the proposed model. The achievements in Table 11.1

TABLE 11.1

The Best Segmentation Performances (%) for the Proposed CNN Models

Model Parameters	ACC	SEN	SPE	IoU	DSC
CB1(conv(3)@32, conv(5)@64)	91.70	91.05	92.35	84.58	0.9164
CB2(conv(10)@64, conv(4)@64)					
CB3(conv(4)@32, conv(5)@32, conv(7)@96)					
CB1(conv(7)@32, conv(5)@32)	93.22	92.66	93.77	87.23	0.9318
CB2(conv(4)@32, conv(4)@96)					
CB3(conv(4)@32, conv(6)@32)					
CB1(conv(3)@96)	95.67	96.78	94.57	91.79	0.9572
CB2(conv(8)@64, conv(7)@32)					
CB3(conv(3)@64, conv(7)@32, conv(7)@64)					
CB1(conv(7)@96)	95.75	96.80	94.69	91.92	0.9579
CB2(conv(9)@96, conv(4)@32)					
CB3(conv(10)@64, conv(4)@32, conv(3)@64)					
CB1(conv(5)@32, conv(6)@64, conv(2)@96)	98.23	96.74	99.71	96.47	0.9820
CB2(conv(8)@64, conv(7)@96)					
CB3(conv(3)@64, conv(4)@64, conv(7)@128)					

CB, Convolution block, conv(3)@64 represents for 3×3 filter dimension with 64 filters.

present the highest classification performances at iterated parameter ranges. We used the softmax output function:

$$\text{Softmax}(\Phi) = e^{\Phi} / \sum e^{\Phi} \qquad (11.6)$$

where $\Phi = W^T X \cdot W$ and X represent for weights and output of segmentation CNN model, respectively.

The highest segmentation accuracy rate for lungs on chest X-rays was achieved using a detailed model with filter sizes. The best CNN model comprises three Conv blocks for two Conv blocks. It is noted that using an increasing number of filters in each sequential Conv provides more sensitive results for segmentation. The highest achievements were obtained using 128 feature maps at the last Conv block. The proposed CNN-based segmentation model had low- and high-level features from the lungs by transferring Conv features between adjacent blocks. The number of classification parameters for the significant number of Conv filters is too high compared to the simplistic models with a lower number of Conv. The proposed segmentation model reached the performance rate of 98.23%, 96.74%, 99.71%, 96.47% and 0.982 for accuracy, sensitivity, specificity, IoU value and DSC value, respectively.

11.4 DISCUSSION

Semantic organ segmentation on chest X-rays has gained importance for enhancing medical image processing, CADx systems and robotic surgery in recent years. Lung segmentation is a common researching topic for developing novel visualization techniques on the lung diseases with increasing popularity. There are many studies focused on using hand-crafted features and advanced image processing techniques for lung segmentation. We assessed the efficacy of DL algorithms with many fusion techniques. Therefore, the proposed model is established using a pruned CNN architecture with our structure in segmentation of lungs. We compared the performances and methods of novel lung segmentation studies with various DL algorithms instead of obtaining hand-crafted analysis. The main idea is using the capability of Conv, feature learning and feature transferring between adjacent layers for chest X-rays with healthy and thoracic pathology.

Various popular DL algorithms were commonly used for semantic segmentation literature (see Table 11.2). Majority of the researches focused on deep generative models with significant analysis capabilities. Zhang et al. analyzed chest X-ray images for both the heart and lung segmentation using dense blocks on GAN. Their proposal established concatenation of each dense layer with a fusion approach with U-Net and DenseNet. They reached a Dice coefficient rate of 89.7% for the lung segmentation using GAN architecture (Zhang et al., 2020). Arbabshirani et al. utilized multi-scale ROIs for training the CNN-based segmentation model. They reached the rates of 98%, 99%, 99%, 91% and 0.96 for accuracy, sensitivity, specificity, IoU and Dice similarity coefficient, respectively (Arbabshirani et al., 2017). Dai et al. fused GAN and CNN models for correcting the segmentation intersections. They

TABLE 11.2

Comparison of the Related DL-Based Lung Segmentation Studies Regarding to Algorithms and Performances

Related Works	Methods	Classifier	Data	ACC	SEN	SPE	IuO	DSC
Zhang et al.	GAN	U-Net + DenseNet	400/100	-	-	-	-	0.897
Arbabshirani et al.	MSA	CNN	311/103	98.00	99.00	99.00	91.00	0.960
Dai et al.	GAN	CNN	209/38	-	-	-	94.70	0.973
Hooda et al.	ROI	CNN	186/61	98.51	-	-	94.76	-
Kalinovsky and Kovalev	SegNet	CNN	354/16-fold CV	96.20	-	-	-	0.974
Ngo and Carneiro	DRLS	DBN	84/123	-	-	-	98.50	0.992
Rashid et al.	U-Net	CNN	147/100	97.10	95.10	98.00	-	0.951
Souza et al.	AlexNet, ResNet	CNN	80/38	96.97	97.54	-	88.07	0.935
This study	Own architecture	CNN	1500/500	98.23	96.74	99.71	96.47	0.982

MSA, Multi-scale Architecture; Data (Train/Test); CV, Cross-validation; DRLS, Distance regularized level set.

improved the performance of the CNN model using a detailed autoencoder kernel on the ground-truth section of the segmentation. They reached IoU rates of 94.70% and dice similarity coefficient of 0.973 for both segmentation of left and right lungs (Dai et al., 2018). Hooda et al. experimented on various up-sampling approaches on CNN-based segmentation. They reported the impact of using low-dimensional up-sampling and achieved the segmentation performance rates of 98.51% and 94.76% for accuracy and IoU, respectively (Hooda et al., 2019). Kalinovsky and Kovalev proposed a CNN-based SegNet model with a detailed encoder and decoder structure. They finalized the convolutional layers by deconvolution-based up-sampling on the encoded segments of the lungs and reported lung segmentation accuracy rate of 96.20% and dice similarity coefficient of 0.974 (Kalinovsky & Kovalev, 2016). Ngo and Carneiro used distance regularized level set as an adaptive procedure for DBN model. They achieved an IoU rate of 98.50% and dice similarity coefficient of 0.992 for lung segmentation (Ngo & Carneiro, 2015). Rashid et al. applied U-Net CNN architecture and adapted post-processing of the segmentation results using the flood-fill algorithm and morphological opening. They reported performance rates of 97.1%, 95.1%, 98% and 0.951 for accuracy, sensitivity, specificity and dice similarity coefficient value, respectively (Rashid et al., 2018). Souza et al. performed a hybrid model using sequential AlexNet-based CNN for initial segmentation, ResNet-based CNN for reconstruction of segmented lungs and a patch-based CNN with resblock architecture. Their proposal has a high time complexity considering the complicated CNN architectures. They reached the accuracy rate of 96.97%, sensitivity rate of 97.54%, IoU rate of 88.07% and Dice similarity coefficient of 0.935 (Souza et al., 2019). The literature focused on small-scale chest X-ray databases for the lung segmentation. Whereas high IoU rates were achieved using many effective DL algorithms, a majority of them comprise multi-stage DL algorithms. The number of the testing chest images is not enough to bear the proposals as a robust model. Comprehensive analysis for the training of DL algorithms requires high workload in training and predictions, and a large database to avoid overfitting. Therefore, we utilized a large-scale database from the state-of-the-art.

The literature shows that the conventional DL algorithms can achieve successful lung segmentation performances using fusion methods and sequential use of popular architecture for correcting the organ regions. The proposed CNN-based model is an effective way to get better results in state-of-art. Significantly, training the DL model using a large-scale of chest X-ray database provides a change-resistant, robust and more general segmentation issues. The proposed model uses the capabilities of advanced deeper models and feature learning by transferring the layer-wise concatenation of each Conv block.

11.5 CONCLUSION

The study contains the novelty of using a large-scale database with routine and thoracic pathology from common ten lung diseases for the training of the segmentation model. The necessity of big data for DL algorithms was exceeded by using a big number of chest X-ray against the state-of-the-art. The proposed model is a basic, pruned and easy-to-integrate architecture for various types of lung diseases to enhance the diagnostic mechanism for clinicians. The achievements indicate that the proposed CNN-based lung segmentation architecture yields significantly higher evaluating metrics than the competing methods. In further analysis, scaling up the number of segmented organs in the chest X-ray will support performing more detailed organ-specific assessments.

REFERENCES

Altan, G. (2019). DeepGraphNet: Grafiklerin Sınıflandırılmasında Derin Öğrenme Modelleri. *European Journal of Science and Technology*, 319–327. Doi: 10.31590/ejosat.638256.

Arbabshirani, M. R., Dallal, A. H., Agarwal, C., Patel, A., & Moore, G. (2017). Accurate segmentation of lung fields on chest radiographs using deep convolutional networks. *Medical Imaging 2017: Image Processing*. Doi: 10.1117/12.2254526.

Brown, M. S., Wilson, L. S., Doust, B. D., Gill, R. W., & Sun, C. (1998). Knowledge-based method for segmentation and analysis of lung boundaries in chest X-ray images. *Computerized Medical Imaging and Graphics*. Doi: 10.1016/S0895-6111(98)00051-2.

Candemir, S., Jaeger, S., Palaniappan, K., Musco, J. P., Singh, R. K., Xue, Z., Karargyris, A., Antani, S., Thoma, G., & McDonald, C. J. (2014). Lung segmentation in chest radiographs using anatomical atlases with nonrigid registration. *IEEE Transactions on Medical Imaging*. Doi: 10.1109/TMI.2013.2290491.

Chen, L. C., Papandreou, G., Kokkinos, I., Murphy, K., & Yuille, A. L. (2018). DeepLab: semantic image segmentation with deep convolutional nets, atrous convolution, and fully connected CRFs. *IEEE Transactions on Pattern Analysis and Machine Intelligence*. Doi: 10.1109/TPAMI.2017.2699184.

Chondro, P., Yao, C. Y., Ruan, S. J., & Chien, L. C. (2018). Low order adaptive region growing for lung segmentation on plain chest radiographs. *Neurocomputing*. Doi: 10.1016/j.neucom.2017.09.053.

Cireşan, D. C., Meier, U., Gambardella, L. M., & Schmidhuber, J. (2011). Convolutional neural network committees for handwritten character classification. *Proceedings of the International Conference on Document Analysis and Recognition, ICDAR*. Doi: 10.1109/ICDAR.2011.229.

Dai, W., Dong, N., Wang, Z., Liang, X., Zhang, H., & Xing, E. P. (2018). Scan: Structure correcting adversarial network for organ segmentation in chest X-rays. *Lecture Notes in Computer Science (Including Subseries Lecture Notes in Artificial Intelligence and Lecture Notes in Bioinformatics)*. Doi: 10.1007/978-3-030-00889-5_30.

Hooda, R., Mittal, A., & Sofat, S. (2019). Lung segmentation in chest radiographs using fully convolutional networks. *Turkish Journal Of Electrical Engineering & Computer Sciences*, 710–722. Doi: 10.3906/elk-1710-157.

Hwang, S., & Park, S. (2017). Accurate lung segmentation via network-wise training of convolutional networks. *Lecture Notes in Computer Science (Including Subseries Lecture Notes in Artificial Intelligence and Lecture Notes in Bioinformatics)*. Doi: 10.1007/978-3-319-67558-9_11.

Kalinovsky, A., & Kovalev, V. (2016). Lung image segmentation using deep learning methods and convolutional neural networks. *International Conference on Pattern Recognition and Information Processing*.

Krizhevsky, A., Sutskever, I., & Hinton, G. E. (2017). ImageNet classification with deep convolutional neural networks. *Communications of the ACM*. Doi: 10.1145/3065386.

Litjens, G., Kooi, T., Bejnordi, B. E., Setio, A. A. A., Ciompi, F., Ghafoorian, M., van der Laak, J. A. W. M., van Ginneken, B., & Sánchez, C. I. (2017). A survey on deep learning in medical image analysis. *Medical Image Analysis*. Doi: 10.1016/j.media.2017.07.005.

Ngo, T. A., & Carneiro, G. (2015). Lung segmentation in chest radiographs using distance regularized level set and deep-structured learning and inference. *Proceedings - International Conference on Image Processing, ICIP*. Doi: 10.1109/ICIP.2015.7351179.

Rajaraman, S., Sornapudi, S., Kohli, M., & Antani, S. (2019). Assessment of an ensemble of machine learning models toward abnormality detection in chest radiographs. *Proceedings of the Annual International Conference of the IEEE Engineering in Medicine and Biology Society, EMBS*. Doi: 10.1109/EMBC.2019.8856715.

Rajpurkar, P., Irvin, J., Zhu, K., Yang, B., Mehta, H., Duan, T., Ding, D., Bagul, A., Langlotz, C., Shpanskaya, K., Lungren, M. P., & Ng, A. Y. (2017). *CheXNet: Radiologist-Level Pneumonia Detection on Chest X-Rays with Deep Learning*. http://arxiv.org/abs/1711.05225.

Rashid, R., Akram, M. U., & Hassan, T. (2018). Fully convolutional neural network for lungs segmentation from chest X-rays. *Lecture Notes in Computer Science (Including Subseries Lecture Notes in Artificial Intelligence and Lecture Notes in Bioinformatics)*. Doi: 10.1007/978-3-319-93000-8_9.

Souza, J. C., Bandeira Diniz, J. O., Ferreira, J. L., França da Silva, G. L., Corrêa Silva, A., & de Paiva, A. C. (2019). An automatic method for lung segmentation and reconstruction in chest X-ray using deep neural networks. *Computer Methods and Programs in Biomedicine*. Doi: 10.1016/j.cmpb.2019.06.005.

Wang, R., Ma, Y., Sun, W., Guo, Y., Wang, W., Qi, Y., & Gong, X. (2019). Multi-level nested pyramid network for mass segmentation in mammograms. *Neurocomputing*, 363, 313–320. Doi: 10.1016/j.neucom.2019.06.045.

Zhang, Y., Miao, S., Mansi, T., & Liao, R. (2020). Unsupervised X-ray image segmentation with task driven generative adversarial networks. *Medical Image Analysis*. Doi: 10.1016/j.media.2020.101664.

Zotin, A., Hamad, Y., Simonov, K., & Kurako, M. (2019). Lung boundary detection for chest X-ray images classification based on GLCM and probabilistic neural networks. *Procedia Computer Science*. Doi: 10.1016/j.procs.2019.09.314.

12 Deep Learning in Healthcare: A Bibliometric Analysis

Said Khalfa Mokhtar Brika,
Abdelmageed Algamdi, and Adam Musa
University of Bisha and University of Oum El Bouaghi

Khalil Chergui and Fethia Yahiaoui
University of Oum El Bouaghi

CONTENTS

12.1 INTRODUCTION

In this chapter, we aim to analyse Deep Learning (DL) in healthcare and present the main challenges and trends related to artificial intelligence (AI) in healthcare; it has been one of the research fields emerging in healthcare. Then, many researchers have started engaging in the domain of developing algorithms (Lancet, 2017, Mahajan, 2018, Lawry, 2020, Bohr & Memarzadeh, 2020, Sisodia, Pachori & Garg, 2020, Catania, 2020, Nordlinger, Villani & Rus, 2020) and others. These in-depth study intelligent agents develop the ability to learn, reason, and react to situations not programmed into the medical machines. This field is another subfield of machine learning. Several authors have attempted to attract inclusion as a branch of AI concerned with designing and developing algorithms and techniques. That allows computers to learn medical issues (Nielsen, 2017, Campion, Carlsson, & Francis, 2017, Solutions, 2018, Hassanien et al., 2019, Medicine, 2019, Panesar, 2019, Jain & Chatterjee, 2020, Agrawal et al., 2020; Mohanty, Nalinipriya, Jena, & Sarkar, 2021) and others.

As a result, a new sub-field of research appeared to find algorithms that allow the machine to learn by simulating the human nervous system, DL. Baldi (2018) notes that DL is a rebranding of neural networks developed and used in the 1980s. Other DL originated with the Neocognitron introduced by Kunihiko Fukushima in 1980. Rina Dechter was familiarizing DL to the machine learning community in 1986; Igor Aizenberg and colleagues adapted DL to artificial neural networks in 2000 (Dechter, 1986, Aizenberg, Aizenberg, & Vandewalle, 2013).

After that, this movement formed a fertile field for research. A large number of literature and research works have been written on DL in healthcare with its various aspects, especially in recent times. Chen & Jain (2019) wrote on medical image detection, segmentation, classification, and enhancement using DL (Dash, Acharya, Mittal, Abraham, & Kelemen, 2019). It has transcribed a book about the advances and techniques for biomedical and health informatics, with three parts: DL for biomedical engineering and health informatics, DL and electronics health records, DL for medical image processing.

Research articles in large numbers (Saba et al., 2019) focus on DL in radiology and their models: supervised (convolution neural network (NN), residual NN) and unsupervised (deep belief NN, autoencoder) (Faes et al., 2019). The DL models and their discriminative performances with statistics expose the arenas using DL (Baldi, 2018): for example, DL in chemoinformatics, proteomics, genomics and transcriptomics, biomedical imaging, and healthcare (Bote-Curiel, Munoz-Romero, Gerrero-Curieses, & Rojo-Álvarez, 2019) tackled DL and big data in healthcare. The DL is playing a vital role in many healthcare areas, improving the quality of diagnoses: electromyogram (EMG), electroencephalogram (EEG), electrocardiogram (ECG), and electro-oculogram (EOG) (Yang, Islam, & Li, 2018).

Many of these research works in DL in healthcare prompted other researchers to look at these studies. Their results, including mainly Liu et al. (2019), prepared a systematic review and meta-analysis of 69 studies among 31,587 studies to compare DL in healthcare professionals in detecting diseases from medical imaging. Ravì et al. (2016) analysed the number of studies that addressed the topic of DL in healthcare from Google Scholar between 2010 and 2015, and indicated the most used DL methods in health informatics: recurrent neural networks (RNNs), deep Boltzmann machines (DBMs), deep belief networks (DBNs), convolutional neural networks (CNNs), deep autoencoder (DAs), and deep neural networks (DNNs).

Also, in this context, there is a bibliometric study of DL for healthcare applications. Faust, Hagiwara, Hong, Lih, & Acharya (2018) prepared a bibliometric analysis of 53 articles published in the period from 01.01.2008 to 31.12.2017, distributed on four clusters: EMG, EEG, ECG, and EOG. They concluded that DL performs better for big and varied data sets than classic analysis and machine classification methods.

The problem of the study appears in this path. Through bibliometric analysis, we are looking for research areas that are most interested in studies and researchers in the field of DL in healthcare.

12.2 METHODS

Bibliometric analysis is one of the theoretical literature review methods (Meta-analysis and Systematic literature review). Science mapping practices bibliometric methods for studying how articles, authors, fields, and resources are related to one another (five methods are using Citation, Co-citation, Bib. coupling, Co-author, and Co-word) and to identify areas of research focus on a specific field of knowledge (Zupic & Čater, 2015).

Depending on the Web of Science (WOS) databases, the research works were filtered between 01.01.2018 and 30.09.2020, 520 studies, including the bibliometric analyses, distributed over 3 years, as shown in Figure 12.1.

Figure 12.1 shows that the number of studies used in the bibliometric analysis distributing as follows: 136 in 2018 (26%), 212 in 2019 (41%), and 172 in 2020 (33%). With a total estimated at 520 studies, these research works are more extensive in number and more comprehensive than the following studies: Faust et al. (2018), Liu et al. (2019), and Ravì et al. (2016). Table 12.1 explains statistical characteristics of these studies.

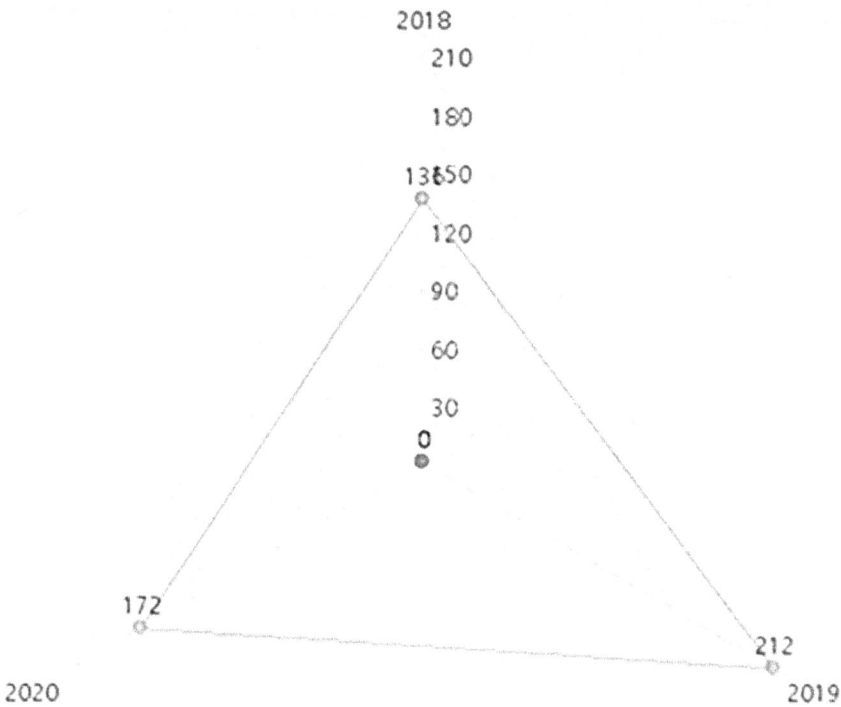

FIGURE 12.1   The number of research works on DL in healthcare published in ISI from 01.01.2018 to 30.09.2020 (KnowledgeMatrix Plus outputs).

TABLE 12.1
**Statistical Characteristics of Study Data (KnowledgeMatrix Plus
Outputs)**

Indicators	Number	Percentage (%)
Abstract	544	98
Article number	169	31
Authors	2,673	100
Authors' full name	2,745	100
Beginning page	298	61
Book digital object identifier (DOI)	1	0
Book group authors	6	9
Book series title	43	12
Conference date	82	19
Conference host	19	3
Conference location	75	19
Conference sponsors	56	14%
Conference title	90	19
Digital object identifier (DOI)	492	89
Document title	550	100
Editors	33	8
Ending page	301	61
Full source title	372	100
Group authors	4	0
ISI unique article identifier	552	100
ISSN	303	83
International Standard Book Number (ISBN)	81	17
Issue	23	51
Part number	2	0
Publication date	106	68
Publication type	3	100
Publication year	3	94
Researcher ID numbers	176	33
Special issue	1	3
Supplement	5	1
Volume	145	79

In all statistics presented in Table 12.1, the reliance is mainly due to the years, titles, abstracts, and keywords for conducting the bibliometric study.

For preparing the bibliometric analysis of studies, two methods have been adopted. First, co-author (connects authors when they co-author the publication to identify key researchers in the field of DL in healthcare). Second, co-word; connects keywords when they seem in a similar title, abstract, or keyword list to identify the main areas of DL in healthcare (Zupic & Čater, 2015).

To extract the statistical analyses of these studies' data, we relied on KnowledgeMatrix Plus (KISTI, 2016); also, to extract the networks and densities of keywords and authors, using the VOSviewer software (Van Eck & Waltman, 2013).

12.3 RESULTS

To carry out the bibliometric analysis, we rely on the outputs of KnowledgeMatrix Plus and VOSviewer software to determine the researchers' clusters and the keyword clusters that define the sub-fields of DL's research topic in healthcare, as specified by Faust et al. (2018).

12.3.1 RESULTS OF THE BIBLIOMETRIC ANALYSIS OF AUTHORS

Figure 12.2 shows researchers who combined the network and density of bibliometric analysis, with their number of publications in the WOS database, during the last 3 years (2018–2020). Many authors have been interested in research in the field of DL in healthcare. The first is Lee, Y., which includes the group of researchers with the same surname (Lee Yeha, Lee Yongbum, Lee Yugyung, and Lee Youngnam) with eight publications. The second is Zhang, L., which contains the following research group (Zhang Le, Zhang Lin, Zhang Lei, and Zhang Ling) with six publications. After that, other authors develop research works that are no less important in

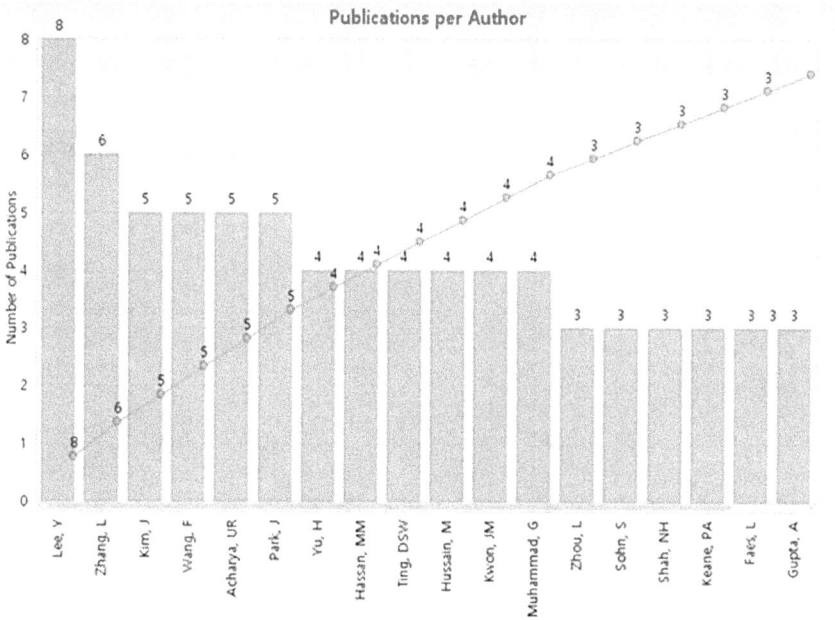

FIGURE 12.2 Publications per authors (KnowledgeMatrix Plus outputs).

numbers than the authors mentioned, which indicates the increased interest in the subject of DL in healthcare by researchers, especially with the emergence of AI and machine learning, as marked (Ravì et al., 2016).

According to their research relevance (co-author), researchers' division into clusters is more critical than dividing them into groups by surnames shown in Figure 12.3., which shows the network and density of the most influential authors in the field of DL in higher education in the WOS database.

Figure 12.3 shows that there are seven researcher clusters well-defined in Table 12.2., which form subgroups in which authors linked to preparing research work in the field of DL in healthcare. Among the works of these authors, we find the studies shown in Table 12.3.

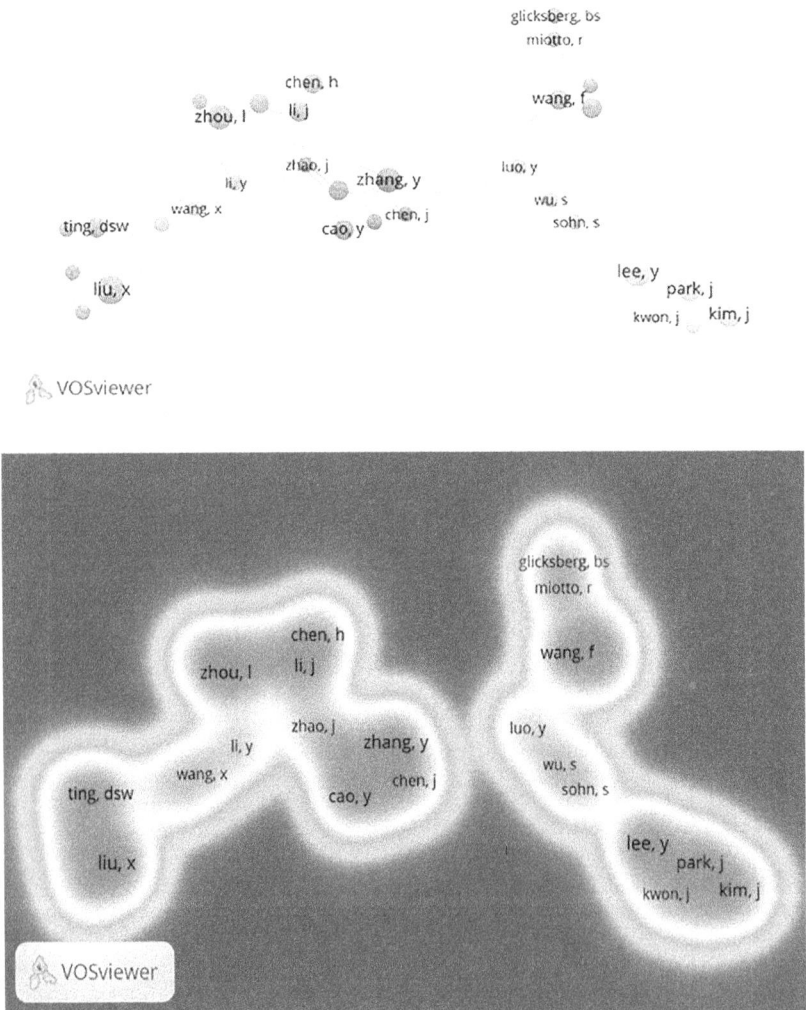

FIGURE 12.3 The network and density of authors (VOSviewer outputs).

TABLE 12.2
Topic Cluster Summary of Authors (VOSviewer Outputs)

Clusters	Authors	Colours
Cluster 1 (6 items)	Cao, Y., Chen, J., Wang, H., Zhang, H., Zhang, Y., Zhao, J.	Red
Cluster 2 (5 items)	Glicksberg, BS., Li, X., Miotto, R., Wang, F., Zhang, X.	Green
Cluster 3 (5 items)	Chen, H., Chen, W., Li, J., Wang, L., Zhou, L.	Blue
Cluster 4 (5 items)	Faes, L., Keane, P., Liu, X., Ting, DSW. Wong, TW.	Dark green
Cluster 5 (4 items)	Kim, J., Kwan, J., Lee, Y., Park, J.	Purple
Cluster 6 (3 items)	Li, Y., Wang, X., Zhang, X.	Light blue
Cluster 7 (3 items)	Luo, Y., Sohn, S., Wu, S.	Orange

TABLE 12.3
Publications of the Most Selected Authors (Researchers' Achievement Depending on VOSviewer Outputs)

Authors	References	Titles	Sub-fields
Lee, Y	Lee et al. (2018)	DL in the medical domain: predicting cardiac arrest using DL	Cardiac arrest and DL
Zhang, L	Zhang et al. (2019)	Improved DL network based in combination with cost-sensitive learning for early detection of ovarian cancer in colour ultrasound detecting system	Cancer and DL
Acharya, UR	Basiri et al. (2020)	A novel method for sentiment classification of drug reviews using a fusion of deep and machine learning techniques	Sentiment classification and DL
Kim, J	Cheon et al. (2019)	The use of DL to predict stroke patient mortality	Mortality and DL
Park, J	Kwon et al. (2020)	A DL algorithm to detect anaemia with ECGs: a retrospective, multicenter study	Anaemia and DL
Wang, F	Miotto et al. (2018)	DL for healthcare: review, opportunities and challenges	DL for healthcare

First, Lee et al. (2018) introduced the DeepEWS (DL-based Early Warning Score), based on a novel DL algorithm, to predict cardiac arrest and decrease mortality. Second, Zhang, Huang, & Liu (2019) offered an image diagnosis system for classifying the ovarian cysts in colour ultrasound images for detecting tumours in the early stage using DL. Third, Basiri, Abdar, Cifci, Nemati, and Acharya (2020) proposed two deep fusion models based on three-way fusion of one DL (3W1DT) and three-way fusion of three deep models (3W3DT) to understand the sentiments of patients. Fourth, Cheon, Kim, and Lim (2019) studied DL in the same direction (Lee et al., 2018). They learned the prediction of mortality using PCA/deep neural network and DNN approach of DL. Fifth, Kwon et al. (2020) found the DL algorithm to predict anaemia screening (ECGs). Finally, Miotto, Wang, Wang, Jiang, and Dudley (2018) talked about DL in healthcare in general and explained its importance in data preferences (electronic health records, imaging, comics, sensor data, and text). Thus, DL's use in predicting mortality, cardiac arrest, cancer, anaemia, and sentiment has recently formed the important sub-fields of research in DL in healthcare.

12.3.2 RESULTS OF THE BIBLIOMETRIC ANALYSIS OF KEYWORDS

Figure 12.4 shows the network and density of keywords and appears that there are many fertile sub-fields of research in DL in healthcare; models, data, electronic health record, neural networks, machine learning, recognition and intervention. Those that appear within three clusters are shown in Table 12.4.

Table 12.4 identifies three significant sub-fields of research in DL in healthcare: the first red cluster or the sub-field of DL and social relationships, recall of the critical studies that have been complete on this aspect (Rafailidis & Crestani, 2017, Guo, Polanía, Garcia-Frias, & Barner, 2019, Eastman, 2019, Georgescu et al., 2020). Collectively, these researchers studied the perception and recognition of social communication and social interaction. The second green cluster reflecting the field of models and domains of DL, among the studies on this site are Purushotham, Meng, Che, & Liu (2018), Yoon (2018), Yazhini and Loganathan (2019), Dash et al. (2019), and Santosh, Das, and Ghosh (2021). These studies deal on the one hand with DL models (supervised (CNN, RNN) and unsupervised (DBNN, autoencoder)), and on the other hand, on the areas of DL use (EMG, EEG, ECG, EOG, medical imaging, mortality, cardiac arrest, cancer, anemia). The third blue cluster was reproducing a new field of big data/virtual data and DL. Among the studies in this field, we find Beam and Kohane (2018), Bote-Curiel et al. (2019), Yu, Li, Liu, Li, and Wang (2019), Ngiam and Khor (2019). This field investigates DL models for using big data to treat patients.

12.4 DISCUSSION

Bibliometric analysis can use to discover research areas in which a researcher must delve into healthcare and DL. This topic has been of great interest to researchers in the recent 3 years (2018–2020). The number of studies selected for analysis reached 520 in the WOS databases (Faust et al., 2018). We used VOSviewer software and, in our research, KnowledgeMatrix Plus software. Two methods have been adopted: co-author and co-word (Keywords). These two methods have resulted in several results, the most important of which has been mentioned below.

The authors were divided into seven research clusters or groups, each group constituting a research sub-field in DL in healthcare, namely, cardiac arrest and DL, cancer and DL, sentiment classification and DL, mortality, and DL, anemia and DL, DL and medical imaging, and DL for healthcare. They appear in Tables 12.2 and 12.3 as

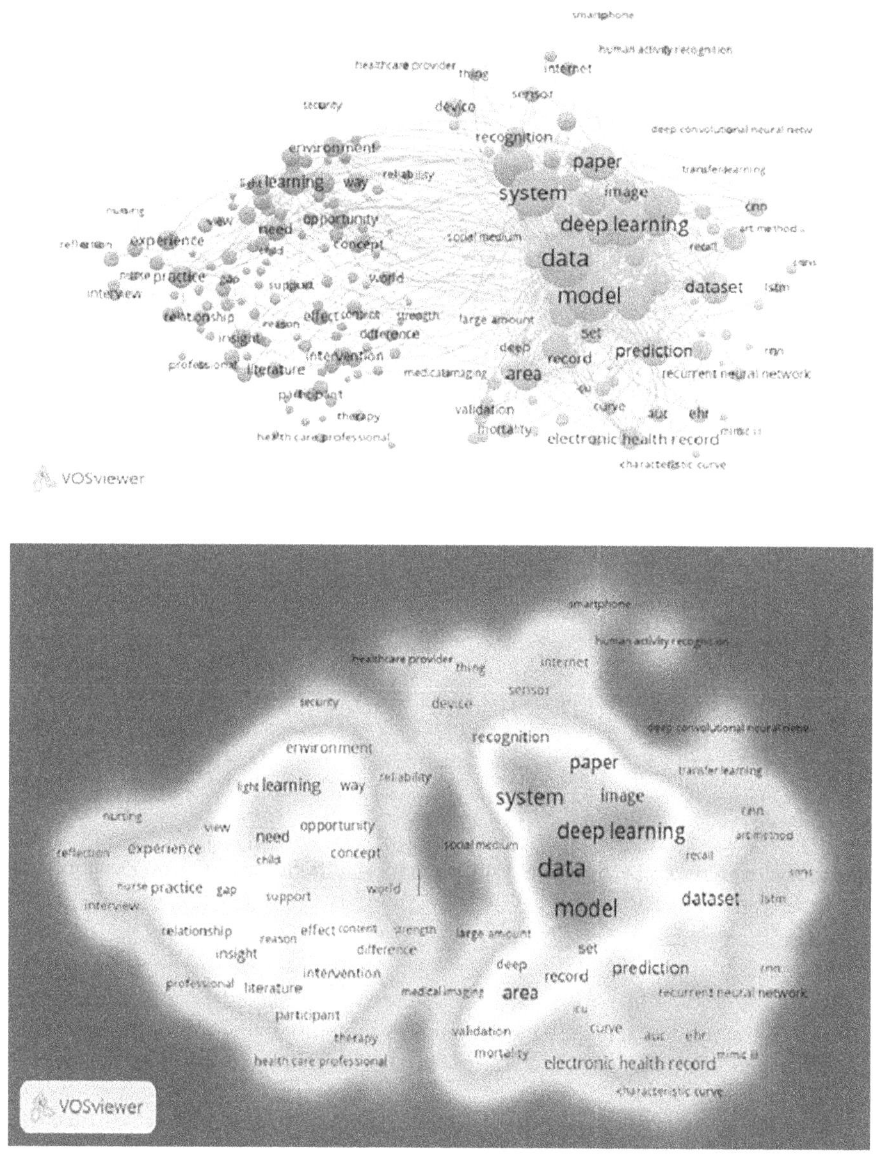

FIGURE 12.4 The network and density of keywords (VOSviewer outputs).

illustrated in the following studies (Lee et al., 2018, Miotto et al., 2018, Zhang et al., 2019, Cheon et al., 2019, Chen & Jain, 2019, Basiri et al., 2020, & Kwon et al., 2020).

The keywords are divided into three clusters or groups that constitute sub-fields of research in DL in healthcare, which are DL and social relationships, models of DL (supervised (CNN, RNN)), unsupervised (DBNN, autoencoder) and DL (EMG, EEG, ECG, EOG, medical imaging, mortality, cardiac arrest, cancer, anaemia), and the new sub-field big data/virtual data and DL; this is what appears in Table 12.4 and

TABLE 12.4

Topic Cluster Summary of Keywords (Researchers' Achievement Depending on VOSviewer Outputs)

Clusters	Keywords	Colours	Sub-fields
Cluster 1 (126 items)	Learning, child, clinical practice, communication, community, country, deeper understanding, education, family, gender, group, health professional, medical imaging, new technology, nursing, students, therapy.	Red	DL and Social Relationship
Cluster 2 (87 items)	DL, models, data, machine learning, neural network, algorithm, architecture, cancer, clinical data, CNN, deep conventional network, electronic health record, mortality, radiologist.	Green	Models and domains of DL
Cluster 3 (15 items)	Application, experiment, healthcare provider, human activity, internet, recognition, scenario, security, smartphone.	Blue	Big data/Virtual data and DL

what researchers have done in many of the previously mentioned studies, such as Rafailidis and Crestani (2017), Purushotham et al. (2018), Bote-Curiel et al. (2019).

These results answer the study;s fundamental problem, which is a determination for research areas that are most interested in studies and authors in the field of DL in Healthcare. Seven sub-fields for researchers and three for keywords, the trend of big data/virtual data, and DL constitute a recent movement of research on DL in healthcare. Thus, the results include scientific value, and the study becomes in the course of the subsequent studies (Ravì et al., 2016, Faust et al., 2018, & Liu et al., 2019).

12.5   CONCLUSION

This chapter's goal is to define the fields of study most concerned by researchers on the topic of deep healthcare education, as they have portrayed DL (CNN, RNN), however, unregulated models DBNN and autoencoder, DL domains, EMG, EEG, ECG, EOG, medical imaging, mortality, cardiac arrest, cancer, anaemia. Social relationships and DL are the sub-fields of large groups of people.

Accordingly, the researchers can choose which approach to research in a DL topic in healthcare and select one of the sub-fields specified in this chapter. They can easily refer to the studies mentioned earlier in each sub-field to determine how to conduct their research.

ACKNOWLEDGMENT

The authors would like to thank the anonymous reviewers and the editor for their insightful comments and suggestions.

REFERENCES

Agrawal, R., Taylor, Group, F., Chatterjee, J. M., Kumar, A., Rathore, P. S., & Le, D. N. (2020). *Machine Learning for Healthcare: Handling and Managing Data*. Taylor & Francis Group.

Aizenberg, I., Aizenberg, N. N., & Vandewalle, J. P. (2013). *Multi-Valued and Universal Binary Neurons: Theory, Learning and Applications*. Springer Science & Business Media.

Baldi, P. (2018). Deep learning in biomedical data science. *Annual Review of Biomedical Data Science*, *1*, 181–205.

Basiri, M. E., Abdar, M., Cifci, M. A., Nemati, S., & Acharya, U. R. (2020). A novel method for sentiment classification of drug reviews using fusion of deep and machine learning techniques. *Knowledge-Based Systems*, *198*, 105949.

Beam, A. L., & Kohane, I. S. (2018). Big data and machine learning in health care. *Jama*, *319*(13), 1317–1318.

Bohr, A., & Memarzadeh, K. (2020). *Artificial Intelligence in Healthcare*. Elsevier Science.

Bote-Curiel, L., Munoz-Romero, S., Gerrero-Curieses, A., & Rojo-Álvarez, J. L. (2019). Deep learning and big data in healthcare: a double review for critical beginners. *Applied Sciences*, *9*(11), 2331.

Campion, F. X., Carlsson, G., & Francis, F. (2017). *Machine Intelligence for Healthcare*. CreateSpace Independent Publishing Platform.

Catania, L. J. (2020). *Foundations of Artificial Intelligence in Healthcare and Bioscience: A User Friendly Guide for IT Professionals, Healthcare Providers, Researchers, and Clinicians*. Elsevier Science.

Chen, Y. W., & Jain, L. C. (2019). *Deep Learning in Healthcare: Paradigms and Applications*. Springer International Publishing.

Cheon, S., Kim, J., & Lim, J. (2019). The use of deep learning to predict stroke patient mortality. *International Journal of Environmental Research and Public Health*, *16*(11), 1876.

Dash, S., Acharya, B. R., Mittal, M., Abraham, A., & Kelemen, A. (2019). *Deep Learning Techniques for Biomedical and Health Informatics*. Springer International Publishing.

Dechter, R. (1986). *Learning While Searching in Constraint-Satisfaction Problems*, AAAI-86 Proceedings, USA.

Eastman, E. M. (2019). *Deep Learning Models for the Perception of Human Social Interactions*. Massachusetts Institute of Technology.

Faes, L., Wagner, S. K., Fu, D. J., Liu, X., Korot, E., Ledsam, J. R., ... Kern, C. (2019). Automated deep learning design for medical image classification by healthcare professionals with no coding experience: a feasibility study. *The Lancet Digital Health*, *1*(5), e232–e242.

Faust, O., Hagiwara, Y., Hong, T. J., Lih, O. S., & Acharya, U. R. (2018). Deep learning for healthcare applications based on physiological signals: a review. *Computer Methods and Programs in Biomedicine*, *161*, 1–13.

Georgescu, A. L., Koehler, J. C., Weiske, J., Vogeley, K., Koutsouleris, N., & Falter-Wagner, C. (2020). Machine learning to study social interaction difficulties in ASD. *Computational Approaches for Human-Human and Human-Robot Social Interactions. Frontiers in Robotics and AI*, *6*, 132.

Guo, X., Polanía, L. F., Garcia-Frias, J., & Barner, K. E. (2019). Social relationship recognition based on a hybrid deep neural network. *Paper presented at the 2019 14th IEEE International Conference on Automatic Face & Gesture Recognition (FG 2019)*, IEEE, Lille.

Hassanien, A. E., Azar, A. T., Gaber, T., Bhatnagar, R., & Tolba, M. F. (2019). *The International Conference on Advanced Machine Learning Technologies and Applications (AMLTA2019).* Springer International Publishing.

Jain, V., & Chatterjee, J. M. (2020). *Machine Learning with Health Care Perspective: Machine Learning and Healthcare.* Springer International Publishing.

KISTI. (2016). *KnowledgeMatrix Plus ver.0.80 for Supporting Scientometric Network Analysis.* Department of Scientometric Research, Korea Institute of Science and Technology Information (KISTI).

Kwon, J.-m., Cho, Y., Jeon, K.-H., Cho, S., Kim, K.-H., Baek, S. D., … Oh, B.-H. (2020). A deep learning algorithm to detect anaemia with ECGs: a retrospective, multicentre study. *The Lancet Digital Health, 2*(7), e358–e367.

Lancet, T. (2017). *Artificial Intelligence in Health Care: Within Touching Distance.* Elsevier.

Lawry, T. (2020). *Artificial Intelligence in Healthcare: A Leader's Guide to Winning in the New Age of Intelligent Health Systems.* Taylor & Francis Group.

Lee, Y., Kwon, J.-m., Lee, Y., Park, H., Cho, H., & Park, J. (2018). Deep learning in the medical domain: predicting cardiac arrest using deep learning. *Acute and Critical Care, 33*(3), 117.

Liu, X., Faes, L., Kale, A. U., Wagner, S. K., Fu, D. J., Bruynseels, A., … Kern, C. (2019). A comparison of deep learning performance against healthcare professionals in detecting diseases from medical imaging: a systematic review and meta-analysis. *The Lancet Digital Health, 1*(6), e271–e297.

Mahajan, P. S. (2018). *Artificial Intelligence in Healthcare.* HarperCollins 360.

Medicine, J. (2019). *Artificial Intelligence and Machine Learning for Business: Approach for Beginners to AI and Machine Learning and Their Revolution of Modern Life, Health Care, Business and Marketing.* Independently Published.

Miotto, R., Wang, F., Wang, S., Jiang, X., & Dudley, J. T. (2018). Deep learning for healthcare: review, opportunities and challenges. *Briefings in Bioinformatics, 19*(6), 1236–1246.

Mohanty, S. N., Nalinipriya, G., Jena, O. P., & Sarkar, A. (2021). *Machine Learning for Healthcare Applications.* Wiley.

Ngiam, K. Y., & Khor, W. (2019). Big data and machine learning algorithms for healthcare delivery. *The Lancet Oncology, 20*(5), e262–e273.

Nielsen, A. (2017). *AI and Machine Learning for Healthcare: An Overview of Tools and Challenges for Building a Health-tech Data Pipeline.* O'Reilly Media.

Nordlinger, B., Villani, C., & Rus, D. (2020). *Healthcare and Artificial Intelligence.* Springer International Publishing.

Panesar, A. (2019). *Machine Learning and AI for Healthcare: Big Data for Improved Health Outcomes.* Apress.

Purushotham, S., Meng, C., Che, Z., & Liu, Y. (2018). Benchmarking deep learning models on large healthcare datasets. *Journal of biomedical informatics, 83,* 112–134.

Rafailidis, D., & Crestani, F. (2017). Recommendation with social relationships via deep learning. Paper Presented at the Proceedings of the ACM SIGIR International Conference on Theory of Information Retrieval, New York, NY.

Ravì, D., Wong, C., Deligianni, F., Berthelot, M., Andreu-Perez, J., Lo, B., & Yang, G.-Z. (2016). Deep learning for health informatics. *IEEE Journal of Biomedical and Health Informatics, 21*(1), 4–21.

Saba, L., Biswas, M., Kuppili, V., Godia, E. C., Suri, H. S., Edla, D. R., … Mavrogeni, S. (2019). The present and future of deep learning in radiology. *European Journal of Radiology, 114,* 14–24.

Santosh, K. C., Das, N., & Ghosh, S. (2021). *Deep Learning Models for Medical Imaging.* Elsevier Science.

Sisodia, D. S., Pachori, R. B., & Garg, L. (2020). *Advancement of Artificial Intelligence in Healthcare Engineering.* Medical Information Science Reference.

Solutions, E. L. (2018). *Machine Learning for Healthcare Analytics Projects: Build smart AI Applications Using Neural Network Methodologies Across the Healthcare Vertical Market.* Packt Publishing.

Van Eck, N. J., & Waltman, L. (2013). VOSviewer manual. *Leiden: Univeristeit Leiden, 1*(1), 1–53.

Yang, H.-C., Islam, M. M., & Li, Y.-C. (2018). Potentiality of deep learning application in healthcare. *Comput. Methods Programs Biomed., 161,* 1.

Yazhini, K., & Loganathan, D. (2019). A state of art approaches on deep learning models in healthcare: an application perspective. *Paper Presented at the 2019* 3rd International Conference on Trends in Electronics and Informatics (ICOEI), Tirunelveli.

Yoon, H. (2018). *New Statistical Transfer Learning Models for Health Care Applications.* Arizona State University.

Yu, Y., Li, M., Liu, L., Li, Y., & Wang, J. (2019). Clinical big data and deep learning: applications, challenges, and future outlooks. *Big Data Mining and Analytics, 2*(4), 288–305.

Zhang, L., Huang, J., & Liu, L. (2019). Improved deep learning network based in combination with cost-sensitive learning for early detection of ovarian cancer in color ultrasound detecting system. *Journal of medical systems, 43*(8), 251.

Zupic, I., & Čater, T. (2015). Bibliometric methods in management and organization. *Organizational Research Methods, 18*(3), 429–472.

13 The Effects of Image Pre-processing in Detection of Brain Tumors Using Faster R-CNN on Magnetic Resonance Scans

Emre Dandıl
Bilecik Seyh Edebali University

Süleyman Uzun
Sakarya University of Applied Science

CONTENTS

13.1 INTRODUCTION

Brain tumors that occur with the abnormal and rapid growth of cells in the brain can adversely affect the lives of people of all ages. The National Brain Tumor Society has emphasized that more than 87,000 new cases of primary brain tumors are expected to be diagnosed in the USA in 2020, and more than 18 thousand people will die due to brain cancer (NBTS, 2020). Similarly, in Global Cancer Statistics collected from 185 different countries, it was stated that approximately 297,000 new brain and central nervous system cases and more than 241,000 deaths would take place in 2018 (Bray et al., 2018). The accurate and precise diagnosis of brain tumors is significant for treatment planning and implementation. The choice of treatment varies depending on the pathological type, grade and time of diagnosis of the brain tumor (Deepak & Ameer, 2019). Therefore, it is very important to precisely determine the type and grade of the brain tumor at an early stage.

According to the World Health Organization (WHO), brain tumors or tumors of central nervous system are divided into four grades ranging from Grade I to Grade IV. Grade I tumors are benign tumors while Grade IV tumors are malign tumors (Sajjad et al., 2019). Although surgery is the most common treatment procedure for brain tumors, there are also other treatment methods such as radiation and chemotherapy used to slow the growth of tumors (Havaei et al., 2017). On the other hand, magnetic resonance imaging (MRI), which helps physicians, is a widely used imaging technique in the diagnosis of brain tumor and provides detailed images of the brain due to its strong resolution in soft tissues. Accurate diagnosis of brain tumors from MRI sequences is very important for effective treatment planning and implementation. Although physicians and radiologists usually diagnose brain tumor using MRI images, computer-aided detection methods can be used as a secondary tool in the diagnosis of some cases (Zhang et al., 2020). However, the excessive raw data generated in MRI scans can prevent manual segmentation in a valid period of time. In addition, it is clear that both experienced physicians and powerful software that would provide manual segmentation are required since manual detection procedures need a lot of time and are unlikely to be repeated. Therefore, automatic or semi-automatic computer-aided systems are needed in the diagnosis of brain tumors on MRI.

Many studies have been proposed for the diagnosis of brain tumors on MRI scans in recent years. In some of these proposed studies, brain tumors are diagnosed by semi-automated methods, and in some of the studies, fully automated methods are used. Most of the semi-automatic and automatic systems apply machine learning algorithm. Besides, semi-automatic and automatic systems used in the diagnosis of brain tumors can be categorized in two sub-categories as generative-based (Menze et al., 2010; Prastawa, Bullitt, Ho, & Gerig, 2004) and discriminative-based models. While the generative-based models require prior information for the diagnosis process, the discriminative-based models can perform classification with different pattern recognition methods using the features of the images (Zhao et al., 2018). Support vector machines (Bauer, Nolte, & Reyes, 2011), decision trees (Zikic et al., 2012), random forests (Tustison et al., 2015) and artificial neural networks (Sharma, Purohit, & Mukherjee, 2018) are among the widely used discriminative algorithms in the detection of brain tumors.

Although a certain level of success has been achieved in the diagnosis of brain tumors especially by automatic methods, it is seen that the problems cannot be solved completely. The fact that brain tumors indicate high variations in terms of shape, size and intensity and tumors from distinct pathological types may show similar appearances are among these problems (Deepak & Ameer, 2019). In recent years, the development of deep learning-based computer-aided diagnosis systems has contributed to overcoming these problems. There are successful studies such as image classification (Krizhevsky, Sutskever, & Hinton, 2012), object detection (Girshick, Donahue, Darrell, & Malik, 2014) and semantic segmentation (Zheng et al., 2015) in the detection of brain tumors using deep learning. It is seen that especially Convolutional Neural Networks (CNN) method is more prominent in the studies conducted on the detection of brain tumors using deep learning techniques (Havaei, Dutil, Pal, Larochelle, & Jodoin, 2015; Zikic, Ioannou, Brown, & Criminisi, 2014). In their study, Ben naceur, Saouli, Akil, & Kachouri, (2018) proposed a fully automated CNN-based method for segmentation of brain tumors on a public data set. In the results, it was emphasized that the proposed model could help the physician experts to reduce the time of diagnosis. In another study, Hussain, Anwar, & Majid (2018) presented an automated brain tumor segmentation algorithm for the detection of brain tumors using deep CNN. Tumors were successfully detected in experimental studies conducted on two different public data sets. In the study suggested for the diagnosis of brain tumors using deep learning approaches, Kumar et al. (2019) proposed feature selection-based Bayesian Multivariate Deep Neural Learning technique for the classification of the brain tumors. Deepak and Ameer (2019) on the other hand presented an approach supported by transfer learning by using CNN features for the classification of brain tumors. Zhao et al. (2018) proposed a Conditional Random Fields- and CNN-based method for the segmentation of brain tumors. Sajjad et al. (2019) proposed multi-grade brain tumor classification using deep CNN with extensive data augmentation. Havaei et al. (2017) proposed a deep learning-based method for the segmentation of brain tumors. In another study, Yang, Song, and Li (2019) proposed a hybrid method for the segmentation of brain tumors by integrating CNN and random forests algorithms.

In summary, the detection of the brain tumors accurately and precisely with the help of a full automatic computer-aided method is crucial in terms of the diagnosis of the disease, treatment planning, and evaluation of the results. Although surgery is the most widely used treatment method for brain tumors, the use of magnetic resonance (MR) scans with a non-invasive approach plays a significant role in the success of clinical practices and the treatment of the patient. In this study, fully automatic detection of brain tumors on MR images in the prepared data set is proposed using faster regional-convolutional neural networks (faster R-CNN). Within the scope of the study, the effect of image pre-processing on detection performance is also investigated with experimental studies both without any pre-processing and with pre-processing by removing noise using a second-order Volterra filter (SOVF) and median filter (MF). In the experimental studies performed on MR images in the test set, it is determined that the performance of the proposed faster R-CNN-based method in the detection of the tumor region is increased since the tumor regions in the image pre-processed brain MR images are more apparent.

The following sections of the study are organized as follows: In Section 13.2, the prepared data set and details of the proposed method are presented. In Section 13.3, experimental studies carried out within the scope of the study are given. In the last section, the discussion and the results obtained are evaluated.

13.2 MATERIALS AND METHODS

13.2.1 Brain MR Data Set

In this study, the images used in the experimental studies were obtained from the MR scanners at Sincan Nafiz Körez State Hospital, and the data set was created from 405 T2-weighted MR images. The images in the data set were scanned using Siemens Magnetom 1.5T MR device. Images were obtained from the scanner in *DICOM* format, then converted to *jpg* format with image processing algorithms and used in experimental studies within the scope of the study. During scanning, 20–70 MRI slices were obtained for each patient. The following parameters were used when acquiring the images: an average of 35 slices/patient, slice thickness of 5 mm, slice gap of 1 mm, field of view of 218×250 mm^2 and image matrix of 448×512 pixels. Pulse sequences were included as the following: T2-weighted (Turbo Spin Echo, TR = 3,600 ms, TE = 116 ms, 15 echoes per TR, flip angle = 1,500, NEX = 1, Ny = 171). The MR images for the data set were obtained from a total of 67 volunteer patients, 17 of whom were female and 50 of whom were male, and who aged between 14 and 71. Of the 405 images with size of 3 and 60 mm in the data set, 215 of them were malignant brain tumors, and 190 of them were benign brain tumors. While malignant brain tumors were glioblastoma multi-forme, oligodendroglioma, anaplastic astrocytoma, metastasis and medulloblastoma, benign brain tumors were meningioma, ganglioglioma, pilocytic astrocytoma, schwannoma and dysembryoplastic neuroepithelial tumor. In Figure 13.1, MR images of some brain tumors acquired in the axial plane and found in the data set are presented.

We manually obtained ground truth segmentations for the each image data set by the aid of a radiologist. The most appropriate slice from each series of the data sets was selected with accompaniment of radiologist. We used a software tool for ground truth segmentation on the data set. The tool marks edges for obtaining boundaries of

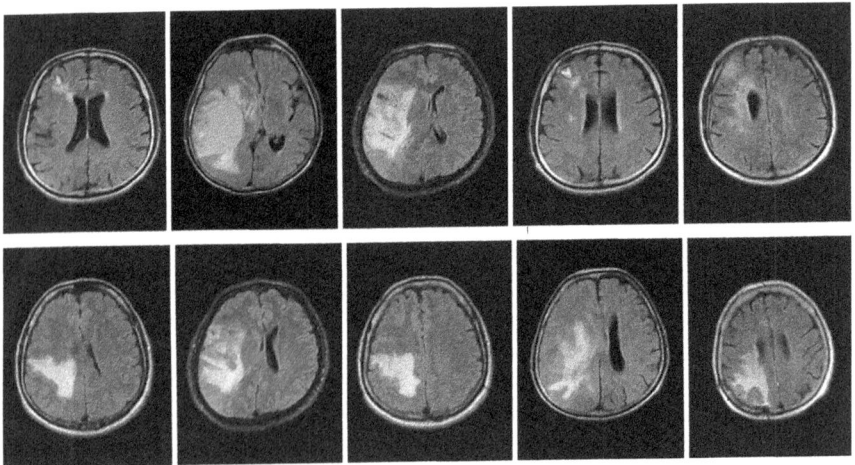

FIGURE 13.1 Some MR images with brain tumors in the data set used in the study.

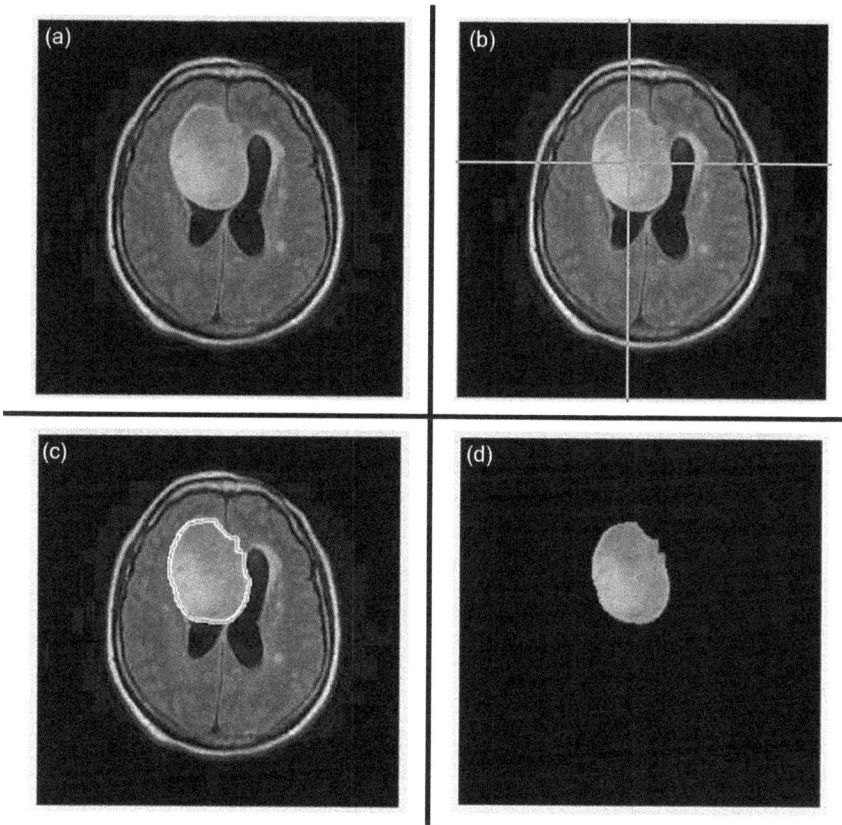

FIGURE 13.2   Developed manual segmentation software tool for radiologists, (a) brain MR image with tumor, (b) determination of tumor region, (c) outlining tumor contours by radiologists, (d) segmentation of brain tumor.

the brain tumor. The developed manual segmentation software tool for radiologists is shown in Figure 13.2.

13.2.2   MEDIAN FILTER

It is seen in image processing that images are often corrupted via positive and negative impulses derived from the errors generated in noise channels. These noises are easily detected by the eye and degrade the image quality (Hwang & Haddad, 1995). The MFs are among the techniques that are widely used to remove or reduce the noise from an image. MF is a non-linear operation technique used with the aim of removing noise from an image or signal, while preserving the edges on the image (Gao, Hu, Gao, & Cheng, 2019). MF removes the noise in the images by using the median value of an image mask such as 3×3, 5×5 and 7×7. Especially, if the generated impulse response is too high, performance may reduce in MF that is very good at removing noise. In addition, non-linear MF cannot remove positive and negative noise impulses simultaneously in images. The application of MF for an X image is shown in Equation (13.1). In this equation, while a and b are values depending on the width and height of the image, W represents the coordinate set in a mask.

$$X_{mf}(a,b) = \text{median} \left\{ X\,(a+u,\, b+t),\,\, (u,t) \in W \right\} \tag{13.1}$$

13.2.3 SECOND-ORDER VOLTERRA FILTERS

SOVFs are preferred since they achieve higher achievement in the field of biomedical image processing, and especially when removing non-linear noises (Meenavathi & Rajesh, 2007). SOVFs also preserve the edges and details in the image while removing noise (Kanamadi, Waghamode, & Bandekar, 2013). SOVFs are a sub-class of discrete non-linear Volterra series (Meenavathi & Rajesh, 2007) and quadratic versions of Volterra filters. The linear filter corresponds to a first-order Volterra filters and cubic filter corresponds to a third-order Volterra filter (Defigueiredo & Matz, 1996; Meenavathi & Rajesh, 2007). The most general form of Volterra filters is shown in Equation (13.2).

$$y(n) = w_0 + \sum_{p=1}^{\infty} w_p[x(n)] \tag{13.2}$$

where y_n is the output, w_0 is the offset value (generally accepted as zero), and w_p represents the pth order of Volterra filters. The most general mathematical equation used for SOVFs is presented in Equation (13.3).

$$y(m,\, n) = y_0 + y_1(m,\, n) + y_2 \tag{13.3}$$

where y_0 represents a constant value (generally accepted as zero), $y(m,\, n)$ represents the output, $y_1(m,\, n)$ represents the linear part of SOVF and $y_2(m,\, n)$ represents the second-order part of Volterra images (Chakrabarty, Jain, & Chatterjee, 2013; Fakhouri, 1980; Nowak & Van Veen, 1994). When $y_1(m,\, n)$ and $y_2(m,\, n)$ are written separately, Equation (13.4) is obtained (Uzun & Akgün, 2018a, b).

$$y_1(m,n) = \sum_{i=-(N-1)/2}^{(N-1)/2} \sum_{j=-(N-1)/2}^{(N-1)/2} w^1_{i,j} x_{m+i,n+j}$$

$$\tag{13.4}$$

$$y_2(m,n) = \sum_{i=-(N-1)/2}^{(N-1)/2} \sum_{j=-(N-1)/2}^{(N-1)/2} \sum_{k=-(N-1)/2}^{(N-1)/2} \sum_{l=-(N-1)/2}^{(N-1)/2} w^2_{i,j,k,l} x_{m+i,n+j} x_{m+k,n+l}$$

where m and n represent the coordinates of the pixels that will be filtered, N represents the size of the filter mask, i and j represent the location of the pixels selected in the filter mask, k and l represent the location of the pixels that selected in the filter mask to obtain second-order derivative.

In previous studies, it is seen that SOVFs are quite successful in noise removal compared to linear filters. In this context, Ramponi (1986) obtained noisy images by adding Gaussian and Gaussian impulse noise on the reference image. Edge-detection process was applied on noisy images using both SOVF and linear filters, and as a result, SOVFs were found to be more successful. Ramponi and Sicuranza (1988) used SOVFs in image enhancement and noise removal processes and achieved better results than other filters. Johilakshmi and Gopinathan (2006) used SOVF to improve the contrast of mammogram images affected by Gaussian, and white noise. They compared the same images with non-linear filters such as low-pass, median, min and max to assess the performance of the filter. They observed that the SOVF produces better results than the others. Meenavathi and Rajesh (2007) used SOVF to enhance the Gaussian and Gaussian impulse noise, and they used a low-pass filter, a high-pass filter and an MF for comparison. According to their results, they achieved much higher performance with SOVFs. Mitra (2012) used SOVF in image contrast enhancement, impulse noise removal and image zooming applications. As a result of the study, it was found that linear filters had low performance in non-linear noise removal, they blurred the image edges and image details were lost. It was also seen that SOVF produced much better results.

In this study, 3×3 size filter mask was used for SOVF. In the pre-processed study, brain MR images were filtered through SOVF one by one as a pre-process. In filtering processes, SOVF weights for each image were recalculated and filtered by training with a genetic algorithm (GA) according to the characteristics of the image. Images with different characteristics were better filtered by calculating the weights of the SOVF after training. Since the calculation of filter weights of SOVF took a very long time, all these operations were performed on the graphical processing unit (GPU).

13.2.4 FASTER REGIONAL-CONVOLUTIONAL NEURAL NETWORK

In recent years, in many studies based on deep CNNs derived from CNNs, successful results and impressive performances have been achieved in object classification and detection. AlexNet, proposed by Krizhevsky et al. (2012), is the first deep CNN that achieved successful results in the ImageNet data set with 1,000 different classes. In the following studies, Ren, He, Girshick, and Sun (2015) proposed the faster R-CNN architecture by combining R-CNN (Girshick et al., 2014) and fast R-CNN (Girshick, 2015) architectures using a Region Proposal Network (RPN) (Huang et al., 2020). Faster R-CNN is one of state-of-art and successful object recognition algorithms (Han, Zhang, Cheng, Liu, & Xu, 2018; Ren et al., 2015). Faster R-CNN represents an upgrade version of fast R-CNN and R-CNN, especially in terms of computation time. Faster R-CNN consists of a single convolutional network composing of two sub-components (Rosati et al., 2020). One of these components is the RPN, and the other performs object recognition in the proposed regions. Unlike R-CNN and faster R-CNN structures, the region proposal process is carried out with RPN in faster R-CNN. In the network used in this study, the ResNet101 architecture was used as a backbone to extract the features, and the COCO data set was used for pre-training of the network. The architecture of the faster R-CNN approach proposed in the study for the detection of brain tumors in MR images is shown in Figure 13.3.

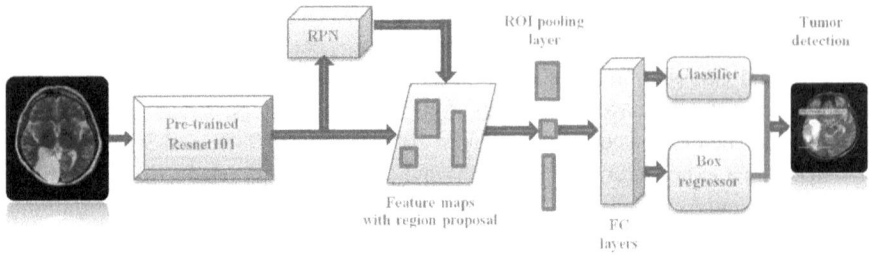

FIGURE 13.3 The architecture of the proposed faster R-CNN approach for the detection of brain tumors on MR scans.

13.3 EXPERIMENTAL RESULTS

The experimental studies were conducted on a desktop computer with an Intel Core i7–3770 3.40 GHz dual-core CPU, 16GB RAM and Nvidia GeForce GTX980 GPU card and a Windows 10 (64-bit) operating system. The GPU card with 4 GB RAM memory used in experimental studies has 75.2 computing capacity and is an external graphics card with 2048 CUDA cores.

In our study, a total of 405 MRI images of brain tumor were used, 305 of these images were used in the training phase and the rest of images were used in the test phase. Within the scope of the study, first, the images were passed through the faster R-CNN-based deep learning system without any pre-processing in the image, and then the training was carried out. Afterward, the performance results were measured on the test set. The same training and test images were pre-processed and used in the proposed system. Two different filters – SOVF and MF – were used for image pre-processing in noise removal. The noise in the images was removed by using a 3×3 mask.

The weights of SOVF for each image were calculated and filtered by training with GA. The mutation rate of GA used in the experimental study for the Volterra filter was 0.05, the crossing rate was 0.3, the upper limit of the second-order derivative was 1.0 and the lower limit of the second-order derivative was determined as −1.0. The number of population was determined as 1,000, the maximum number of iterations was determined as 300 and the stopping criterion of GA was determined as the maximum number of iterations. The grey levels of all images were taken in order to calculate the error rate during the training phase. The reference images were moved to SOVF, and calculations were conducted by comparing the filtered image with the grey-level image while calculating the error. Mean Absolute Error (MAE) and Mean Squared Error (MSE) image quality assessment metrics were used to determine the image quality of the images for both with pre-processing and without pre-processing. While MAE gives the MAE of the corresponding pixels in source and fused images, MSE measures the error calculated by averaging the sum of squares of the error between the two images (Kavitha & Thyagharajan, 2016). Low MAE and MSE values represent high image quality. The equation of MAE is shown in Equation (13.5), and the equation of MSE is denoted in Equation (13.6). In these equations, N is the number of data, x_i is the predicted value, and x is the real value.

$$MAE = \frac{1}{N} \sum_{i=1}^{N} |x_i - x| \qquad (13.5)$$

$$MSE = \frac{1}{N} \sum_{i=1}^{N} (x_i - x)^2 \qquad (13.6)$$

In Figure 13.4, some samples of training and test images used in experimental studies with and without image pre-processing (original) using MF and SOVF are shown.

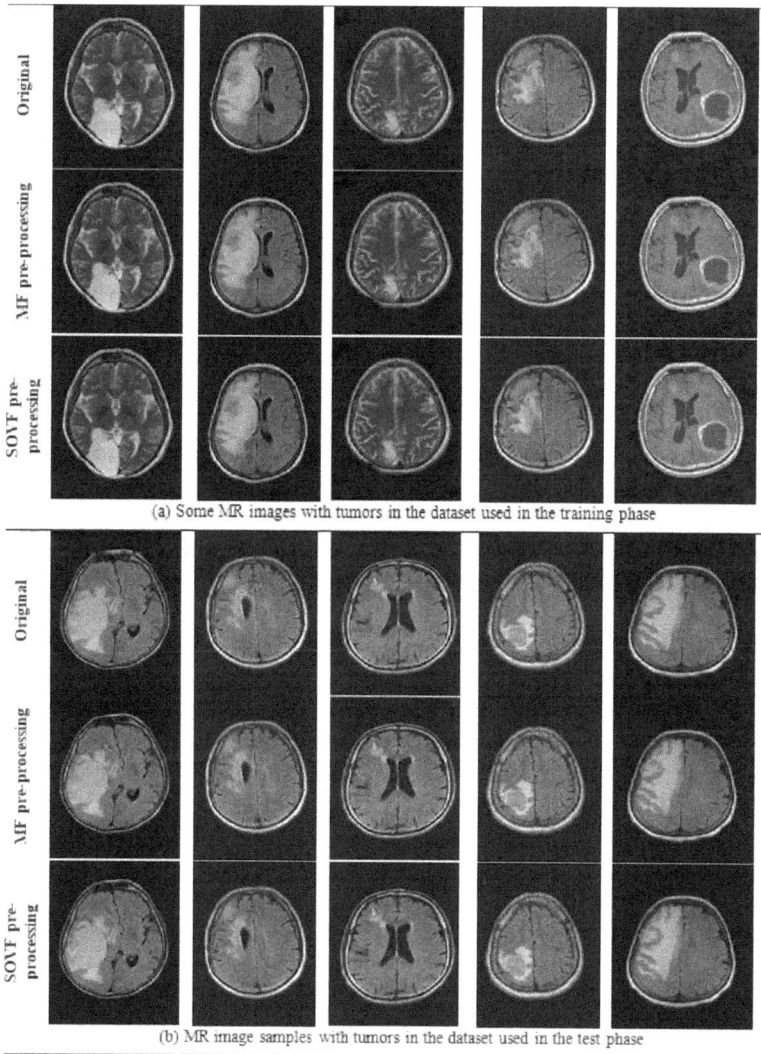

(a) Some MR images with tumors in the dataset used in the training phase

(b) MR image samples with tumors in the dataset used in the test phase

FIGURE 13.4   Image pre-processing using MF and SOVF on some original training and test MR images in the data set.

The original MR images shown in Figure 13.4 were used without any image pre-processing. The images preprocessed by MF show the images obtained after passing the original images through a MF, and the images preprocessed by SOVF show the images obtained by using a second-order Volterra image filter.

Table 13.1 shows the performance results obtained on images with and without image pre-processing during the training phase of the faster R-CNN based system proposed in this study. While the training accuracy performance in experimental studies conducted without pre-processing was 98.35%, the average training accuracy for images pre-processed by MF was 98.51%, and the average training accuracy was 98.63% for images pre-processed by SOVF.

The brain tumor detection performance of the proposed faster R-CNN method both with image pre-processing and without image pre-processing was compared by the experimental studies conducted on 105 test images, and the results are presented in Table 13.2. The results show that the accuracy of the deep learning system in the detection of the tumor regions was higher when the images were pre-processed compared to the without pre-processing step. In the pre-processed experimental studies, it was seen that the accuracy of detecting the tumor region was higher when the images were preprocesses by SOVF compared to the images preprocessed by MF.

Table 13.3 shows the average MAE and MSE values of the results obtained from 30 times running of some of the images in the data set on the GTX980 GPU card. Since GTX980 GPU card has more cores than CPUs, it completes the training faster. Although MAE, MSE and calculation time parameters were evaluated on different images after the images were passed through SOVF to remove the noise in the images, it was seen that the results were very close to each other when the image quality metrics were examined. This shows that the proposed method is successful without damaging image quality. In addition, as seen in Table 13.4, while the MAE value of the noisy image obtained by adding noise to the reference image was 23.250687, this value was on average 7.842018 as a result of denoisinig by SOVF. This means that most of the noises were removed.

Images of sample brain tumors successfully detected on MR images using the faster R-CNN based deep learning approach proposed in this study are presented in Figure 13.5. In this experimental study, after the images were pre-processed by removing the noise by SOVF, training and test processes were carried out with faster R-CNN. These images in the test set were determined with 100% accuracy. In the experimental studies performed without applying any pre-processing to the images in the test set, only 8% of the total image in the test set was detected with 100% accuracy. After pre-processing the images in the test set by MF, the image rate in the test set detected with 100% accuracy increased to 28%, while this rate increased to 57% when the images were pre-processed by SOVF.

Figure 13.6 shows sample images where the tumor region was detected incorrectly using the proposed faster R-CNN as a result of the experimental studies. One of the reasons for this is that regions such as skull bone and eyes are very similar to the color tones of the tumor region on brain MRI images. Another reason is that the number of tumor regions marked on the images is less. In addition, training the faster R-CNN network with more MR images would contribute to reducing the number of incorrectly detected brain tumors on MR images.

TABLE 13.1

Results Obtained in Experimental Studies Conducted with and Without Pre-processing During the Training Phase for Detection of Brain Tumors with the Proposed Faster R-CNN-Based Approach

Number of Epoch	Number of Iteration	Learning Rate	without Image Pre-processing			With Image Pre-processing			Pre-processing via VF		
			Time (s)	Loss	Accuracy (%)	Time (s)	Loss	Accuracy (%)	Time (s)	Loss	Accuracy (%)
90	50	0.001000	227.37	0.0090	99.22	227.57	0.0201	99.22	229.28	0.0031	100.00
91	50	0.001000	229.98	0.0007	100.00	229.63	0.0261	99.22	231.38	0.0014	100.00
92	50	0.001000	231.41	0.0024	100.00	231.71	0.006	100.00	235.50	0.0335	99.21
93	50	0.001000	235.29	0.0318	99.22	233.91	0.003	100.00	237.53	0.0422	98.44
94	50	0.001000	237.52	0.0442	99.22	236.10	0.0034	100.00	239.56	0.0018	100.00
95	50	0.001000	239.68	0.0066	100.00	240.21	0.0009	100.00	241.58	0.0005	100.00
96	50	0.001000	241.68	0.0683	98.44	242.25	0.0040	100.00	245.63	0.0049	100.00
97	50	0.001000	245.58	0.0025	100.00	244.37	0.0136	99.22	247.62	0.0008	100.00
98	50	0.001000	247.54	0.0090	100.00	246.47	0.0065	100.00	249.66	0.0021	100.00
99	50	0.001000	249.52	0.0006	100.00	248.52	0.0285	99.22	251.68	0.0021	100.00
100	50	0.001000	253.41	0.0007	100.00	252.60	0.0019	100.00	255.71	0.0009	100.00

TABLE 13.2

Performance Comparison in Detection of the Tumor Region on Brain MRI Images by the Proposed Method

Image Enhancement Procedure	Accuracy (%)
Without pre-processing	85.87
Pre-processing via MF	88.70
Pre-processing via SOVF	91.06

TABLE 13.3

MAE, MSE and Calculation Time Values Obtained After Denoising by SOVF on the Images in the Data Set

Image ID	MAE	MSE	Computation Time (s)
IMG_MRI_b1	7.811954	102.737000	103.091320
IMG_MRI_b2	8.348015	121.223326	103.035306
IMG_MRI_b3	7.734155	99.741165	98.551440
IMG_MRI_b4	7.793245	101.038412	98.536374
IMG_MRI_b5	7.672215	97.931055	98.479003
IMG_MRI_b6	7.851873	102.349969	98.521361
IMG_MRI_b7	7.657575	97.586883	98.503886
IMG_MRI_b8	7.799071	100.934488	98.499178
IMG_MRI_b9	7.892844	108.588825	98.448810
IMG_MRI_b10	7.477479	96.394677	98.506008

TABLE 13.4

Initial and Final MAE and MSE Values Measured on Reference Images by VF Filtering

Reference Image	Initial MAE – MSE Values		Final MAE – MSE Values		Computation Time (s)
	MAE	MSE	MAE	MSE	
ref_img_mri_b1	23.250687	748.022949	7.842018	103.491310	11312.480736
ref_img_mri_b2	21.052839	708.676208	9.162480	124.571678	36812.528912
Subtraction	−2.197848	−39.346741	1.320462	21.080368	25500.048176

13.4 DISCUSSION AND CONCLUSIONS

In this study, a method was proposed for the detection of brain tumors using faster R-CNN on MR images in the axial plane in the data set. Within the scope of the study, the effect of image pre-processing on the detection performance was also investigated by removing the noise through pre-processing the images by SOVF and MF, and without any pre-processing. In the experimental studies performed on 105 test images,

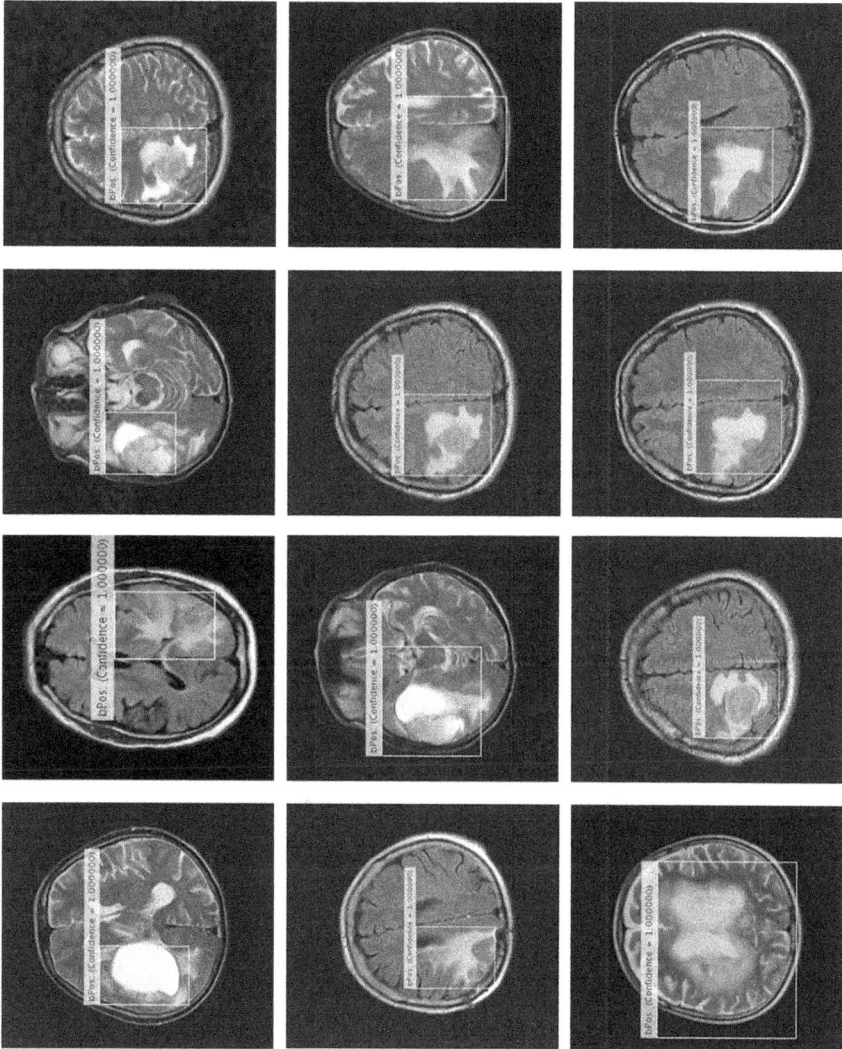

FIGURE 13.5 Detection of brain tumors using the proposed faster R-CNN method after pre-processing the images in the data set via SOVF.

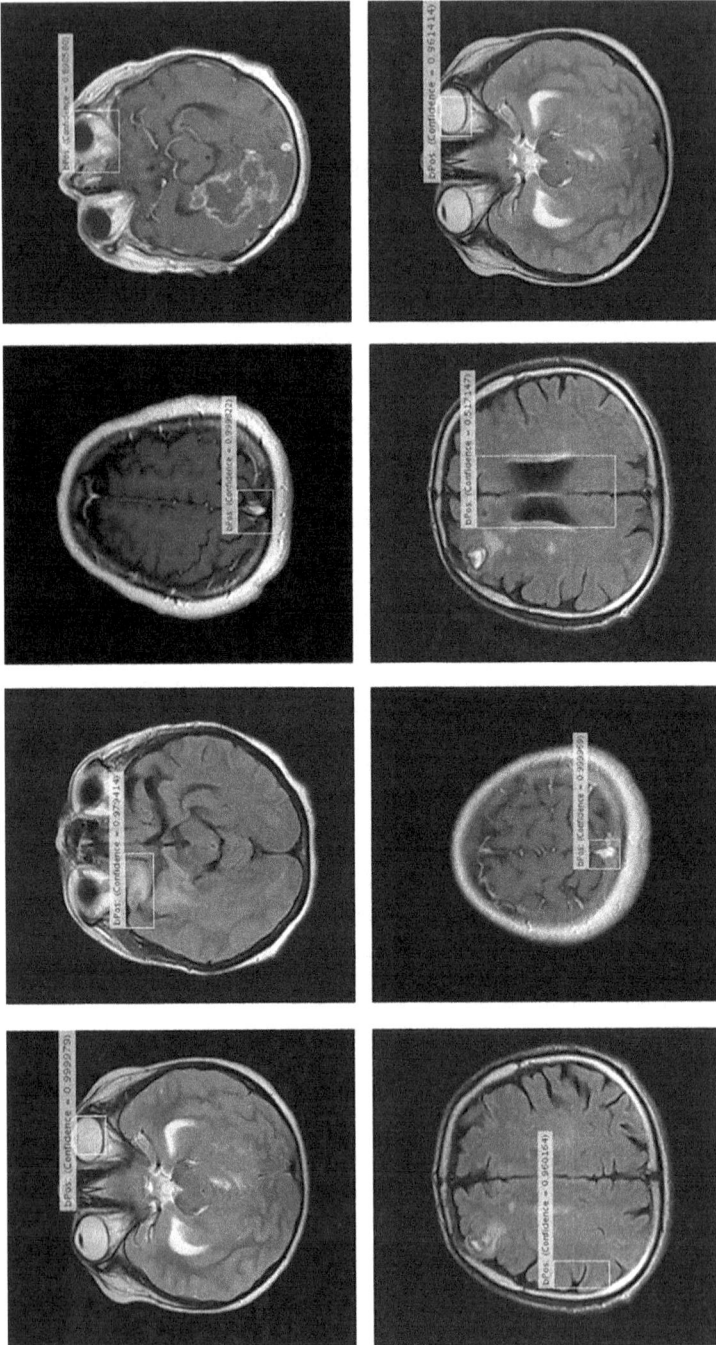

FIGURE 13.6   Image samples in which the brain tumor region detected incorrectly in the data set.

brain tumors were diagnosed with 85.87% accuracy without any pre-processing, while 88.70% and 91.06% diagnosis accuracy rates were obtained when the images were preprocessed by MF and SOVF, respectively. Therefore, it was determined that the proposed faster R-CNN-based method produced higher accuracy in the detection of the brain tumors since the tumor regions in the pre-processed brain MR images became more apparent. One of the main reasons for the high performance of the proposed method in the detection of the tumor region, especially when pre-processed by SOVF, is that Volterra image filters contain both low-pass and high-pass filters, which protect the edges of the tumor regions while filtering images.

In the experimental studies without pre-processing, the number of MR images where the tumor region could not be detected at all was 12% of the test images. While the number of images in which the tumor region could not be detected in the pre-processing by MF was 8% of the test images, the number of the images in which the tumor region could not be detected in the pre-processing by SOVF was 6% of the test images. In addition, in the tests conducted without pre-processing, the number of images in which the tumor region was detected with 100% accuracy or less was 78% of the test images. When image pre-processing was performed by MF, the number of images in which the tumor region was detected with 100% accuracy or with less rates was 85% of the test images, while this rate was 87% by SOVF.

In the following studies, which would be a continuation of the study, images can be pre-processed using different image processing techniques and comparative analyses can be presented by measuring the performance of deep learning in classification. In addition, the accuracy of the proposed method can be evaluated on more data sets.

REFERENCES

Bauer, S., Nolte, L.-P., & Reyes, M. (2011). Fully automatic segmentation of brain tumor images using support vector machine classification in combination with hierarchical conditional random field regularization. *Paper Presented at the International Conference on Medical Image Computing and Computer-Assisted Intervention*, Springer, Toronto.

Ben naceur, M., Saouli, R., Akil, M., & Kachouri, R. (2018). Fully automatic brain tumor segmentation using end-to-end incremental deep neural networks in MRI images. *Computer Methods and Programs in Biomedicine, 166*, 39–49.

Bray, F., Ferlay, J., Soerjomataram, I., Siegel, R. L., Torre, L. A., & Jemal, A. (2018). Global cancer statistics 2018: GLOBOCAN estimates of incidence and mortality worldwide for 36 cancers in 185 countries. *CA: A Cancer Journal for Clinicians, 68*(6), 394–424.

Chakrabarty, A., Jain, H., & Chatterjee, A. (2013). Volterra kernel based face recognition using artificial bee colonyoptimization. *Engineering Applications of Artificial Intelligence, 26*(3), 1107–1114.

Deepak, S., & Ameer, P. (2019). Brain tumor classification using deep CNN features via transfer learning. *Computers in Biology and Medicine, 111*, 103345.

Defigueiredo, R. J., & Matz, S. C. (1996). *Exponential nonlinear Volterra filters for contrast sharpening in noisy images. Paper Presented at the 1996 IEEE International Conference on Acoustics, Speech, and Signal Processing Conference Proceedings*, IEEE, Atlanta, GA.

Fakhouri, S. (1980). *Identification of the Volterra kernels of nonlinear systems. Paper Presented at the IEE Proceedings D-Control Theory and Applications*, IET Digital Library, USA.

Gao, H., Hu, M., Gao, T., & Cheng, R. (2019). Robust detection of median filtering based on combined features of difference image. *Signal Processing: Image Communication, 72,* 126–133.

Girshick, R. (2015). *Fast R-CNN. Paper Presented at the Proceedings of the IEEE International Conference on Computer Vision*, Santiago.

Girshick, R., Donahue, J., Darrell, T., & Malik, J. (2014). Rich feature hierarchies for accurate object detection and semantic segmentation. *Paper Presented at the Proceedings of the IEEE Conference on Computer Vision and Pattern Recognition*, Columbus, OH.

Han, J., Zhang, D., Cheng, G., Liu, N., & Xu, D. (2018). Advanced deep-learning techniques for salient and category-specific object detection: A survey. *IEEE Signal Processing Magazine, 35*(1), 84–100.

Havaei, M., Davy, A., Warde-Farley, D., Biard, A., Courville, A., Bengio, Y., ... Larochelle, H. (2017). Brain tumor segmentation with deep neural networks. *Medical Image Analysis, 35,* 18–31.

Havaei, M., Dutil, F., Pal, C., Larochelle, H., & Jodoin, P.-M. (2015). A convolutional neural network approach to brain tumor segmentation. *Paper Presented at the BrainLes, Switzerland.*

Huang, H., Wang, C., Liu, S., Sun, Z., Zhang, D., Liu, C., ... Xu, R. (2020). Single spectral imagery and faster R-CNN to identify hazardous and noxious substances spills. *Environmental Pollution, 258,* 113688.

Hussain, S., Anwar, S. M., & Majid, M. (2018). Segmentation of glioma tumors in brain using deep convolutional neural network. *Neurocomputing, 282,* 248–261.

Hwang, H., & Haddad, R. A. (1995). Adaptive median filters: New algorithms and results. *IEEE Transactions on Image Processing, 4*(4), 499–502.

Jothilakshmi, G., & Gopinathan, E. (2006). Mammogram enhancement using quadratic adaptive Volterra filter—A comparative analysis in spatial and frequency domain. *ARPN Journal of Engineering and Applied Sciences, 10*(13), 5512–5517.

Kanamadi, M., Waghamode, V., & Bandekar, S. (2013). Alpha weighted quadratic filter based enhancement for mammogram. *Paper presented at the Proceedings of International Conference on "Emerging Research in Computing, Information, Communication and Applications" (ERCICA)*, Bangalore, India.

Kavitha, S., & Thyagharajan, K. (2016). A survey on quantitative metrics for assessing the quality of fused medical images. *Research Journal of Applied Sciences, Engineering and Technology, 12*(3), 282–293.

Krizhevsky, A., Sutskever, I., & Hinton, G. E. (2012). Imagenet classification with deep convolutional neural networks. *Paper Presented at the Advances in Neural Information Processing Systems*, Nevada, USA.

Kumar, A., Ramachandran, M., Gandomi, A. H., Patan, R., Lukasik, S., & Soundarapandian, R. K. (2019). A deep neural network based classifier for brain tumor diagnosis. *Applied Soft Computing, 82,* 105528.

Meenavathi, M., & Rajesh, K. (2007). Volterra filtering techniques for removal of Gaussian and mixed Gaussian-impulse noise. *International Journal of Electrical, Computer, Energetic, Electronic and Communication Engineering, 1*(2), 176–182.

Menze, B. H., Van Leemput, K., Lashkari, D., Weber, M.-A., Ayache, N., & Golland, P. (2010). A generative model for brain tumor segmentation in multi-modal images. *Paper Presented at the International Conference on Medical Image Computing and Computer-Assisted Intervention*, Berlin, Germany.

Mitra, S. K. (2012). Image processing using quadratic volterra filters. *Paper presented at the 2012 5th International Conference on Computers and Devices for Communication (CODEC)*, India.

NBTS. (2020). Quick brain tumor facts. Retrieved from https://braintumor.org/brain-tumor-information/brain-tumor-facts/.

Nowak, R. D., & Van Veen, B. D. (1994). Random and pseudorandom inputs for Volterra filter identification. *IEEE Transactions on Signal Processing, 42*(8), 2124–2135.

Prastawa, M., Bullitt, E., Ho, S., & Gerig, G. (2004). A brain tumor segmentation framework based on outlier detection. *Medical Image Analysis, 8*(3), 275–283.

Ramponi, G. (1986). Edge extraction by a class of second-order nonlinear filters. *Electronics Letters, 22*(9), 482–484.

Ramponi, G., & Sicuranza, G. L. (1988). Quadratic digital filters for image processing. *IEEE Transactions on Acoustics, Speech, and Signal Processing, 36*(6), 937–939.

Ren, S., He, K., Girshick, R., & Sun, J. (2015). Faster R-CNN: Towards real-time object detection with region proposal networks. *Paper Presented at the Advances in Neural Information Processing Systems*, Montreal, Quebec, Canada.

Rosati, R., Romeo, L., Silvestri, S., Marcheggiani, F., Tiano, L., & Frontoni, E. (2020). Faster R-CNN approach for detection and quantification of DNA damage in comet assay images. *Computers in Biology and Medicine, 123*, 103912.

Sajjad, M., Khan, S., Muhammad, K., Wu, W., Ullah, A., & Baik, S. W. (2019). Multi-grade brain tumor classification using deep CNN with extensive data augmentation. *Journal of Computational Science, 30*, 174–182.

Sharma, M., Purohit, G., & Mukherjee, S. (2018). Information retrieves from brain MRI images for tumor detection using hybrid technique K-means and artificial neural network (KMANN) *Networking Communication and Data Knowledge Engineering* (pp. 145–157): Springer.

Tustison, N. J., Shrinidhi, K., Wintermark, M., Durst, C. R., Kandel, B. M., Gee, J. C., … Avants, B. B. (2015). Optimal symmetric multimodal templates and concatenated random forests for supervised brain tumor segmentation (simplified) with ANTsR. *Neuroinformatics, 13*(2), 209–225.

Uzun, S., & Akgün, D. (2018a). An accelerated method for determining the weights of quadratic image filters. *IEEE Access, 6*, 33718–33726.

Uzun, S., & AkgÜn, D. (2018b). A literature review on quadratic image filters. *Paper Presented at the 2018 2nd International Symposium on Multidisciplinary Studies and Innovative Technologies (ISMSIT)*, IEEE, Ankara, Turkey.

Yang, T., Song, J., & Li, L. (2019). A deep learning model integrating SK-TPCNN and random forests for brain tumor segmentation in MRI. *Biocybernetics and Biomedical Engineering, 39*(3), 613–623.

Zhang, M., Young, G. S., Chen, H., Li, J., Qin, L., McFaline-Figueroa, J. R., … Xu, X. (2020). Deep-learning detection of cancer metastases to the brain on MRI. *Journal of Magnetic Resonance Imaging.*

Zhao, X., Wu, Y., Song, G., Li, Z., Zhang, Y., & Fan, Y. (2018). A deep learning model integrating FCNNs and CRFs for brain tumor segmentation. *Medical image analysis, 43*, 98–111.

Zheng, S., Jayasumana, S., Romera-Paredes, B., Vineet, V., Su, Z., Du, D., … Torr, P. H. (2015). Conditional random fields as recurrent neural networks. *Paper Presented at the Proceedings of the IEEE International Conference on Computer Vision*, Santiago, Chile.

Zikic, D., Glocker, B., Konukoglu, E., Criminisi, A., Demiralp, C., Shotton, J., … Price, S. J. (2012). Decision forests for tissue-specific segmentation of high-grade gliomas in multi-channel MR. *Paper Presented at the International Conference on Medical Image Computing and Computer-Assisted Intervention*, Springer, Nice.

Zikic, D., Ioannou, Y., Brown, M., & Criminisi, A. (2014). Segmentation of brain tumor tissues with convolutional neural networks. *Proceedings MICCAI-BRATS*, 36–39, Boston, MA.

14 Evaluation of Deep Neural Network and Ensemble Machine Learning Methods for Cesarean Data Classification

A. Karacı
University of Kastamonu

CONTENTS

14.1 INTRODUCTION

Cesarean section is the most common operation performed at birth (Kan, 2020). In recent years, cesarean rates have been increasing in low-, middle- and high-income countries. Cesarean delivery is medically effective in preventing negative consequences (Yisma, Smithers, Lynch, Mol, 2019). Most women who have had a cesarean before want to have a normal birth. However, this is not possible. Because doctors do not take the risk of normal delivery after cesarean. Newborns have anesthesia problems and breathing problems. Children born with cesarean are more likely to have asthma, allergies and diabetes. The risk of asthma is 79% higher than normal birth, and the risk of diabetes is 20% higher (Sana, Razzaq and Ferzund, 2012).

Deep Neural Networks (DNNs) are Artificial Neural Networks that are formed by multiple layers of neural networks with a high number of nonlinear neurons per layer. DNN is similar to shallow neural network in structure but has more hidden layers and more obvious hierarchy structure. DNN has received a considerable deal of attention by performing better than the alternative ML methods in several significant applications (Karaci et al. 2019; Feng, Zhou and Dong, 2019; Karacı, 2020a). DNNs have become important with the advancement of GPUs and the storage of big data. DNNs are parametric models that achieve sequential operations on their input data. Each operation, called a layer, consists of a linear transformation followed by a pointwise linear or nonlinear activation function (Bouwmans, Javed and Sultana, 2019). Although DNNs are the most suitable solution for large data sets, they can also be a reasonable choice in small data sets if large data sets are not available (Feng, Zhou and Dong, 2019).

Multiple classifier systems, also called ensemble systems, have attracted increasing attention in the computational intelligence and machine learning (ML) community. They have also proven to be very effective and versatile in a wide range of problem areas and in real-world applications (Polikar, 2012). An ensemble is a group of predictors; accordingly, this technique is named as Ensemble Learning, and an Ensemble Learning algorithm is named as an Ensemble method (Géron, 2017). Ensemble learning is a method that combines multiple learning algorithms (Sagi and Rokach, 2018). The purpose of the approach of the ensemble classifier is to combine multiple individual classifiers to create a new high-accuracy classifier (Qi and Tang, 2018).

According to the literature review, there are very few studies that perform cesarean classification with ML. No study has been encountered that classifies cesarean data using DNN. Alsharif et al. (2019) classified the cesarean data set used in this study with Support Vector Machines (SVM), K-Nearest-Neighbors, Naive Bayes (NB), Decision Tree (DT) and Random Forest ML algorithms. They achieved the highest classification performance in SVM (accuracy: 58.33%, recall: 90.9%) and NB (accuracy: 70.83%, recall: 87.50%) algorithms. Sana et al. (2012) classified a different cesarean data with DT and Artificial Neural Networks (ANN) ML algorithms. The highest classification performance achieved in this study was 80% accuracy and 84% recall.

The purpose of this study is to classify the normal birth or cesarean status of the individuals who will give birth by using DNN and Ensemble models with age, delivery number, delivery time, blood pressure and heart problem attributes, and compare the performance of these models on this data set. In the second part of the study, structures and parameters of the DNN and the Ensemble models, data set; in the third section, the classification performances of these models are explained.

14.2 MATERIALS AND METHODS

14.2.1 Data Set

The data set used in the study was taken from the University of California at Irvine (UCI) ML repository (Uci, 2020). The data set consists of five attributes. These attributes are age, delivery number, delivery time, blood pressure and heart problem. The data set also contains information on cesarean section decision (1: cesarean or 0: normal birth). In the creation of DNN, Ensemble and Individual ML models, five attributes are used as input and cesarean section decision information is used as output. The attributes and value ranges are shown in Table 14.1.

TABLE 14.1

Inputs of Machine Learning Models

Attribute Number	Inputs	Value Ranges
1	Age	[17–40]
2	Delivery number	[1,2,3,4]
3	Delivery time	0 = timely, 1 = premature, 2 = latecomer
4	Blood pressure	0 = low, 1 = normal, 2 = high
5	Heart problem	0 = apt, 1 = inept

14.2.2 MACHINE LEARNING METHODS

The flow chart shown in Figure 14.1 was used to create and evaluate the models. First of all, the model parameters were determined and training and test procedures were carried out by creating the models in accordance with these parameters. Two methods were used for training and testing. In the first method, the data set was randomly divided into 70% education and 30% test data. With these data sets, training and testing of DNN-1 and Ensemble-1 ML methods were performed. The second method

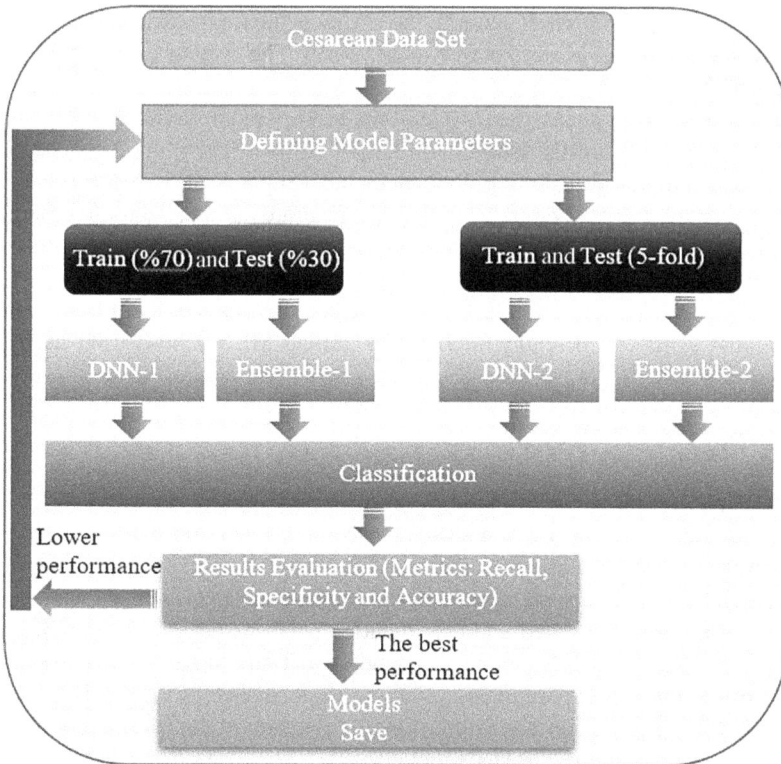

FIGURE 14.1 Creation of DNN and ensemble models.

is 5-fold cross-verification. With this method, DNN-2 and Ensemble-2 models were trained and tested. After each test operation, comparison was made with the classification performance obtained from the previous model. If the performance of the new model is worse than the previous ones, the new parameters were defined and the models were reconstructed. When a model with a better performance was obtained, the model was saved.

Sklearn and Keras Library were used on the Python programming language to create the models. Different hidden layer and neuron numbers were used in the creation of DNN models. In addition, different parameters have been tried in the training of DNN and Ensemble models. The best models have been recorded. Five attributes were given as input to models. These attributes and their values were described in the data set section. The models have two outputs and the models perform classification. The first output represents the "cesarean" decision, while the second output represents the "normal birth" decision. The structures of the DNN-1 and DNN-2 models are shown in Figure 14.2.

ANN, XGBoost and NB individual classifiers were used in the creation of Ensemble models. Ensemble classifiers are a method that combines multiple learning algorithms in supervised ML. When combining individual classifiers, different combining methods can be used. In this study, weighted majority voting (soft voting) method was used. In this method, after calculating the weights of each classifier decision, the class with the highest score in the voting is the final class predict (Moreno-Seco, Iñesta, León and Micó, 2006; Karacı, 2019). The structures of the Ensemble models are shown in Figure 14.3.

The ANN individual classifier is one of the most popular methods of ML used in many scientific fields. ANN usually consists of an input layer, one or more hidden layers and an output layer (Rezaee, Jozmaleki and Valipour, 2018). Naïve Bayes algorithms were earlier explained to be amazingly accurate on many classification duties even when the limited autonomy assumption on which they are based is disrupted (Alsharif, et al., 2019). XGBoost is a package of gradient tree booster algorithms that are scalable, portable and capable of distributed computing. Gradient tree booster is a prominent technique in many applications among ML methods used in practice (Güzel and Önder, 2018).

14.2.3 TRAINING OF DNN AND ENSEMBLE MODELS

While DNN-1 and Ensemble-1 models are trained with 70% of the data, they are tested with 30%. The DNN-2 and Ensemble-2 models were trained and tested with 5-fold cross-validation. Different activation function, optimization algorithm, loss function and epoch values were used in the training of DNN models. Models with the best results were recorded and classification performances were presented. The parameters of the best DNN models were shown in Table 14.2.

One of the important parameters affecting performance in the training of DNN models is the optimization algorithm. One of the important parameters affecting performance in the training of DNN models is the optimization algorithm. The optimization algorithm defines how the parameters in the DNN model are updated (An et al., 2018). That is, the learning algorithm defines how training will take place. In

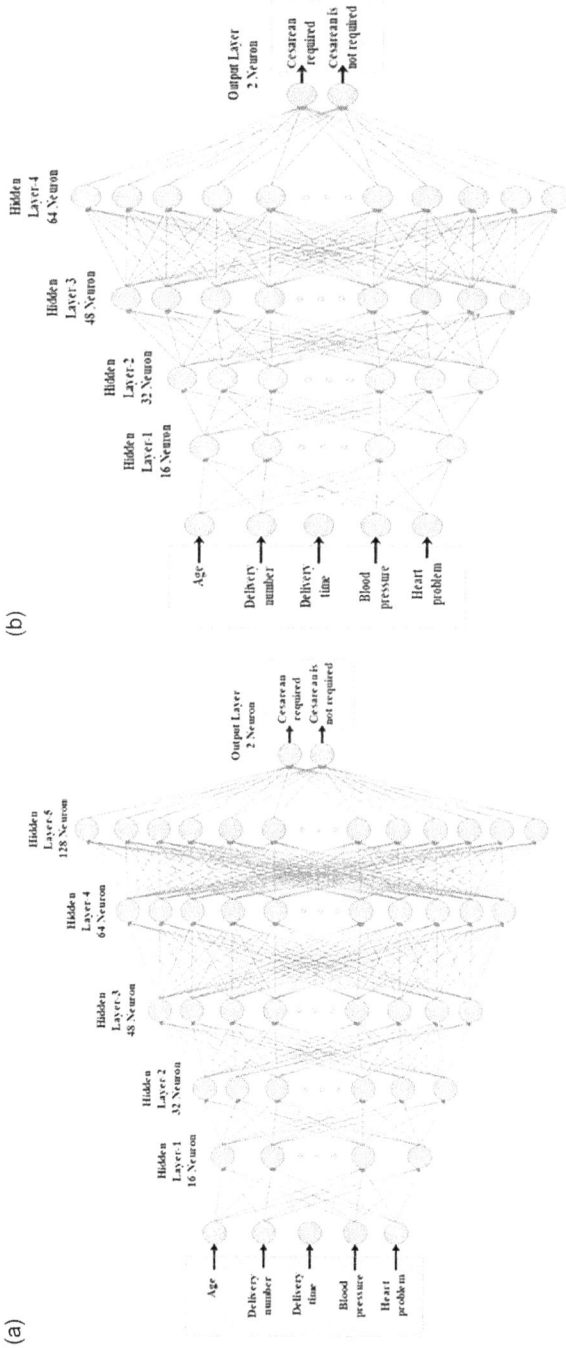

FIGURE 14.2 Structure of DNN models: (a) DNN-1. (b) DNN-2.

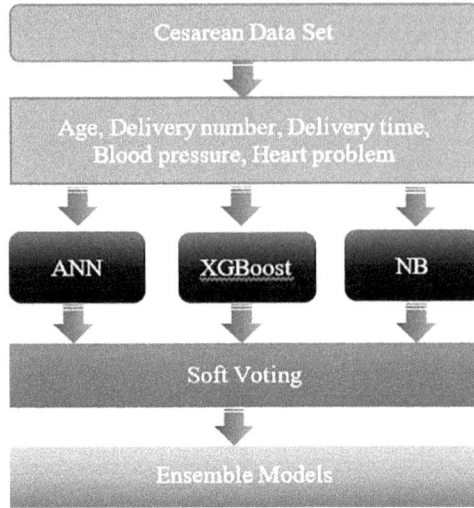

FIGURE 14.3 The structure of the ensemble models.

TABLE 14.2
Parameters of DNN Models

	DNN-1	DNN-2
Parameters	**Value**	**Value**
Optimizer algorithm	Adamax	Nadam
Learning rate	0.002	0.0002
Hidden layer activation function	Elu	Elu
Output layer activation function	Softmax	Softmax
Number of input layer neurons	5	5
Number of hidden layers	5	4
Number of hidden layers neurons	16,32,48,64,128	16,32,48,64
Number of output layers neuron	2	2
Learning cycle	100 Epochs	75 Epochs
Loss function	MSE	MSE

the training of DNN models, six different optimization algorithms (Adam, Adadelta, Sgd, Rmsprop, Adamax and Nadam) have been tried. The best classification performance was obtained in Adamax and Nadam algorithms. Learning rate is another parameter that affects model performances. It determines to what extent the link weights between neurons are updated. In the models, 0.002 and 0.0002 learning rates are used, respectively.

Loss function is used in calculating model error and affects model performance. The value of this function is desired to approach 0 with various optimization techniques (Kızrak and Bolata, 2018). In DNN, binary cross-entropy and mean-squared error (MSE) are the two main loss functions. For this reason, these two loss functions were tried while the models were trained. However, the best classification performance was achieved by MSE.

Another important parameter that needs to be determined for training of DNN models is the activation function. This function is used to simulate the response state of the biological neuron and obtain the neuron output (Karacı, 2020b). Elu, tanh, relu activation functions were tried in the training of DNN models. The best classification performance was obtained in the Elu activation function. Softmax activation function was used in the output layer since the models perform classification. Softmax is generally preferred in the output layer of DNN models that perform two or more classification operations. The number of hidden layers and neurons is another important parameter. The DNN-1 and DNN-2 models consist of five (16, 32, 48, 64, 128) and four (16, 32, 48, 64) hidden layers, respectively.

It is important to adjust the parameters of individual classifiers in the training of Ensemble models. The following parameters are used in the Ensemble-1 model:

- *XGBoost*: booster = 'gblinear,' learning_rate = 0.01, n_estimators = 200, max_depth = 6, normalize_type = 'tree,' subsample = 1
- *ANN*: solver = 'sgd,' alpha=1e-5, activation= 'tanh,' learning_rate= 'constant,' learning_rate_init = 0.00001, hidden_layer_sizes = (30), random_state = 1, max_iter = 500
- *NB*: Used with default parameters.

In Ensemble-2 model, only ANN model parameters were changed. This change is hidden_layer_sizes = (47).

Recall (sensitivity), specificity and accuracy (ACC) metrics were used to evaluate the classification performance of the models. Recall reveals how accurately the models classify those who need to have a cesarean section, and specificity reveals how accurately they classify those who need to have a normal delivery. That is, Recall gives the correct classification rate of true positives, while specificity gives the correct classification rate of true negatives. Recall, specificity and accuracy are defined as in Equation (9.1) (Karacı, 2020a; Karacı, 2020b; Darmawahyuni, Nurmaini and Firdaus, 2019).

$$\text{Recall}(R) = \frac{TP}{TP+FN}, \text{Specificity}(S) = \frac{TN}{TN+FP}, \text{Acuracy}(ACC)$$

$$= \frac{TP+TN}{TP+TN+FP+FN} \tag{14.1}$$

14.3 RESULTS

This section explains the classification performances of all models as comparative. The R, S and ACC metrics of the DNN-1, Ensemble-1, ANN-1, XGB-1 and NB-1 models are shown in Table 14.3. These metrics show the performance of the models on 30% test data. In evaluating the classification performance of models, evaluating the R and S parameters together is important for making a more accurate decision.

TABLE 14.3
Performance Values for 30% Test Data of Models

Metrics	DNN-1	ANN-1	XGB-1	NB-1	Ensemble-1
R	0.92	0	1	0.85	0.92
S	0.82	1	0	0.73	0.73
ACC	0.88	0.46	0.54	0.79	0.83

The fact that both the *R* and *S* metrics are very high indicates that the model classifies both true positives and true negatives highly accurately.

According to Table 14.3, the best classification performance belongs to the DNN-1 model. The DNN-1 model correctly classifies those who should have a cesarean section by 92%, and those who should have a normal birth by 82%. The DNN-1 model classifies both true positives and true negatives at a high accuracy rate compared to other models. The Ensemble-1 model correctly classifies those who should have a cesarean section by 92%, and those who should have a normal birth by 73%. The XGB-1 model correctly classifies those who need to have a cesarean section at a rate of 100% and those who need to have a normal birth at a rate of 0%. This model classifies true positives without errors. It can therefore be used to verify the "cesarean" result obtained from DNN-1 and Ensemble-1 models. ANN-1 model, on the contrary of XGB-1 model, classifies those who should have normal birth by 100% correctly. This model classifies true negatives without errors. It can therefore be used to verify the "normal birth" result obtained from DNN-1 and Ensemble-1 models. According to accuracy values, model performances are as follows: (a) DNN-1, (b) Ensemble-1, (c) NB-1, (d) XGB-1 and (e) ANN-1. Another point of note here is that the Ensemble-1 model has higher classification performance than individual classifiers. Since Ensemble classifiers combine the best results of individual classifiers, overall they also have a better classification performance.

The R, S and ACC metrics of the DNN-2, Ensemble-2, ANN-2, XGB-2 and NB-2 models are shown in Table 14.4. These models are models trained and tested with 5-fold cross-validation. Model performances are from large to small according to ACC metric: (a) DNN-2, (b) Ensemble-2, (c) NB-2, (d) XGB-2 and (e) ANN-2. Model performance decreased slightly in 5-fold cross-validation. However, the ranking has not changed. Again, the model with the highest classification performance is the

TABLE 14.4
5-Fold Cross-Validation Performance Values of Models

Metrics	DNN-2	ANN-2	XGB-2	NB-2	Ensemble-2
Mean R	0.77	0	1	0.68	0.77
Mean S	0.83	1	0	0.60	0.60
Mean ACC	0.80	0.43	0.58	0.65	0.70

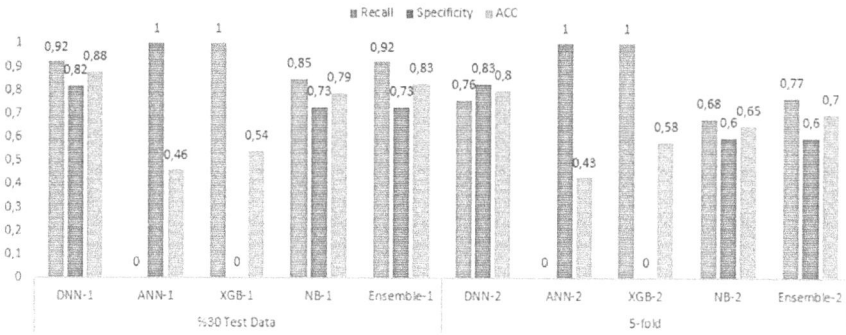

FIGURE 14.4 Performance metrics graph of models.

DNN-2 model. This model correctly classifies those who need to have a cesarean section by 77% and those who need to have a normal birth by 83%. The ANN-2 and XGB-2 models have classification performance similar to the ANN-1 and XGB-1 models. The ANN-2 model classifies true negatives without errors, while the XGB-2 model classifies true positives without errors. The ANN-2 model can therefore be used to confirm the "normal birth" result obtained from the DNN-2 model, while the XGB-2 model can be used to confirm the "cesarean section" result. Ensemble-2 model has lower performance as classification performance than DNN-2 model. However, it can be used to validate both the "cesarean" and "normal birth" result obtained from the DNN-2 model.

The comparison of R, S and ACC metrics for all models is shown in Figure 14.4. As seen in this figure, the most stable models in terms of accurate classification of both true negatives and true positives are the DNN-1 and DNN-2 models. Second place is Ensemble-1 and Ensemble-2 models.

Table 14.5 shows the R, S and ACC values of the models for each fold. In the DNN-2 model, the largest R value (0.9) was obtained in the Fold-4 step, and the largest S value (0.9) was obtained in the Fold-1 step. In the Ensemble-2 model, the largest R (1) and S (0.88) were obtained in the Fold-1 step.

The confusion matrix is an effective method used to show the numbers of True Positive, False Positive, True Negative and False Negative in model prediction. In Figure 14.5, the complexity matrices obtained from the test data of the models are shown.

DNN models developed in this study have higher classification performance than SVM (accuracy: 58.33%, recall: 90.9%) and NB (accuracy: 70.83%, recall: 87.50%) models developed by Alsharif et al. (2019) and tested with 30% test data. When the number of data and attributes is low, it is said that DNN models will not have sufficient prediction and classification performance. However, the DNN model showed higher classification performance in the cesarean data set than Ensemble, ANN, XGBoost, SVM and NB models. In addition, the DNN models in this study have higher classification performance than ANN model (80% accuracy and 84% recall) developed by Sana et al. (2012) on a different cesarean data set.

TABLE 14.5

R, S and ACC Values for Each Fold of the Models

Models	Fold-1			Fold-2			Fold-3			Fold-4			Fold-5		
	R	S	ACC	R	S	ACC	R	S	ACC	R	S	ACC	R	S	ACC
DNN-2	0.67	0.9	0.81	0.78	0.71	0.75	0.83	1	0.88	0.9	0.84	0.88	0.67	0.71	0.69
Ensemble-2	1	0.88	0.94	0.5	0.5	0.5	0.67	0.57	0.62	0.78	0.71	0.75	0.9	0.34	0.69
NB-2	0.88	0.88	0.88	0.5	0.5	0.5	0.56	0.57	0.56	0.56	0.71	0.62	0.9	0.33	0.69
XGB-2	1	0	0.5	1	0	0.62	1	0	0.56	1	0	0.56	1	0	0.62
ANN-2	0	1	0.5	0	1	0.38	0	1	0.44	0	1	0.44	0	1	0.38

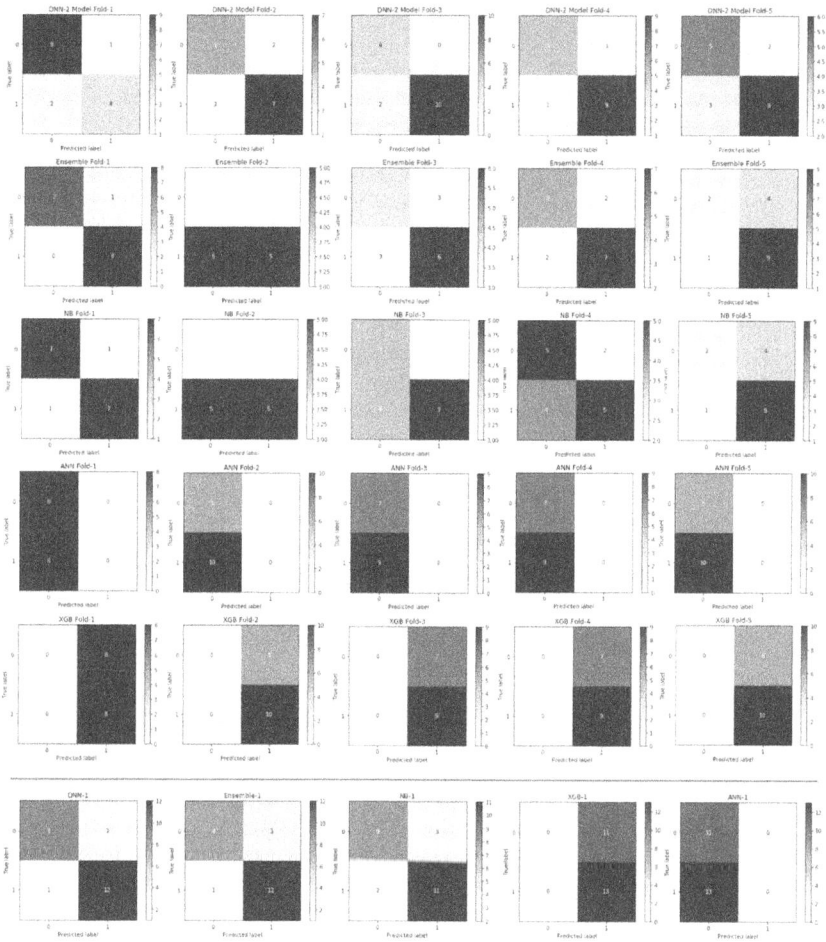

FIGURE 14.5 Confusion matrix of models.

14.4 CONCLUSION

In this study, the performances of different DNN and Ensemble models were tested on cesarean data set. Model performances are demonstrated by both 30% test data and 5-fold cross-validation method. It has been determined that DNN models classify both true positives and true negatives more accurately than other models. The second highest classification performance was obtained in the Ensemble models. In addition, XGBoost models can be used to verify the true positives obtained from DNN and Ensemble models, while ANN models can be used to verify the true negatives. Rather than developing a single model, it is more effective to verify the classification results of models through these models by developing more than one suitable model. DNN models have higher classification performance than similar studies in the literature. Contrary to common belief, DNN models can also have effective classification and prediction performance on data sets where the number of data and attributes is low.

REFERENCES

Alsharif, O.S.S., Elbayoudi, K.M., Aldrawi, A.A.S., Akyol, K., Evaluation of different machine learning methods for caesarean data classification. *International Journal of Information Engineering and Electronic Business*, 5, 19–23, (2019).

An, W., Wang, H., Sun, Q., Xu, J., Dai, Q., & Zhang, L., A PID controller approach for stochastic optimization of deep networks. Proceedings of the IEEE Computer Society Conference on Computer Vision and Pattern Recognition, Salt Lake City, 8522–8531, (2018). Doi: 10.1109/CVPR.2018.00889.

Bouwmans, T., Javed, S., Sultana, M., Jung, S. K., Deep neural network concepts for background subtraction: A systematic review and comparative evaluation, *Neural Networks*, 117, 8–66, (2019). Doi: 10.1016/j.neunet.2019.04.024.

Darmawahyuni, A., Nurmaini, S., Firdaus, F., Coronary heart disease interpretation based on deep neural network. *Computer Engineering and Applications*, 8(1), 1–12, (2019).

Feng, S., Zhou H., Dong, H., Using deep neural network with small dataset to predict material defects. *Materials & Design*, 162, 300–310, (2019). Doi: 10.1016/j.matdes.2018.11.060.

Géron, A. *Hands-On Machine Learning with Scikit-Learn and TensorFlow: Concepts, Tools, and Techniques to Build Intelligent Systems*. O'Reilly Media, (2017), Sebastopol, USA.

Güzel, B.E., Önder, D., Performance comparision of boosting classifiers on breast termography images. *2018* 26th Signal Processing and Communications Applications Conference (SIU), 1–4, (2018), IEEE, İzmir, Turkey.

Kan, A., Classical cesarean section, precision surgery in obstetrics and gynecology, 2020. Doi: 10.1055/s-0039-3402072.

Karacı A., Fiziksel ve motor engelli çocukların öz bakım problemlerinin derin sinir ağları ile sınıflandırılması, *Politeknik Dergisi*, 23(2): 333–341, (2020b).

Karacı, A, Hibrit Topluluk Sınıflandırıcı İle Parkinson Hastalığının Tespit Edilmesi, 2nd International Turkish World Engineering and Science Congress, November 7–10, 153–158, (2019), Antalya, Turkey.

Karacı, A., Predicting breast cancer with deep neural networks. In: Hemanth D., Kose U. (eds) *Artificial Intelligence and Applied Mathematics in Engineering Problems. ICAIAME 2019. Lecture Notes on Data Engineering and Communications Technologies*, vol 43. Springer, Cham, (2020a)

Karaci, A., Yaprak, H., Ozkaraca, O., Demir, I., & Simsek, O., Estimating the properties of ground-waste-brick mortars using DNN and ANN, *CMES*, 118(1), 207–228, (2019).

Kızrak M. A., Bolata B., Comprehensive survey of deep learning in crowd analysis, *International Journal of Informatics Technologies*, 11(3), 263–286, (2018).

Moreno-Seco F., Iñesta J.M., de León P.J.P., Micó L., Comparison of classifier fusion methods for classification in pattern recognition tasks, *Lecture Notes in Computer Science*, 4109, 705–713, (2006).

Polikar, R., Ensemble learning, in Cha Zhang and Yunqian Ma (Eds.), "*Ensemble Machine Learning Methods and Applications*. Springer US, 1–34, (2012).

Qi, C., & Tang, X., A hybrid ensemble method for improved prediction of slope stability. *International Journal for Numerical and Analytical Methods in Geomechanics*, 42(15), 1823–1839, (2018).

Rezaee, M. J., Jozmaleki, M., Valipour, M., Integrating dynamic fuzzy C-means, data envelopment analysis and artificial neural network to online prediction performance of companies in stock Exchange, *Physica A: Statistical Mechanics and its Applications*, 489, 78–93, (2018).

Sagi, O, Rokach, L., Ensemble learning: A survey, *WIREs Data Mining and Knowledge Discovery*, 8:e1249, 2–18, (2018). Doi: 10.1002/widm.1249.

Sana, A., Razzaq, S., and Ferzund, J., Automated diagnosis and cause analysis of cesarean section using machine learning techniques, *International Journal of Machine Learning and Computing*, 2(5), 677–680, (2012). Doi: 10.7763/ijmlc.2012.v2.213.

Uci, https://archive.ics.uci.edu/ml/datasets/Caesarian+Section+Classification+Dataset, Son Erişim Tarihi: (2020, February 18).

Yisma, E., Smithers, L. G., Lynch, J. W., Mol, B. W., Cesarean section in Ethiopia: prevalence and sociodemographic characteristics, *The Journal of Maternal-Fetal & Neonatal Medicine*, 32(7), 1130–1135, (2019). Doi: 10.1080/14767058.2017.1401606.

15 Transfer Learning for Classification of Brain Tumor

Prajoy Podder and Subrato Bharati
Bangladesh University of Engineering and Technology

Mohammad Atikur Rahman
Ranada Prasad Shaha University

Utku Kose
Suleyman Demirel University

CONTENTS

15.1 INTRODUCTION

Brain is the most complex and essential organ constructed by billions of cells. A brain tumor emerges when there is the uncontrolled division of cells shaping an uncommon gathering of cells inside or around the brain. That gathering of cells can influence the regular use of the mind movement and obliterate the healthy cells (Bahadure, Ray, & Thethi, 2018; Havaei et al., 2017; Pereira, Pinto, Alves, & Silva, 2016). Brain tumors ordered to high-grade or malignant tumors and low-grade or benign tumors. The cancer is occurred by malignant tumors where the benign is non-cancerous. Nevertheless, malignant tumors increase rapidly with uncontrolled boundaries. These tumors can be started in the cerebrum itself which is known as originated or primary malignant (Bharati, Podder, & Mondal, 2020a; Bharati, Rahman, & Podder, 2018; Gordillo, Montseny, & Sobrevilla, 2013; Sharma, Kaur, & Gujral, 2014).

The imaging technique including magnetic resonance imaging (MRI) is depends on displaying tumor evolution and identifying the brain tumors in both the treatment phases and detection. Medical imaging system such as MRI has a major effect on the diagnosis and detection for its capacity to give information about the brain abnormalities and structure inside the brain tissues owing to the high-resolution MRI images (Amin, Sharif, Yasmin, & Fernandes, 2017; Cabria & Gondra, 2017; Zhang & Xu, 2016). Indeed, researchers introduced various automated methods for classification and detection of brain tumors conducting brain MRI since it has developed probably to load and scan medical images. Nevertheless, neural networks and support vector machines (SVM) are usually applied for their efficient performance throughout the recent years (Bharati, Podder, & Mondal, 2020c; Bharati, Podder, Mondal, Mahmood, & Raihan-Al-Masud, 2018; Bharati, Robel, Rahman, Podder, & Gandhi, 2019; Pan et al., 2015). However, nowadays, transfer learning approaches set a related trend in machine learning (ML) as the transfer learning model can proficiently offer complex relationships apart from considering a massive number of nodes such as shallow models, for example, K-nearest neighbor and SVM. Hence, they produced quickly to develop the model in various health informatics sections like medical informatics, bioinformatics and medical image evaluation (Crum, Camara, & Hill, 2006; Haux, 2010; Min, Lee, & Yoon, 2017).

The role of this work is employing the transfer learning concepts like VGG to present an automated classification of brain tumors from brain MRI and observe its performance. The suggested methodology is proposed to differentiate between different sorts of brain tumors including sarcoma, glioblastoma, etc., and normal brain employing brain MRI. We propose VGG model for detection and classification of brain MRI.

15.2   BACKGROUND

Deep learning (DL) is effective in multiple level classification of images from a large image data set by building a hierarchy of features. In this case, higher level features are defined from lower level features (Bharati, Khan, Podder, & Hung, 2020; Bharati, Podder, & Mondal, 2020b; Menze et al., 2014). Traditional neural network models have been extended by various DL architectures due to the addition of more hidden layers to the NN architecture between the input and output layers. Researchers have got a huge interest on DL in the recent years because of it having good performance capability and accuracy. It can be considered comparatively the best solution in various problems in medical image (X-ray, CT, MRI, ultrasound) related applications such as image segmentation, image noise removing, registration and classification (Ahmed, Hall, Goldgof, Liu, & Gatenby; Anuse & Vyas, 2016; Bharati, Podder, et al., 2020c). Many researchers have already worked on the brain tumor detection. Both ML and DL methods have been applied in order to classify the brain tumor (binary classification or multilevel classification).

Sonu Sohag et al. proposed FCM (Fuzzy C-means) segmentation of MRI images in order to handle the data set and identify the tumor region as well as classify the type of tumors accurately (Suhag & Saini, 2015). They also used multi-SVM (Suhag & Saini, 2015) for classifying three type of tumors such as Metastasis, Gliomas and Astrocytoma. The data set used in Suhag & Saini (2015) had 130 images only. Dogra,

Jain, & Sood (2019) proposed a hybrid technique consisting of fuzzy segmentation and ML classifiers (SVM and K Nearest Neighbour(KNN)) in order to classify the Glioma tumors (High grade type and low grade type) from the MRI image. They used a data set of 300 images and 10-fold cross-validation. Arun Kumar et al. used a nature-inspired optimization algorithm named Grey Wolf Optimization as a feature selection technique on MR images (3,064) of T1 type (Kumar, Ansari, & Ashok, 2019). They selected only 315 images after pre-processing. They used multi-SVM (Jayachandran & Sundararaj, 2015; Kumar et al., 2019) for classifying the type of tumors. A Reema Mathew applied a filter named anisotropic diffusion for pre-processing the brain MRI image and then used discrete wavelet transform (DWT) for extracting the features from the images (Mathew & Anto 2017). SVM was used for tumor classification (Mathew & Anto 2017).

Another methodology was proposed in Tarkhaneh and Shen (2019) utilizing the evolutionary procedure Differential Evolution called ALDE (Adaptive Differential Evolution with Lévy Distribution). In multi-level thresholding, differential evolution is utilized for keeping up the harmony between exploitation and exploration. The multi-level thresholding technique had been utilized for MRI image segmentation. For the segmentation, a DL technique (Thaha et al., 2019) utilizing convolutional neural network (CNN) had been utilized. This technique utilized 3×3 little kernels for the structure of CNN. A new technique offered in paper Hu et al. (2019) according to multi-cascade CNN for maintaining multi-scale features and various local pixels of 3D MRI and improving the achieved results. It had excluded the false positives and smoothens the edges of tumor images.

The results of brain MRI have been verified on different BRATS 2013, 2015 and 2018 data sets. A tumor might be detected as either benign or malignant. In Rajam, Reshmi, Suresh, Suresh, and Sindhuja (2018), the researchers proposed a technique with two phases to detect the tumor. A two-pathway-group-based CNN model offered in Razzak, Imran, and Xu (2018) also included the global and local contextual features. They achieved a CNN model to moderate the problem of over-fitting and instabilities parameter sharing.

The authors of Kamnitsas et al. (2017) used segmentation technique for brain lesion detection. This technique refers to two key parts such as dual pathway structure. The performances of MRI had been implemented on the two data sets including ISLES 2015 and BRATS 2015. A new method approach such as Cuckoo Search Algorithm had been proposed in Rajinikanth, Fernandes, Bhushan, and Sunder (2018) on MRI images. In Ain, Jaffar, and Choi (2014), the ensemble method was used for classification and used ensemble of SVM after the feature extraction and noise removal stage. Fuzzy c-means is also used for segmentation. Conversely, CNN is commonly applied for the brain tumor prediction, classification and segmentation (Rother, Kolmogorov, & Blake, 2012; Top, Hamarneh, & Abugharbieh, 2011; Vaidhya, Thirunavukkarasu, Alex, & Krishnamurthi; Wang et al., 2016). CNNs provided good result for prediction, classification and segmentation among all methods. Both 2D-CNNs (Havaei et al., 2017; Havaei, Dutil, Pal, Larochelle, & Jodoin, 2015) and 3D-CNNs (Kamnitsas et al., 2017; Mlynarski, Delingette, Criminisi, & Ayache, 2019;

Trivizakis et al., 2018) were implemented to develop brain tumor prediction, classification and segmentation methods. Segmentation approaches categorize the MRI image patch into various classes, including healthy tissues, necrosis, enhancing core, edema and nonenhancing core.

15.3 METHODOLOGY AND PROPOSED MODELS

The MRI data set applied for tumor detection and classification has been described in this part. Essential parameters for implementing optimized VGG model and predicting the classification accuracy (CA) have also been illustrated here. The MRI image data set used to train and test the transfer learning architectures is available in Rajam et al. (2018). 85% of image data, i.e., 215 images, are used for testing purpose and 15% of image data, i.e., 38 images, are used for testing purpose.

Figures 15.1 and 15.2 illustrate the model summary of VGG-16 and VGG-19, respectively. The number of non-trainable parameters of VGG-16 and VGG-19 is 14714688 and 20024384, respectively.

Table 15.1 presents the performance of VGG-16 for the brain tumor detection. A loss function can determine the performance of a given predictor for classifying the input data points in a data set. The smaller the loss, the better the job of the classifier is at modelling the relationship between the input data and the output targets. When the epoch is 2, the loss in the training stage is 0.6613. But when it is 12, the loss is 0.3584.

In the data augmentation stage, the value of the rotation range is 15. It is the range of random rotations. No horizontal or vertical flipping is applied. The input size at the time of loading the base VGG-19 network is $224 \times 224 \times 3$. The base model is pre-trained on Imagenet. The transfer learning-driven networks are trained by Adam optimization algorithm with 0.001 initial learning rate. The value of batch size is 16, and epoch is 25.

The CA denotes typically the capability to predict the target class correctly and guess the amount of predicted attribute for new data. CA of 0.8683 (86.83%) is achieved in the training stage at 23rd epoch when VGG-16 is deployed. On the other hand, CA of 0.8662 (86.62%) is acquired in the validation stage at 24th epoch for the same architecture.

94.47% area under the curve (AUC) is achieved in the training stage at 15th epoch when VGG-16 is deployed. On the other hand, 86.24% AUC is acquired in the validation stage at 24th epoch for the same architecture.

Figures 15.3 and 15.4 show the performance of loss and AUC for training and validation stage when VGG-16 is applied. The values of TP, FP, TN and FN are 19, 3, 3 and 1, respectively. Here TP and FP refer to true positive and false positive, respectively, while TN and FN refer to true negative and false negative, respectively. The achieved precision and recall for VGG-16 is 87% and 95%, respectively. In addition to the overall CA, receiver operating characteristic (ROC) curves are evaluated during analysis. Figure 15.5 represents the ROC curves obtained after applying optimized VGG-16 model.

Layer (type)	Output Shape	Param #
input_2 (Input Layer)	[(None, 224, 224, 3)]	0
block1_conv1 (Conv2D)	(None, 224, 224, 64)	1792
block1_conv2 (Conv2D)	(None, 224, 224, 64)	36928
block1_pool (MaxPooling2D)	(None, 112, 112, 64)	0
block2_conv1 (Conv2D)	(None, 112, 112, 128)	73856
block2_conv2 (Conv2D)	(None, 112, 112, 128)	147584
block2_pool (MaxPooling2D)	(None, 56, 56, 128)	0
block3_conv1 (Conv2D)	(None, 56, 56, 256)	295168
block3_conv2 (Conv2D)	(None, 56, 56, 256)	590080
block3_conv3 (Conv2D)	(None, 56, 56, 256)	590080
block3_pool (MaxPooling2D)	(None, 28, 28, 256)	0
block4_conv1 (Conv2D)	(None, 28, 28, 512)	1180160
block4_conv2 (Conv2D)	(None, 28, 28, 512)	2359808
block4_conv3 (Conv2D)	(None, 28, 28, 512)	2359808
block4_pool (MaxPooling2D)	(None, 14, 14, 512)	0
block5_conv1 (Conv2D)	(None, 14, 14, 512)	2359808
block5_conv2 (Conv2D)	(None, 14, 14, 512)	2359808
block5_conv3 (Conv2D)	(None, 14, 14, 512)	2359808
block5_pool (MaxPooling2D)	(None, 7, 7, 512)	0
average_pooling2d_1 (Average	(None, 1, 1, 512)	0
flatten (Flatten)	(None, 512)	0
dense_2 (Dense)	(None, 256)	131328
dropout_1 (Dropout)	(None, 256)	0
dense_3 (Dense)	(None, 2)	514

Total params: 14,846,530
Trainable params: 131,842
Non-trainable params: 14,714,688
None

FIGURE 15.1 Model summary of VGG-16.

Layer (type)	Output Shape	Param #
input_1 (InputLayer)	[(None, 224, 224, 3)]	0
block1_conv1 (Conv2D)	(None, 224, 224, 64)	1792
block1_conv2 (Conv2D)	(None, 224, 224, 64)	36928
block1_pool (MaxPooling2D)	(None, 112, 112, 64)	0
block2_conv1 (Conv2D)	(None, 112, 112, 128)	73856
block2_conv2 (Conv2D)	(None, 112, 112, 128)	147584
block2_pool (MaxPooling2D)	(None, 56, 56, 128)	0
block3_conv1 (Conv2D)	(None, 56, 56, 256)	295168
block3_conv2 (Conv2D)	(None, 56, 56, 256)	590080
block3_conv3 (Conv2D)	(None, 56, 56, 256)	590080
block3_conv4 (Conv2D)	(None, 56, 56, 256)	590080
block3_pool (MaxPooling2D)	(None, 28, 28, 256)	0
block4_conv1 (Conv2D)	(None, 28, 28, 512)	1180160
block4_conv2 (Conv2D)	(None, 28, 28, 512)	2359808
block4_conv3 (Conv2D)	(None, 28, 28, 512)	2359808
block4_conv4 (Conv2D)	(None, 28, 28, 512)	2359808
block4_pool (MaxPooling2D)	(None, 14, 14, 512)	0
block5_conv1 (Conv2D)	(None, 14, 14, 512)	2359808
block5_conv2 (Conv2D)	(None, 14, 14, 512)	2359808
block5_conv3 (Conv2D)	(None, 14, 14, 512)	2359808
block5_conv4 (Conv2D)	(None, 14, 14, 512)	2359808
block5_pool (MaxPooling2D)	(None, 7, 7, 512)	0
average_pooling2d (AveragePo	(None, 1, 1, 512)	0
flatten (Flatten)	(None, 512)	0
dense (Dense)	(None, 256)	131328
dropout (Dropout)	(None, 256)	0
dense_1 (Dense)	(None, 2)	514

Total params: 20,156,226
Trainable params: 131,842
Non-trainable params: 20,024,384

None

FIGURE 15.2   Model summary of VGG-19.

TABLE 15.1

Performance of VGG-16 for Brain Tumor Detection

Epoch	Training Stage			Validation Stage		
	Loss	Accuracy	AUC	Loss	Accuracy	AUC
1	0.6980	0.6256	0.6514	0.5899	0.8462	0.8373
2	0.6613	0.6209	0.6888	0.5331	0.7308	0.8033
3	0.5796	0.6777	0.7625	0.5094	0.8077	0.8506
4	0.4749	0.7867	0.8547	0.4967	0.8462	0.8491
5	0.5213	0.7204	0.8160	0.4973	0.7692	0.8373
6	0.5230	0.7299	0.8182	0.5580	0.6538	0.7648
7	0.4717	0.7725	0.8599	0.5070	0.7308	0.8210
8	0.4165	0.8009	0.8973	0.4935	0.8077	0.8425
9	0.4018	0.8057	0.9032	0.4884	0.8177	0.8402
10	0.3895	0.8678	0.9111	0.5581	0.6154	0.7618
11	0.4378	0.7867	0.8767	0.4984	0.8077	0.8351
12	0.3584	0.8531	0.9338	0.4738	0.8077	0.8402
13	0.3840	0.8214	0.9102	0.5220	0.7308	0.7781
14	0.4050	0.8199	0.8961	0.5172	0.8077	0.8351
15	0.3234	0.8626	0.9447	0.4960	0.8462	0.8373
16	0.3429	0.8673	0.9288	0.4889	0.8077	0.8388
17	0.3337	0.8436	0.9334	0.5050	0.7308	0.8151
18	0.3680	0.8199	0.9154	0.5164	0.8662	0.8358
19	0.3697	0.8389	0.9178	0.4857	0.8592	0.8373
20	0.3508	0.8246	0.9229	0.4682	0.8077	0.8491
21	0.3595	0.8483	0.9209	0.4832	0.7308	0.8306
22	0.3665	0.8246	0.9176	0.4722	0.8277	0.8516
23	0.3399	0.8683	0.9329	0.4655	0.8077	0.8565
24	0.3341	0.8389	0.9347	0.4643	0.8077	0.8624
25	0.3345	0.8673	0.9317	0.4828	0.8462	0.8580

Table 15.2 describes the performance of VGG-19 for the brain tumor detection with respect to the loss, accuracy and AUC. The chosen optimizer is "Adam." When the epoch is 2, the training loss is 0.3947. But when it is 12, the loss is 0.3584. The validation loss is 0.4680 at 19th epoch. Highest training accuracy of 0.8636 (86.36%) is achieved at 20th epoch. Highest testing accuracy of 0.8532 (85.32%) is performed at 20th epoch. Highest AUC of 0.8482 (84.82%) is obtained in the validation stage at 20th epoch.

Figures 15.6 and 15.7 show the performance of loss and AUC for training and validation stage when VGG-19 is applied. The values of TP, FP, TN and FN are 17, 4, 4 and 1, respectively. Here TP and FP refer to true positive and false positive, respectively, while TN and FN refer to true negative and false negative, respectively. The achieved precision and recall for VGG-19 is 81% and 94%, respectively.

Epoch vs. Loss

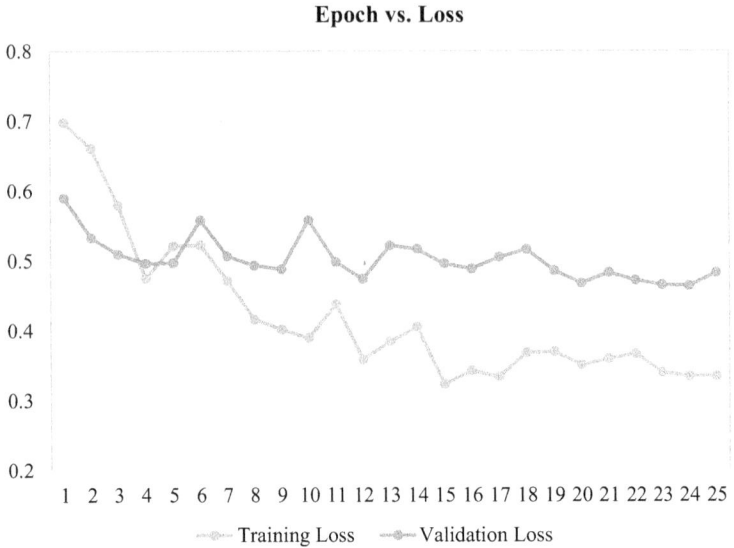

FIGURE 15.3 Training and validation loss using VGG-16.

Epoch vs. AUC

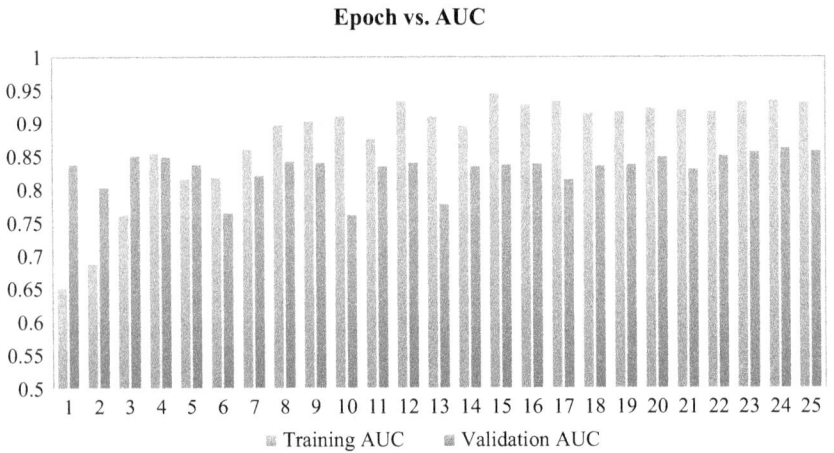

FIGURE 15.4 Training and validation AUC using VGG-16.

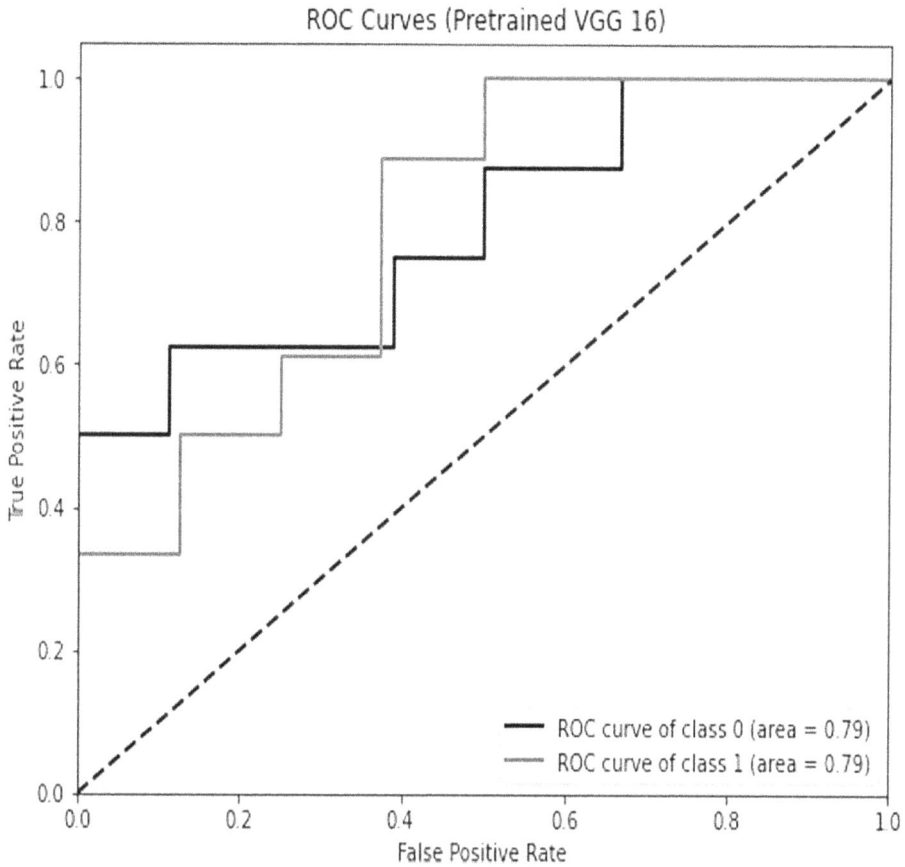

FIGURE 15.5 Receiver operating characteristic curves of classifier.

15.4 CONCLUSION

This paper presents the transfer learning models like VGG-16 and 19 for detection, prediction and classification of the brain MRI. The VGG-16 provides the highest training and validation accuracy of 86.73% and 85.80%, respectively. Moreover, the achieved recall and precision for VGG-19 is 94% and 81%, respectively. Thus, these models can be detected brain tumor on MRI images. Furthermore, this paper depicts the ROC plot for these algorithms. The obtained AUC in the validation and training stage is 85% and 83.73%, respectively, when optimized VGG-19 is applied.

TABLE 15.2
Performance of VGG-19 for Brain Tumor Detection

Epoch	Training Stage			Validation Stage		
	Loss	Accuracy	AUC	Loss	Accuracy	AUC
1	0.738	0.5972	0.5746	0.5987	0.7692	0.8217
2	0.6669	0.5924	0.6558	0.6206	0.6538	0.7330
3	0.5952	0.6493	0.7432	0.5387	0.7308	0.8033
4	0.5479	0.7393	0.7974	0.5617	0.7692	0.8018
5	0.5497	0.7411	0.8012	0.5220	0.7692	0.8136
6	0.5428	0.7441	0.8051	0.5111	0.7692	0.8210
7	0.5110	0.7583	0.8300	0.5234	0.8077	0.8077
8	0.4786	0.7773	0.8617	0.5312	0.7692	0.8077
9	0.4885	0.7962	0.8508	0.5169	0.7692	0.8107
10	0.4877	0.7946	0.8516	0.5131	0.7692	0.8136
11	0.4608	0.7867	0.8660	0.5236	0.7692	0.8180
12	0.4374	0.8057	0.8893	0.5882	0.6923	0.8092
13	0.4490	0.7915	0.8696	0.5408	0.6923	0.7929
14	0.4234	0.8104	0.8902	0.5222	0.7692	0.8254
15	0.4164	0.8389	0.8963	0.5096	0.7692	0.8314
16	0.4656	0.7962	0.8615	0.5020	0.7692	0.8284
17	0.4258	0.8199	0.8921	0.4871	0.7692	0.8482
18	0.4233	0.8152	0.8889	0.4867	0.7692	0.8351
19	0.4259	0.8057	0.8892	0.4680	0.8532	0.8417
20	0.3947	0.8636	0.9058	0.5239	0.6923	0.8062
21	0.4328	0.7867	0.8813	0.5167	0.7692	0.8388
22	0.4348	0.8294	0.8790	0.5238	0.7692	0.8402
23	0.4069	0.8246	0.8956	0.5119	0.6538	0.8151
24	0.4000	0.8199	0.9022	0.4870	0.8077	0.8284
25	0.4039	0.8294	0.9005	0.4939	0.8077	0.8373

Epoch vs. Loss

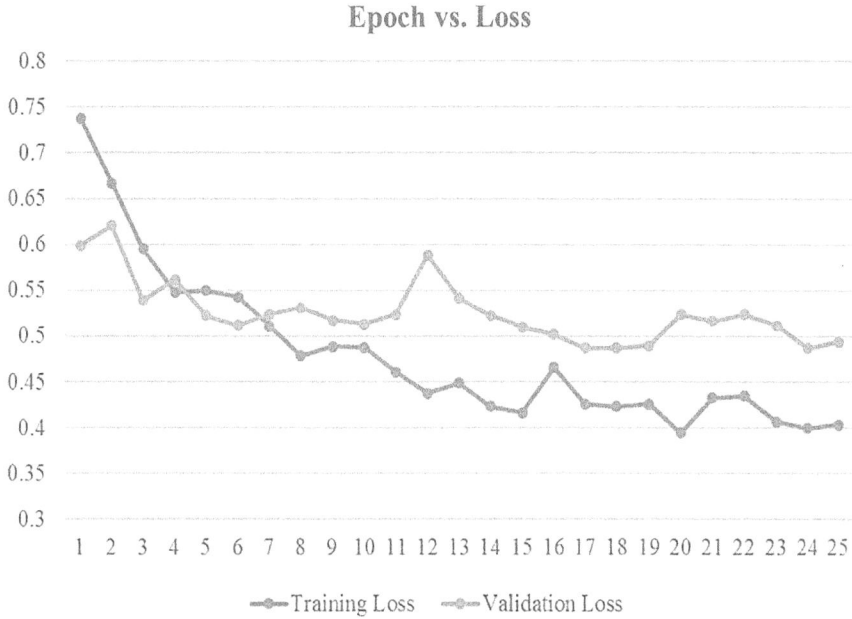

FIGURE 15.6 Training and validation loss using VGG-19.

Epoch vs. Accuracy

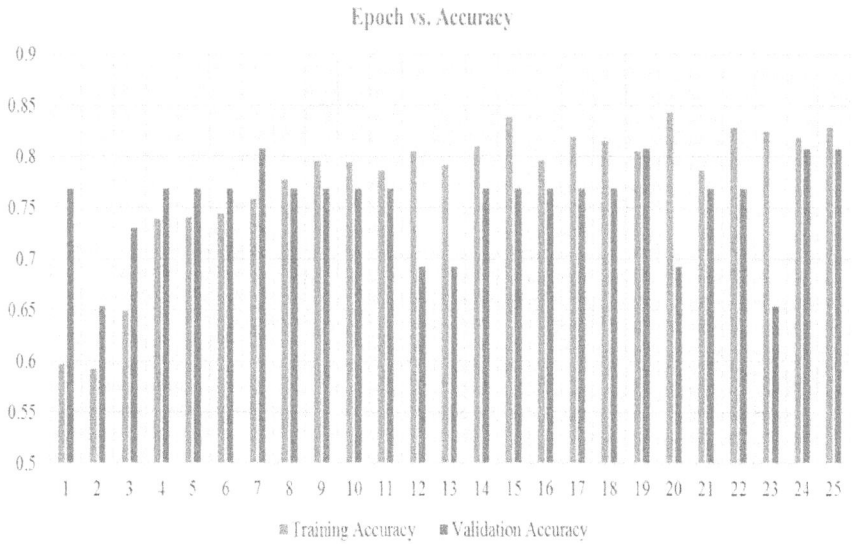

FIGURE 15.7 Training and validation accuracy using VGG-19.

REFERENCES

Ahmed, K. B., Hall, L. O., Goldgof, D. B., Liu, R., & Gatenby, R. A. (2017). *Fine-Tuning Convolutional Deep Features for MRI Based Brain Tumor Classification.* In *Medical Imaging 2017: Computer-Aided Diagnosis* (Vol. 10134, p. 101342E). International Society for Optics and Photonics, Bellingham, WA.

Ain, Q., Jaffar, M. A., & Choi, T.-S. (2014). Fuzzy anisotropic diffusion based segmentation and texture based ensemble classification of brain tumor. *Applied Soft Computing, 21,* 330–340.

Amin, J., Sharif, M., Yasmin, M., & Fernandes, S. L. (2020). A distinctive approach in brain tumor detection and classification using MRI. *Pattern Recognition Letters,* 139, 118–127.

Anuse, A., & Vyas, V. (2016). A novel training algorithm for convolutional neural network. *Complex & Intelligent Systems, 2*(3), 221–234.

Bahadure, N. B., Ray, A. K., & Thethi, H. P. (2018). Comparative approach of MRI-based brain tumor segmentation and classification using genetic algorithm. *Journal of Digital Imaging, 31*(4), 477–489.

Bharati, S., Khan, T. Z., Podder, P., & Hung, N. Q. (2020). A comparative analysis of image denoising problem: Noise models, denoising filters and applications. *Cognitive Internet of Medical Things for Smart Healthcare* (pp. 49–66), Springer, Cham.

Bharati, S., Podder, P., & Mondal, M. R. H. (2020a). Artificial neural network based breast cancer screening: A comprehensive review. *International Journal of Computer Information Systems and Industrial Management Applications, 12,* 125–137.

Bharati, S., Podder, P., & Mondal, M. R. H. (2020b). *Diagnosis of Polycystic Ovary Syndrome Using Machine Learning Algorithms,* In *2020 IEEE Region 10 Symposium (TENSYMP)* (pp. 1486–1489), IEEE, Dhaka, Bangladesh.

Bharati, S., Podder, P., & Mondal, M. R. H. (2020c). Hybrid deep learning for detecting lung diseases from X-ray images. *Informatics in Medicine Unlocked, 20,* 100391.

Bharati, S., Podder, P., Mondal, R., Mahmood, A., & Raihan-Al-Masud, M. (2018). Comparative performance analysis of different classification algorithm for the purpose of prediction of lung cancer. *Paper presented at the International Conference on Intelligent Systems Design and Applications,* Vellore, India.

Bharati, S., Rahman, M. A., & Podder, P. (2018). Breast cancer prediction applying different classification algorithm with comparative analysis using WEKA. *Paper presented at the 2018 4th International Conference on Electrical Engineering and Information & Communication Technology (iCEEiCT),* Dhaka, Bangladesh.

Bharati, S., Robel, M. R. A., Rahman, M. A., Podder, P., & Gandhi, N. (2019). Comparative performance exploration and prediction of fibrosis, malign lymph, metastases. *Normal Lymphogram Using Machine Learning Method.*

Cabria, I., & Gondra, I. (2017). MRI segmentation fusion for brain tumor detection. *Information Fusion, 36,* 1–9.

Crum, W. R., Camara, O., & Hill, D. L. G. (2006). Generalized overlap measures for evaluation and validation in medical image analysis. *IEEE Transactions on Medical Imaging, 25*(11), 1451–1461.

Dogra, J., Jain, S., & Sood, M. (2019). Glioma classification of MR brain tumor employing machine learning. *International Journal of Innovative Technology and Exploring Engineering (IJITEE), 8*(8), 2676–2682.

Gordillo, N., Montseny, E., & Sobrevilla, P. (2013). State of the art survey on MRI brain tumor segmentation. *Magnetic Resonance Imaging, 31*(8), 1426–1438.

Haux, R. (2010). Medical informatics: past, present, future. *International Journal of Medical Informatics, 79*(9), 599–610.

Havaei, M., Davy, A., Warde-Farley, D., Biard, A., Courville, A., Bengio, Y.,... Larochelle, H. (2017). Brain tumor segmentation with deep neural networks. *Medical Image Analysis, 35,* 18–31.

Havaei, M., Dutil, F., Pal, C., Larochelle, H., & Jodoin, P.-M. (2015). *A Convolutional Neural Network Approach to Brain Tumor Segmentation.*

Hu, K., Gan, Q., Zhang, Y., Deng, S., Xiao, F., Huang, W., … Gao, X. (2019). Brain tumor segmentation using multi-cascaded convolutional neural networks and conditional random field. *IEEE Access, 7,* 92615–92629.

Jayachandran, A., & Sundararaj, G. K. (2015). Abnormality segmentation and classification of multi-class brain tumor in MR images using fuzzy logic-based hybrid kernel SVM. *International Journal of Fuzzy Systems, 17*(3), 434–443.

Kamnitsas, K., Ledig, C., Newcombe, V. F. J., Simpson, J. P., Kane, A. D., Menon, D. K., … Glocker, B. (2017). Efficient multi-scale 3D CNN with fully connected CRF for accurate brain lesion segmentation. *Medical image analysis, 36,* 61–78.

Kumar, A., Ansari, M. A., & Ashok, A. (2019). A hybrid framework for brain tumor classification using grey wolf optimization and multi-class support vector machine. *International Journal of Recent Technology and Engineering (IJRTE), 8*(3), 7746–7752.

Mathew, A. R., & Anto, P. B. (2017). *Tumor Detection and Classification of MRI Brain Image Using Wavelet Transform and SVM,* In *2017 International Conference on Signal Processing and Communication (ICSPC)* (pp. 75–78), IEEE, Tamilnadu, India.

Menze, B. H., Jakab, A., Bauer, S., Kalpathy-Cramer, J., Farahani, K., Kirby, J., … Wiest, R. (2014). The multimodal brain tumor image segmentation benchmark (BRATS). *IEEE Transactions on Medical Imaging, 34*(10), 1993–2024.

Min, S., Lee, B., & Yoon, S. (2017). Deep learning in bioinformatics. *Briefings in bioinformatics, 18*(5), 851–869.

Mlynarski, P., Delingette, H., Criminisi, A., & Ayache, N. (2019). 3D convolutional neural networks for tumor segmentation using long-range 2D context. *Computerized Medical Imaging and Graphics, 73,* 60–72.

Pan, Y., Huang, W., Lin, Z., Zhu, W., Zhou, J., Wong, J., & Ding, Z. (2015). *Brain Tumor Grading Based on Neural Networks and Convolutional Neural Networks.* In *2015 37th Annual International Conference of the IEEE Engineering in Medicine and Biology Society (EMBC)* (pp. 699–702). IEEE, USA.

Pereira, S., Pinto, A., Alves, V., & Silva, C. A. (2016). Brain tumor segmentation using convolutional neural networks in MRI images. *IEEE Transactions on Medical Imaging, 35*(5), 1240–1251.

Rajam, R. A., Reshmi, R., Suresh, A., Suresh, A., & Sindhuja, S. (2018). *Segmentation and Analysis of Brain Tumor using Meta-Heuristic Algorithm.* In *2018 International Conference on Recent Trends in Electrical, Control and Communication (RTECC)* (pp. 256–260), IEEE, USA.

Rajinikanth, V., Fernandes, S. L., Bhushan, B., & Sunder, N. R. (2018). *Segmentation and Analysis of Brain Tumor Using Tsallis Entropy and Regularised Level Set.* In *Proceedings of 2nd International Conference on Micro-electronics, Electromagnetics and Telecommunications* (pp. 313–321). Springer, Singapore.

Razzak, M. I., Imran, M., & Xu, G. (2018). Efficient brain tumor segmentation with multiscale two-pathway-group conventional neural networks. *IEEE Journal of Biomedical and Health Informatics, 23*(5), 1911–1919.

Rother, C., Kolmogorov, V., & Blake, A. (2012). Interactive foreground extraction using iterated graph cuts. *ACM Transactions on Graphics, 23,* 3.

Sharma, K., Kaur, A., & Gujral, S. (2014). Brain tumor detection based on machine learning algorithms. *International Journal of Computer Applications, 103*(1), 7–11.

Suhag, S., & Saini, L. M. (2015). *Automatic Brain Tumor Detection and Classification Using SVM Classifier.*

Tarkhaneh, O., & Shen, H. (2019). An adaptive differential evolution algorithm to optimal multi-level thresholding for MRI brain image segmentation. *Expert Systems with Applications, 138,* 112820.

Thaha, M. M., Kumar, K. P. M., Murugan, B. S., Dhanasekeran, S., Vijayakarthick, P., & Selvi, A. S. (2019). Brain tumor segmentation using convolutional neural networks in MRI images. *Journal of Medical Systems, 43*(9), 294.

Top, A., Hamarneh, G., & Abugharbieh, R. (2011). *Active Learning for Interactive 3D Image Segmentation.*

Trivizakis, E., Manikis, G. C., Nikiforaki, K., Drevelegas, K., Constantinides, M., Drevelegas, A., & Marias, K. (2018). Extending 2-D convolutional neural networks to 3-D for advancing deep learning cancer classification with application to MRI liver tumor differentiation. *IEEE Journal of Biomedical and Health Informatics, 23*(3), 923–930.

Vaidhya, K., Thirunavukkarasu, S., Alex, V., & Krishnamurthi, G. (2015). *Multi-Modal Brain Tumor Segmentation Using Stacked Denoising Autoencoders.* In *BrainLes 2015* (pp. 181–194). Springer, Cham.

Wang, G., Zuluaga, M. A., Pratt, R., Aertsen, M., Doel, T., Klusmann, M., … Ourselin, S. (2016). Slic-Seg: A minimally interactive segmentation of the placenta from sparse and motion-corrupted fetal MRI in multiple views. *Medical Image Analysis, 34*, 137–147.

Zhang, S., & Xu, G. (2016). A novel approach for brain tumor detection using MRI Images. *Journal of Biomedical Science and Engineering, 9*(10), 44–52.

16 Comparative Study on Analysis of Medical Images Using Deep Learning Techniques

R. S. M. Lakshmi Patibandla
Vignan's Foundation for Science, Technology, and Research

V. Lakshman Narayana and Arepalli Peda Gopi
Vignan's Nirula Institute of Technology & Science
for Women

B. Tarakeswara Rao
Kallam Haranadha Reddy Institute of Technology

CONTENTS

16.1 INTRODUCTION

Deep learning (DL) is a significant supporter of contemporary artificial intelligence (AI) in virtually different backgrounds. This is an immediate product of ongoing research due to its application across a wide range of rational research fields along with computer visualisation, natural language processing, molecular materials science, DNA exams, intelligence circuits and the central constitution, investigation and so on. Recently, it has also pulled into a popular joint. The structure of DL makes it possible to train technology in multi-faceted numerical methods for information portrayals which can be used to conduct accurate information testing. These methods gradually process irregular or potentially direct knowledge capabilities to be precisely biased by replica borders. If this ability is dealt with 'layers' knowledge privilege, the incremental use of countless such layers often transfers the term DL. The shared objective of DL strategies is to know iteratively the limits of the computational model through the use of an information index preparation, with the purpose of improving the model in performing, for example, the perfect task of grouping over this information under a specified measure. The calculation model itself tends to be an artificial neural network (ANN) consisting of different layers of neurons and the fundamental computational places of perception, while its boundaries demonstrate the consistency of the connections between the neurons of different layers. When prepared for a given business, the DL models are also prepared to make a similar errand by using a range of already unspeakable details (for example, testing information). Right now this strong DL speculation ability stands apart from the other AI methods. A deep model is learned using a back-proliferation framework that enables some forms of the mainstream inclination drop method to display iteratively at the ideal boundary estimates. Refresh model limits using the full knowledge as known as the solitary organisational age/model planning. Contemporary DL models may typically be transmitted for several ages before. While DL was born in the 1940s, the sudden late increase in its use to deal with complex questions from the cutting edge culminated in three big wonderful developments.

1. Accessibility of a lot of preparational information: a lot of information is available for the preparation of complex computational models with late digitization of data. DL has the inherent potential to demonstrate complex capabilities by piling different layers of its basic computing squares. It is also an advantageous choice to handle tough problems. Oddly enough, this deep-model potential has been documented for a few years now (Lundervold et al., 2019). The bottleneck of moderately modest knowledge index training, however, restricted up to this point DL's usefulness.
2. Access to innovative computing equipment: Mastering complex skills over massive knowledge measures produces massive computational requirements. These criteria can be fulfilled by linked exploration networks as of late.
3. Accessibility of public libraries that update DL calculations: In different exploration networks late development trends are used to distribute open-stage source codes. The use of this technique in various application spaces was exploded by simple group to DL calculation.

Since the 1960s, the field of clinical imaging has violated AI (Poplin et al., 2018). In any case, during the 1990s, Clinical Imaging showed its most prominent commitments which associate with today's DL procedures (Ravi et al., 2017). The correlation of these methods with contemporary DL is accomplished by the use of ANNs to achieve clinical imaging. Restricted to the calculation of information preparation and computer properties, all these works created networks that are only a few layers deep. This is not considered 'deep' in cutting edge time at this stage. In most contemporary DL models, the quantity of layers varies from 12 to more than 100. For the picture exam, such models have usually begun writing in PC Vision.

In dissecting advanced images, the field of PC visualisation closely identifies with Clinical Imaging. Clinical Imaging has a long convention to take advantage of PC Vision findings. In 2012, DL gave a big leap forward in PC Vision by performing an incredibly hard picture grouping task with remarkable precision. The PC visualisation community has steadily shifted its primary concentration to DL from then on. Clinical imaging also started to see techniques misusing deep neural networks roughly in 2013, and now those methods are gradually being used. Sahiner et al. (Raissi et al., 2018) found that friends had considerably increased distributions using DL for radiological images from 2016 (100) to 2017 (300), while more than hundred such distributions have occurred alone in the main quarter of 2018. In 2018, the regular Clinical Imaging Gathering, for example, distributed over 120 papers using DL for Clinical Picture Investigation in its fundamental procedures for 'Clinical picture figuring and PC-Assisted Intercession' (MICCAI). The large influx of DL commitments in clinical imaging has also contributed to the 2018 Global Meeting on 'Clinical Imaging with Deep Learning' (MIDL). We note that there are also a few audit papers at this distribution hour for strongly relevant review headings. Among them are just X-ray highlights when primarily talking about writing until 2017. Nevertheless, DL's rapid growth and findings have only disproved a few perceptions made in those audits. Furthermore, there are a large number of later procedures for clinical imaging using DL innovations which were not (or maybe not) coined at the time of those studies. Apart from the later assessment, our analysis also offers an outstanding PC Vision and AI point of view on clinical imaging in comparison to current audits. Restricted by their thin point of view, the latest surveys often miss the mark about the key drivers of DL in Clinical Imaging difficulties.

Moreover, they cannot offer bits of information to use the findings in various fields to solve problems. These concerns are specifically discussed in our audit. In this paper we present a systematic survey of ongoing DL procedures in Clinical Imaging, with an outline of existing techniques distributed in 2018 or later. We categorise these strategies into different examples and sub-order them according to a scientific classification that is based on human life structures (Jiang et al., 2018). After the examined writing has been broken down, we identified the lack of adequately explained large data sets for the Clinical Imaging orders as the critical test (among various difficulty) to misuse DL for such companies. We then use the writing of PC Vision, Example Transparency and AI in general to establish guidance to handle this and various difficulties in a clinical study using profound learning. This audit also discusses publicly available data sets to prepare DL models for clinical imaging tasks. In the absence of a deep appreciation of DL by the broader clinical community, this article also provides a suitable interpretation of the centre's advanced ideas associated with DL.

16.2 MACHINE LEARNING, ARTIFICIAL NEURAL NETWORKS, DEEP LEARNING

In machine learning, techniques are developed and studied that allow PCs to tackle problems through meetings. The goal is to produce numerical models to produce useful results while taking care of data. Machine learning models come together through knowledge planning and are designed to establish accurate expectations for preparation information by measuring improvements. The main purpose of the models is to have the opportunity, to summarise their skills and to express the right expectation of fresh, concealed knowledge. The speculative ability of a model is generally evaluated in preparation using a separate data set, approval set and used as critique for further tuning of the model. After some preparations and tuning, the last model is analysed on a test range, which will redefine how the model will work in the face of new, unknown information (Yukun et al., 2019).

Some types of machine learning are defined roughly by the way the models use their knowledge in training. In strengthening learning, specialists are established who benefit from their environment through experiments, while improving their target function. A well-known use of reinforcement is AlphaGo and AlphaZero (Abadi, et al., 2016). DeepMind's generated Go-Playing machine learning system. In unregulated learning, the PC is charged with revealing examples without our guidance. Clustering is a perfect picture. The vast majority of today's machine learning structures have a place in the directed learning class (Kamnitsas.et al., 2017). Here a collection of effective marked or clarified information is given to the PC and the PC is asked to establish the right names for new previously unexpected data sets based on the concepts contained in the so-called information gathering. The whole model is prepared to conduct explicit information handling undertakings using a bunch of information yield models (Yuan et al., 2017). Comments using human knowledge such as characterising skin injuries as a threat and discovering cardiovascular hazard factors in retinal fundus photographs are two instances of the enormous number of medical imaging problems assaulted by direct learning (Rao et al., 2020). The machine learning has a long history and is part of several sub-fields, the main subject of which is DL from now on. There are several impressive, transparent contours and DL studies. For short, general awareness of DL, we shall only specify a few simple necessities in the field, trusting that these will fill the territories, which are currently the most impressive in medical imaging, with support.

The ANN is a gradual arrangement of basic computational components called neurons (or perceptrons). Various neurons live in a solitary succession, framing the organization's solitary layer (Patibandla et al., 2020). The use of multiple layers in an ANN makes it deep. A neuron plays the corresponding basic calculation:

$$a = f\left(w^T x + b\right), \qquad (16.1)$$

where $x \in Rm$ is the information signal, $w \in Rm$ contains the neuron's loads and $b \in R$ is a predisposition term. The image $f(.)$ signifies an enactment work, and the figured $a \in R$ is the neuron's initiation signal or essentially its actuation. For the most part, $f(.)$ is kept non-straight to permit an ANN to instigate complex non-direct computational models. The exemplary decisions for $f(.)$ are the notable 'sigmoid' and 'exaggerated digression' capacities.

A neural organization must become familiar with the weight and inclination terms in Equation (16.1). The system used to get familiar with these boundaries (for example, back-spread) requires $f(.)$ to be a differentiable capacity of its data sources. In the cutting edge DL time, the Rectified Linear Unit (ReLU) is broadly utilized for this capacity, particularly for non-standard ANNs, for example, CNNs. ReLU is characterized as $a = \max (0, w^T x + b)$. For the subtleties past the extent of this conversation, ReLU permits more productive and for the most part more compelling learning of complex models when contrasted with the exemplary sigmoid and exaggerated digression enactment capacities.

It is conceivable to minimalistically speak to the loads related with all the neurons in a solitary layer of an ANN as a lattice $W \in Rp \times m$, where 'p' is the absolute number of neurons in that layer. This permits us to register the initiations of the apparent multitude of neurons in the layer without a moment's delay as follows:

$$a = f (Wx + b) \tag{16.2}$$

where $a \in Rp$ presently stores the initiation estimations of the apparent multitude of neurons in the layer viable. Taking note of the various levelled nature of ANNs, it is anything but difficult to see that the practical type of a model incited by an L-layer organization can be given as

$$M(x, 2) = fL\left(WLfL - 1\left(WL - 1fL - 2...(W1x + b1) + \cdots + bL - 1\right) + bL\right) \tag{16.3}$$

where the addendums indicate the layer numbers. We all in all signify the boundaries $Wi, bi, \forall i \in \{1,..., L\}$ as 2.

A model can be framed using a substitute number of layers, with a substitute number of neurons in each layer, and irrespective of their capacity for starting with various layers. In combination, these options choose the neural association strategy. The design components and those of the study estimate are defined as hyperboundaries of the association. While model boundaries are usually discovered, a manual iterative cycle is often the most sensitive assessment of the hyperbound. Standard ANNs are often consistently called multi-layer perceptions because their layers consistently consist of standard neurons/perceptions. An unmistakable exception to this layer fusion is, for example, the Softmax layer used together in the last layer. Softmax neurons test principles that are standardised in all institutional evaluations of that layer, instead of 'free' activation in each neuron in the standard layer of the perceptron. Mathematically, the ith neuron for a softmax layer tests the establishment which is seen as the upside of normalisation of the sanction sign is that the output of the softmax layer can be interpreted as a probability vector that ensures that a specific model has a position in a certain class. This understanding of softmax layer yields is a commonly used idea in related composition (Patibandla and Narayana 2021).

AI models are usually optimised for accommodation tasks subject to truly arranged features that are isolated from rough data or that other direct AI models learn. Unimportant learning, the PCs that learn to change representations and features normally bypass this manual and problematic growth, clearly from unrefined data. By far, different forms of false neural correlations have become the most prominent models of significant learning, but there are others. The key feature of important learning processes is their consideration of integrating learning: later learning data depictions. This is the fundamental difference between significant learning approaches and anything from this point on 'conventional' AI is possible.

Finding and playing a role is a problem and both are strengthened during a comparable calculation. The primary in meaningful learning in clinical imaging is typically decided by convolutional neural networks (CNNs), a powerful way to deal with the learning of essential images and other co-ordinated info (Krishna et al., 2020). These features should typically be planned by hand or produced by less astonishing AI models before it is possible to use CNN successfully. At the point where features actually taken from the data could be included; countless handcrafted drawings were usually left by the way as they seemed to be useless differently in integrating discoverers discovered by CNNs. There are some clear trends in CNN's output which make us understand why they are so inconceivable. Let us therefore examine the structural squares of CNNs.

16.3 MACHINE LEARNING AND DEEP LEARNING IN MEDICAL IMAGING

AI calculations are particularly incredible to think about express contaminations in clinical imaging. Different kinds of components cannot be adequately seen, for instance, by a simple mathematical course of action (Patibandla, 2020), wounds and organs in the preparation of clinical scenes. The manufacturer used the pixel-based evaluation to evaluate clinical illnesses. The pixel test in AI was performed in clinical planning, which uses such characteristics in images directly instead of extracting features from abnormalities as data. This approach can be better endorsed than simple segment-based classifiers in unambiguous matters (Altaf, 2019). The low separation picture is a moving problem in the study of its properties. In contrast to ordinary classifiers which avoid bumbles created by misdivision and feature calculation, the evaluation and separation of the component is not important for pixel-based AI (Hu, 2018). The pixel exam uses long preparation time due to the high dimensionality of data in the creator (a large number of pixels in a picture) which is zeroed in on the clinical images for evaluation. The Histogram Equalization is the most capable method for optimising contrast. The creators proposed a method called 'Changed Histogram-Based Contrast Enhancement using Homomorphism Filtering' (MHFIL). It used two phases that deal with the cycle; overall contrast is improved with histogram shift in the critical level. In addition, homomorphic second-stage filtering is foreseen for sharpening of the image. Ten low-contrast X-shaft chest clinical images are studied. The MH-FIL has limited features in each of the 10 image PCs with different strategies. The clinical clarification is the radiologist's most important commitment, with organisations introducing higher quality comparative images and their evaluation. The PC upheld the CAD proposal for a considerably longer time (Patibandla et al., 2020).

Various AI techniques are divided between them by clinical pictures, for example, the direct discrimination test, vector machine maintenance, decision-making trees, etc., in the clinical picture assessment process used by the manufacturer (Patibandla et al., 2020). Unmistakably, they used double-model neighbourhoods commonly considered among surface descriptors; in addition, an evaluation of new principles using a couple of small double-model descriptors of biomedical images and the data set of neonatal facial images for the application of torture from facial portrayals. Particularly the results on the 2D-HeLa data set were generally arranged and the descriptor proposed gets the most outrageous application including all surface descriptors. The 2D-HeLa data set and the PAP data set have a straight support vector with machining classifier. The precision of 92.4% is the most imperative consistency among all different descriptors on the data set. In clinical images, the neural association technique is used to analyse the complexities of the ailment. The neural association packs are held for the disclosure of infections. It is used to denounce when a cell is natural and ludicrous where any unquestionable interaction has conceivably just two effects, so it would be a regular cell or harm cell. The wishes for these cell associations are connected by a prevailing method, for example, by the provision of a vote. The findings showed that in general the neural interaction refined the high-precision movement and the low evaluation of false negative tests (Naresh, 2020).

The AI as frameworks provides the creation of premises from knowledge for patients. Different criteria are drawn up from the bosses' knowledge to the authority structure viewpoint. The social affair of clinical questions can be used as express representations and data from knowledgeable networks can be accomplished by AI gestures that can be used to deliver a deliberate representation of clinical characteristics that certainly show clinical conditions. Knowledge may adequately be expressed as a decision tree in the operation of simple guidelines, or as much as possible (Rao, 2020). CARDIO, which is programmed to decode ECGs, is a typical instance of this characterisation of the structure. The extraordinary standard for the inspection of the picture is a quantifiable test in the clinical image assessment. The hotel observator channelized (CHO) is typically used unambiguously in nuclear imaging. The canals are excited about the fun subjects in the human visual structure. This approach is used to interpret the consistency of the image and the CHO also affects clinical imagery. The following approximation is called a channelled SVM. Two clinical physicists have tested the observable quality in 100 noisy images and then a six-point assessment of the responsive contemporary fact. From now on and into the near future, a training course will include an additional 60 pictures. The human viewers accomplished this undertaking in six community conclusions of the levelling channel with two varying choices about the number of priorities in the OS-EM restoration calculation (Figure 16.1).

Many of the image assurance tasks require a fundamental interest in identifying contradictions, evaluating and modifying over time. Automated image evaluation gadgets based on AI figures are the main impacts to enhance the idea of image

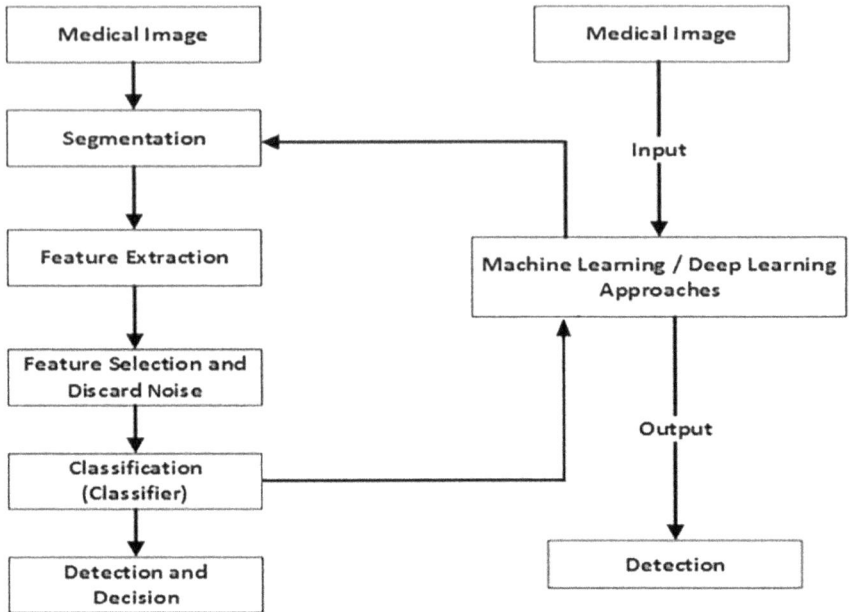

FIGURE 16.1 Machine and DL algorithms workflow in medical image.

investigation and understanding by allowing conspicuous confirmation of findings. Profound learning is a method that is completely implemented and gives a condition of it towards the back precision. It opened new doors not already in the clinical picture review. The application of DL for clinical purposes covers a wide range of concerns ranging from adverse developmental screening and infection to ready treatment recommendations (Latif, et.al, 2020). Various sources of today's data – radiological imaging (X-ray, computed tomography (CT) and magnetic resonance imaging (MRI)), pathology imagery and late-coming genomic growth have led to a vast amount of data available to experts. Nevertheless, we are not yet able to turn these data into accommodating details. In the discussion below we included the use of in-depth learning in the clinical review. In either case, the once-over does not give an absolute indication of the long-lasting profound impact of learning in today's clinical imaging industry (Pouyanfar, et al, 2018).

To direct PCs to learn features that show data for the specific problem, this concept is the basis of a variety of in-depth learning methods. The models which contained different layers adjusting input pictures to provide results on specific diseases by pressing one small step at a time increased level characteristics (Rastogi et al., 2018). The best form of these image evaluation models is CNN. The CNNs have a few layers that transform the commitment to channels of convolution. The initiative to systematically use in-depth clinical learning methods adapt to existing models to obvious data courses, such as three-dimensional data. The inspirations that push CNNs to massive details, complete 3D convolutions and the resulting enormous number of goals are done whatever the volume of interest is not divided into allocations.

16.3.1 GROUPING

1. Set of photographs

The compilation of the clinical image is the key activity in order to thoroughly examine clinical problems for the early therapy of the patient. The portrait can be general or different images as an engagement with a single, inconsistent feature (contamination yes or no). In these instances, every test is a model and data set sizes are clearly smaller than those in the PC Vision. The fine adjustment eclipsed function extraction, achieving 57.6% precision in multi-class knee-arthritis evaluation against 53.4%. However, they showed that CNN function recovery has changed cytopathology's depiction accuracy by 70.5% versus 69.1%.

2. Demand for object

The event focuses on the tiny interesting parts of the clinical image. These protuberances can be extended into two groups in any case. The local information of these items and the hypothesis overall information are important for greater precision. The creator used three CNN methodologies to thoroughly understand how to set the image to a substitute scale. The delayed effects of these three systems eventually mirrored the structure of the overall image features.

16.3.2 ID: ORGAN AND COUNTRY ORGAN

The area of concern and limitation is the accompanying point. It is a big development in the division, where we can literally remove the toughness of any article and concentrate on the interesting thing and discard the chaos. A 3D data parsing approach uses in-depth learning counts to challenge this issue. The manufacturer used three self-sufficient 2D and 3D MRI instruments in clinical images. It is used to discover regions of various related objects dealing with such unique pollutants, such as the nucleus, aortic bend and sliding aorta.

16.3.3 PART SECTION

The period of division is extended to the organs and bases of the clinical images. It is used for objective examination of clinical characteristics (Akhtar and Mian, 2018), for example, heart or brain evaluation. It is also used for limits in CAD. The object of interest is the perception of express pixels. The U-net is the combination of plans of up-samples and down-samples. It mixed the convolution relationship and the deconvolutional layer trial.

16.3.4 SELECTION

Selection is the way to change various data plans into a single coordinate system. It is a major development of clinical images in order to analyse or combine data from a particular perspective, time, importance, sensors, etc. This is the iterative cycle in which we choose a certain form of boundary as normal. The similitude limits of two images are determined using DL estimates. The registration is used in prescriptions such as PC tomography (CT) and nuclear magnetic resonance (NMR) data (Haarburger et al., 2018). This is highly useful in order to get open-minded information, track tumour growth, remedy claims and to link information about the patient to anatomical diagram books. The common data are that Powell's and Brent's approaches are used to recruit magnetic resonance (MR); CT is not quite the same as in chest MR images.

DL calculations are a subset of AI counts that hope to learn important factors in the data through the use of different levels of representation. DL is completed by a deep association, which for the most part is a neural association with many covered layers and reflects on promising particular centre points. The most recent AI counts are labelled 'shallow' since there are many progressions to the information before they are translated into an output. Then, estimates are again considered to be 'profound' since the data witnessed a shift movement until they were converted into a yield (Norris et al., 2018). It is a propulsion technique which has been applied extensively in a few customary areas of human brain power, including falsified vision, characteristic language handling and learning movements, etc. The three main purposes of this profound learning effect today are the evolution of chip preparation limits (e.g. GPU), the unpredictable cost decrease of PC equipment and the avoidable growth. While this is a growing area, late examinations reveal that DL is extensively concentrated and has proven effective in tasks like PC Vision. Different similar ideologies have therefore been developed. The different systems of in-depth research estimates are – CNN, Boltzmann Restricted Machines and auto coders and sparse coding.

CNN is one of the most common methods for deeply realising the arrangement of different layers. It was exploited in multiple clinical picture evaluation procedures, which began too late (Antony et al., 2016). A CNN includes three neural layers, specifically the convolutional layer, the pooling layer and the associated layer, if in question. These various types of layers have wavering tasks.

Zhang (2018) kept an eye on the imperative for specific cell division in the cervical test covering collections and cell pathologies. Pap Smear and liquid-based cytology (LBC) are normal and fruitful infection screening instruments. The previous methods were focused primarily on extracting hand-made features, such as morphology and surface from cell data sets. The manufacturers suggested a technique 'DeepPap' for organising cells with deep-rooted neural organisations (ConvNets). A ConvNet was pre-arranged using the ImageNet data set during the readiness process. Next the pre-set association with the behaviour of cervical cell data has been updated with the aid of movement learning including extended, re-examined image fixes usually based around the centres. In the test process, the test images were taken beforehand for the finely tuned ConvNet. The oddity score was obtained by applying the rates of ConvNet. For Papanicolaou and LBC, the proposed strategy was investigated. The results showed that the device beats previous measurements with a selection accuracy of 98.3%. With a distinction of 98.3%, the pedagogical spectrum is measured by five times over for the Herlev Papanicolaou. The H&E stained manual liquid-based cytology (HEMLBC) educational spectrum offered comparable unmatched presentations (H and E recoloured manual LBC).

Han et al. (2017) proposed a multi-classification method on the BreaKHis enlightening record, a histopathologic data set, for eight classes of chest harm using a profound convolutional-neuronal interaction subject to a class structure (CSDCNN). The proposed method is a planned work measure comprising three stages: planning, acceptance and evaluation. The purpose of the readiness stage is to comfortably demonstrate the sufficient limits and to improve the separation of the space of the different groups. The inspiration for the approval stage is to adjust the limits and pick models from each time. The test stage is supposed to analyse the CSDCNN show. They achieved 93.2% accuracy. They used this technique as the extraction of task-related characteristics by a clinical master with an enormous machine weight was inefficient and problematic. Furthermore, the presentation and treatment of management preparation limits are equally dim and repetitive. The strategy also discussed concerns related to the analysis of intra-class and inter-class histopathological images (Kim et al., 2016).

Havaei (2017) has another CNN-subject architecture, the Deep neural network, which separates cerebral tumours (gliomas and glioblastomas), which would be difficult in one direction or another for the region by the powerless separation and loosen the structures like the members. The closely kept credits and the more general legitimate features of the MR pictures were exploited. They suggested that the two-stage philosophy that was discovered is important to track lopsided impression movements. They have used the 2013 MACAI Brain Tumour Segmentation (BRATS) illuminating assortment to plan and test the relation. Their methodologies were second to most of frontline tactics in the 2013 BRATS scoreboard.

Gulshan et al. (2016) built in-depth learning counts for robotic acknowledgment of diabetic retinopathy (DR) and macular diabetic use of the EyePACS-1 and Messidor-2 instructional lists for retinal fundus images. From the outset, the limits in the neural interaction were subjective characteristics. The association is preparing itself for DR depending on the powers of the pixel in the preparation range of the fundus images. The affectability and expressions of the figures for the identification of insinuated diabetic retinopathy or of the inferable diabetic macular oedema is referenced as normal. They suggested that a thorough examination was needed in order to select the viability of applying this count in the clinical setting, as well as to see if the use of the measure could lead to a better psyche. The abstract of the study of clinical photos with DL has shown up in Table 16.1.

16.4   MEDICAL IMAGE ANALYSIS USING DEEP LEARNING

CNN has been put in charge of organising, containing, recognising, separating and enlisting the image analysis. AI research draws a qualification between containment (draws a hop around the solitary object of the picture) and identification (draw bounding boxes around various articles, which might be from various classes). Division sketches and marks diagrams along the edges of the goals (semantic division). The listing refers to fitting an image into another (which may be 2- or 3-dimensional). This division of orders depends on different AI methods and is preserved below. This division of orders is not overly important to the clinician, and the developers believe that an AI system down to earth will integrate some or all of the tasks into a

TABLE 16.1

Analysis of Medical Images using DL

Machine Learning Challenges	Data Set	Results	Applications
Inefficient feature engineering Gulshan et al (2016)	Retinal fundus photographs (EyePACS-1 Data set and Messidor-2 data set)	Deep Learning	Diabetic Retinopathy Detection
Accurate Segmentation Havaei (2017)	BRATS 2013 Data set	Deep Neural Network	BRATS
Inefficient feature engineering; high intra-class and low inter-class variations Han et al. (2017)	BreaKHis data set (Histopathological images)	Deep convolutional neural network based on class-structure (CSDCNN)	Breast Cancer Classification
Accurate Cell Segmentations	Pap Smear (Herlev Data Set) LBC (HEMLBC Data Set) ImageNet data set (pre-training)	ConvNets	Cervical cancer screening

consolidated framework. Also in a solo work process, it is desirable to diagnose and ultimately restrict and fragment a lung tumour in a CT chest sweep, and to forecast various alternative therapies such as chemotherapy or a surgical procedure. A part of these activities obscures in the papers discussed here. From a clinic point of view, does order learn whether or not an illness is available, i.e., does blood on this MRI test indicate a haemorrhagic stroke? Limitation implies that typical structure of life is differentiated; for example, where is the kidney in this ultrasound image? This is instead of identifying a strange neurosis; for example, where are the lung tumours largely in this lung CT output? Fragmenting the blueprint of a lung tumour allows a clinician to assess its good ways from significant anatomical structures and helps to respond to a questionnaire; for example, if this is a patient and if so, what should the resection amount be?

16.4.1 GROUPING OF GOODS

The meeting is often referred to as computer-assisted diagnosis. Lo et al. portrayed CNN in 1995 to describe chest X-radiate lung handles. They used 55 chest X-radiates and a CNN with two covered layers to assess the long handle of a territory. The availability of chest X-pillar images overall has possibly facilitated profound learning development. Rajkumar et al. extended 1850 photographs of chest X-shaft into 150,000 ready for test. Using a modified prearranged GogLeNet CNN, they showed the heading of the images in frontal or flat views with almost 100% accuracy. While the task of seeing the path of the chest X-bar is of minimal clinical value, it illustrates the feasibility of pre-preparation and data creation to learn the corresponding image metadata, as an integral part of an inevitably modernised illustrative work process. Pneumonia or defilement of the chest is an ordinary health condition which is visibly treatable worldwide.

In the use of 112,000 images from the ChestXray14 data set, Rajpurkar et al. used a modified DenseNet with 121 convolutional layers called ChenNet to represent 14 extraordinary diseases seen on chest X-radiates. The pneumonia depiction clearly cultivated a 0.7632 area under curve score with the evaluation of the Receiver Operating Characteristics. In addition, CheXNet composed or enhanced the introduction of four individual radiologists on the test collection of 420 images and the presentation of a board comprising three radiologists.

In the case of 1,010 stamped CT lung checks from the Lung Image Database Consortium (LIDC-IDRI) data set, Shen et al. used CNN's classified with Support Vector Machine (SVM) and Random Forest classifiers for the representation of lung handle as Liberal or Dangerous. They used three similar CNNs with two convolutional layers each and each CNN took photo patches at various scales to eliminate the characteristics. The informed features were used to assemble a vector-integrated input, which was represented in a heart-conscious or hurtful way using either an SVM with extended justification work (radial basis function (RBF)) or an RF classification. They assembled 86% precision handles and also found good against various levels of uproar inputs.

Li et al. used three-dimensional CNNs to integrate missing imagery data into MRI and positron emission tomography (PET) images. The Alzheimer Disease Neuroimaging Initiative (ADNI) database inspected 830 patients with MRI and PET. The 3-D CNNs were generated separately of MRI and PET images for knowledge and return, and were used to alter the PET images of patients who had them not. Their PET photos' change almost predicted the reality of potential outcomes from the selection of contamination, but one stipulation is that overfitting problems were not discussed, restricting the likely generality of their process. Hosseini-Asl et al. managed to achieve frontline diagnosis of 99% of patients with Alzheimer's disease versus normal. They used 3-D CNNs in a self-encoder plan, which were pre-prepared for normal brain aids in the CADDementia data collection. The educated section findings were then correlated with higher layers where profound supervision techniques changed the count's ability to isolate between rates of traditional brain patients, responsive scientific deficiency and Alzheimer's disease in the ADNI database.

Korolev et al. investigated the implementation of VOXCNN and ResNet, which exclusively depended upon the architectures of the VGGNet and residual neural connections. They also used the ADNI database to isolate normal patients and patients with Alzheimer's disease. Although their accuracy of 79% for Voxnet and 80% for ResNet was lower than that achieved by Hosseini-Asl, Korolev said his computations required no manual manufacturing features and were easier to execute. Similarly, CNNs can break down DR. Pratt et al. developed a CNN with 10 convolutional layers and three associated layers on about 90,000 fundus images with their advanced photographs of the eye fundus. They asked DR for 5 DR clinically used game plans with 75% accuracy.

Abramoff et al. tested the IDx-DR interpretation X2.1 (IDx LLC, Iowa City, Iowa) for the purpose of perceiving DR. CNN plans are not uncovered but Alexnet and VGGNet charge it. The unit has a score of 0.98 area under the ROC curve (AUC) on up to 1.2 million DR images.

Independent learning approaches are also a field of evaluation. In addition, Deep Belief Networks was used to delete features from utilitarian (fMRI) images and MRI results of Huntington and Schizophrenia patients. Suk et al. collected fMRI images for completion sound or mild cognitive disability by using a stacked RBMs plan to learn common hierarchical connections between various areas of the brain. Externally looking at traditional CNN models, Kumar et al. have specifically broken down the visual bag of Visual words (BOVW) and local binary patterns, thus showing striking CNN's Alexnet and VGGNet in different techniques (LBP). Oddly enough the BOVW technique was best used for requiring histopathological images in 20 distinct tissue types.

16.4.2 RESTRICTION

Impediment to standard life frames is less likely to interest the practitioner, while applications may occur in the preparation of life structures. There will obviously be a restriction in the mechanised application from beginning to end, whereby the radiological picture is self-supervised and recorded without human interference. Yan et al. looked at a cross-CT image cut and created a two-stage CNN where the chief stage saw fixes closely and in the subsequent stage, different body organ misunderstood the local patches, achieving ideal results with a regular CNN. A CNN with five convolutional layers was arranged by Roth et al. to isolate about 4,000 CT pictures at the middle in one of five classes: neck, lung, liver, pelvis and legs. Following data increase methodology, he had the option to obtain a 5.9% order screw and an AUC score of 0.998. Shin et al. used stacked autoencoders in 78 separations to distinguish areas for the liver-, heart-, kidney- and spleen-enhanced MRI rates of the local stomach containing liver or kidney metastatic tumours. Hierarchical features have been discovered across space and common areas, giving recognition of accuracy, depending on the organ, of 62% and 79%.

16.4.3 LOCATION

The area, commonly referred to as Computer-Aided Detection, is a sharp field of study because the lack of a yield problem can have remarkable effects both on the patient and the clinician. The mission for the 2017 Kaggle Data Science Bowl recalled the disclosure of vulnerable lung handles for CT lung channels. Around 2,000 CT resistance inspections were carried out and the Fangzhou victor received a logarithmic incident score of 0.399. Their response was a 3-D CNN powered by U-Net designed to isolate fixes first for the disclosure of the handle. At that time, this return was dealt with in a later stage with two linked layers for the harm likelihood game plan. Shin et al. surveyed five excellent CNN plans for the identification of thoracoabdominal lymph centre points and interstitial lung disease in CT scans. The awareness of lymph centres is enormous because it may be a sign of defilement or risk. They obtained an AUC mediastinal point AUC score of 0.95, with 85% affectability with

Google LeNet, the top rank. They also reported the benefits of movement learning and the use of profound learning models up to 22 layers as opposed to less layers, the standard of clinical review. Overfeat was a CNN prepared for features which won the limitation task of ILSVRC 2013. Ciompi et al. used 2-dimensional cutbacks of CT lung control in the coronal, central and sagittal planes to anticipate the presence of handles both inside and outside the lung hole. They combined this philosophy with classifier direct SVM and RF, like a Frequencies Bag, which is a new three-dimensional descriptor of their own. Other than lung wounds, a variety of different applications are similar, like separating compromise cells of the skin.

Esteva et al. used 130,000 dermatological and dermoscopic photos to create a Google LeNet Inception V3CNN, with no hand-made features. The CNN has beaten human dermatologists to say the images as welcoming, dangerous or non-neoplastic wounds and showed 72% accuracy, which varied by approximately 65% and 66% to two people. The CNN again strengthened the picking of 21 human dermatologists for two forms of skin disease: carcinoma and melanoma. This work included 376 biopsy-exhibited photographs, and AUC values between 0.91 and 0.96 were achieved by CNN.

Histopathological photographs are dynamically digitised and numerous papers in this area have been prompted. The images of human pathologists who are searching for danger indicators are currently troublingly studied, for instance, extended centre to cytoplasm, expanded mitotic figures with expanded cell reproduction, the atypical cell strategy, the signs of cell depletion, high-level cell extension records from sub-nuclear markers such as Ki-67. A histopathological slide can contain hundreds to thousands of cells and the risk of lack of variation in neoplastic districts can be increased via them. Ciresan et al. used 11–13 layer CNNs to collect mitotic figures from 50 MITOS data set chest histology photographs. Their methodology obtained accuracy and independent sample ratings of 0.88 and 0.70.

Further, from late on, Yang et al. achieved 97%–98% accuracy in collecting kidney dangerous histopathological pictures into tumour or non-tumour, using deep five to seven layers CNNs. In any event, Sirinukunwattana et al. have also used the CNNs to perceive cell centres in 100 photos of the histology of colorectal adenocarcinoma. To get ready, about 30,000 centres have to be tested by hand. The interest in their technique was the use of their spatially limited CNN, which recognised the focal points of centres using spatial backlashes and spatial environments. Centres for chest infection histological slides were also recognised by Xu et al. but in light of all he uses the Stacked Sparse Autoencoder. Their model obtained reliable and independent survey scores of 0.89 and 0.83, showing that performance learning methods can also be properly employed in this area. Albarquoni et al. are concerned with the question of the non-checking of clinical pictures by 'freely supporting' the naming of mitosis in histology photographs of chest harm to non-experts on the Internet. The openly retained data marks were treated in CNN, addressing a captivating inspection of reasoning that can cope with the permanent problem of lack of naming in clinical scenarios evaluation.

16.4.4 Part Section

Work on CT and MRI picture division includes a combination of organs such as the liver, prostate and knee tendon, while a great deal of work has been done on brain division, including tumour division. The latter is very careful to select the farthest reaches of the tumour in order to have a precautionary resection. Renunciation of a lot of understandable brain regions during surgery will cause neurological retrogressions, such as insufficient membership, death and mental impediments. The division of the clinical anatomy was created by hand, with a clinician drawing diagram separated by a slice around the whole MRI or CT volume stack, so it is desirable to complete a response that updates this laborious task. Akkus et al. formed a remarkable summary of the brain MRI division, which analysed the distinctive CNN structures and figures used in the division.

16.5   CONCLUSION

This chapter addressed an analysis of the advancement of DL in medical imaging. It contributed by three monumental headings closely. We particularly knew a brilliant presentation of the core considerations of DL. With the general lack of knowledge among medical imaging specialists of the DL structure, we kept our conversation instinctively. This fragment can be regarded as DL reflections commonly used in medical imaging. The third basic piece assessed the enormous difficulties and explored the potential direction of DL in Medical Image Analysis. We can decide that medical imaging can benefit entirely from DL through synergical assessments with the collaborations of computer vision and machine learning researchers.

REFERENCES

Abadi, M., Barham, P., Chen, J., Chen, Z., Davis, A., Dean, J., Devin, M., (2016). Tensorflow: A system for large-scale machine learning. In 12th USENIX Symposium on Operating Systems Design and Implementation OSDI 16), 265–283.

Akhtar, N. and Mian, A. (2018). Threat of adversarial attacks on deep learning in computer vision: A survey. *IEEE Access*, 6, 14410–14430.

Altaf, F., Islam, S.M.S., Akhtar N., Janjua, N.K. (2019). Going deep in medical image analysis: Concepts, methods, challenges, and future directions, *IEEE Access*, 7, 99540–99572.

Antony, J., McGuinness, K., O'Connor, N.E. and Moran, K (2016). Quantifying radiographic knee osteoarthritis severity using deep convolutional neural networks. In *Pattern Recognition (ICPR)*.

Haarburger, C., Schock, J., Baumgartner, M., Rippel, O. and Merhof, D., (2019). Delira: A high-level framework for deep learning in medical image analysis. *Journal of Open Source Software*, 4, 1488.

Hu, Z., Tang, J., Wang, Z., Zhang, K., Zhang, L., Sun, Q. (2018). Deep learning for image-based cancer detection and diagnosis Ñ A survey, *Pattern Recognition*, 83, 134–149.

Jiang S., Chin K.-S., Tsui K.L. (2018). A universal deep learning approach for modeling the flow of patients under different severities. *Computer Methods and Programs in Biomedicine* 154,191–203.

Kamnitsas, K., Ledig, C., Newcombe, V.F., Simpson, J.P., Kane, A.D., Menon, D.K., Rueckert, D. and Glocker, B, (2017). Efficient multi-scale 3d CNN with fully connected CRF for accurate brain lesion segmentation. *Medical Image Analysis*, 36,61–78.

Ker, J., Wang, L., Rao J., Lim, T. (2018). Deep learning applications in medical image analysis, *IEEE Access*, 6, 9375–9389.

Kim, E., M. Corte-Real, and Z. Baloch, (2016). A deep semanticmobile application for thyroid cytopathology. In Medical Imaging 2016: PACS and Imaging Informatics: Next Generation and Innovations. International Society for Optics and Photonics.

Krishna, P.S., Reddy, U.J., Patibandla, R.L. Khadherbhi, S.R. (2020). Identification of lung cancer stages using efficient machine learning framework. *Journal of Critical Reviews*, 7, 385–390.

Latif, J., Xiao, C., Imran, A. and Tu, S. (2019).Medical imaging using machine learning and deep learning algorithms: A review. *2nd International Conference on Computing, Mathematics and Engineering Technologies (iCoMET)*, Sukkur, Pakistan, 1–5.

Lundervold, A.S., Lundervold, A. (2019). An overview of deep learning in medical imaging focusing on MRI. *Zeitschrift für Medizinische Physik*, 29,102–127.

Naresh, A. (2020). Unsupervised text classification for heart disease using machine learning methods, *Test Engineering and Management*, 11005–11016.

Norris, D.J., (2017). Machine learning: Deep learning. *Beginning Artificial Intelligence with the Raspberry Pi.*Springer. 211–247.

Patibandla, R.S.M.L. (2020). Prediction of pneumonia disease by using deep convolutional neural networks, *Journal of Engineering Sciences*, 9, 393–399.

Patibandla R.S.M.L., Narayana V.L. (2021) Computational intelligence approach for prediction of COVID-19 using particle swarm optimization. In: Raza K. (eds) *Computational Intelligence Methods in COVID-19: Surveillance, Prevention, Prediction and Diagnosis. Studies in Computational Intelligence*, Vol. 923. Springer, Singapore.

Patibandla, R.L., Rao, B.T., Krishna, P.S. and Maddumala, V.R. (2020). Medical data clustering using particle swarm optimization method. *Journal of Critical Reviews*, 7, 363–367.

Poplin R., Chang P.-C., Alexander D., Schwartz S., Colthurst T., Ku A. (2018). A universal SNP and small-indel variant caller using deep neural networks. *Nature Biotechnology*, 36, 983–987.

Pouyanfar, S., Sadiq, S., Yan, Y., Tian, H., Tao, Y., Reyes, M.P., Shyu, M.L., Chen, S.C. and Iyengar, S.S. (2018). A survey on deep learning: Algorithms, techniques, and applications. *ACM Computing Surveys*. 51, 1–36.

Rao, B.T. (2020). Performance analysis of deep learning models using bagging ensemble, *Journal of Xi'an University of Architecture & Technology*, XII, 1682–1687.

Rao, B.T., Patibandla, R.L. and Murty, M.R. (2020). A comparative study on effective approaches for unsupervised statistical machine translation. In V. Bhateja, S. Satapathy, H. Satori (Eds.), *Embedded Systems and Artificial Intelligence. Advances in Intelligent Systems and Computing*, Vol. 1076. Singapore: Springer.

Raissi M., Karniadakis G.E. (2018). Hidden physics models: Machine learning of nonlinear partial differential equations. *Journal of Computational Physics*, 357, 125–41.

Rastogi, P., Singh, V. and Yadav, M. (2018). Deep learning and big datatechnologies in medical image analysis. *Fifth International Conference on Parallel, Distributed and Grid Computing (PDGC)*, Solan Himachal Pradesh, India, 60–63.

Ravi D., Wong C., Deligianni F., Berthelot M., Andreu-Perez J., Lo B. (2017). Deep learning for health informatics. *IEEE Journal of Biomedical and Health Informatics*, 21, 4–21.

Yuan, Y. and Meng, M.Q.-H. (2017). Deep learning for polyp recognition in wireless capsule endoscopy images. *Medical Physics*, 44, 1379–1389.

Yukun, S. (2019). Deep learning applications in medical image recognition. *American Journal of Computer Science and Technology*, 2, 22–26.

Index

347

For Product Safety Concerns and Information please contact our EU
representative GPSR@taylorandfrancis.com
Taylor & Francis Verlag GmbH, Kaufingerstraße 24, 80331 München, Germany